Developmental and
Therapeutic Interventions in the NICU

Developmental and Therapeutic Interventions in the NICU

by

Elsie R. Vergara, Sc.D., OTR, FAOTA
Boston University

and

Rosemarie Bigsby, Sc.D., OTR, FAOTA
Brown University, Providence, Rhode Island
Women & Infants' Hospital, Providence, Rhode Island

with invited contributors

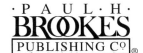
·P·A·U·L·H·
BROOKES
PUBLISHING C⁰ ®

Baltimore • London • Sydney

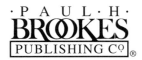

Paul H. Brookes Publishing Co.
Post Office Box 10624
Baltimore, Maryland 21285-0624

www.brookespublishing.com

Typeset by International Graphic Services, Inc., Newtown, Pennsylvania.
Manufactured in the United States of America by
Versa Press, Inc., East Peoria, Illinois.

The information provided in the book is in no way meant to substitute for a
medical practitioner's advice or expert opinion. Readers should consult a medical practitioner if they are interested in more information. This book is sold
without warranties of any kind, express or implied, and the publisher and
authors disclaim any liability, loss, or damage caused by the contents of this
book.

The stories in this book are based on the authors' experiences. Some of the
vignettes represent actual people and circumstances. Individuals' names and
identifying details have been changed to protect their identities. Other vignettes
are composite accounts that do not represent the lives or experiences of specific
individuals, and no implications should be inferred.

Learn more about the concepts in this book through Brookes On Location,
a program that connects you with the experts behind Brookes books for
seminars tailored to specific needs. Seminars can be conducted in English or
Spanish. For more information, visit www.brookespublishing.com, e-mail
rights@brookespublishing.com, or call 410-337-9580.

Library of Congress Cataloging-in-Publication Data

Vergara Elsie.
   Developmental and therapeutic interventions in the NICU / by Elsie R.
Vergara and Rosemarie Bigsby.
      p.   cm.
   Includes bibliographical references and index.
   ISBN 1-55766-675-X
   1. Neonatal intensive care.   2. Infants (Newborn)—Development.   3. Infants
(Newborn)—Diseases—Treatment.   I. Bigsby, Rosemarie.   II. Title.
RJ253.5.V47 2003
618.92'01—dc22   2003060651

British Library Cataloguing in Publication data are available from the British
Library.

Contents

About the Authors

Elsie R. Vergara, Sc.D., OTR, FAOTA, Associate Professor of Occupational Therapy, Sargent College of Health and Rehabilitation Sciences, Boston University, 635 Commonwealth Avenue, Boston, Massachusetts 02215

Dr. Vergara received a bachelor of science degree in physical and occupational therapy in 1968 and a master of public health degree in maternal and infant health in 1977 from the University of Puerto Rico. Her interest in neonatal care emerged during her clinical experiences in Puerto Rico. These experiences took place when major medical and technological advances in neonatal practice were occurring in the United States. Dr. Vergara moved to Boston to pursue a doctoral degree that would expand on the knowledge and skills in neonatal intervention that she had acquired through intensive self-study and her master's-level experiences. Dr. Vergara received training from respected neonatal care scholars such as Dr. Kevin Nugent and Dr. Heidelise Als, and in 1987 she earned a doctor of science degree from Boston University.

Following the reauthorization of the Education of the Handicapped Act Amendments of 1986 (PL 99-457) as the Individuals with Disabilities Education Act Amendments of 1991 (PL 102-119), states began to develop educational resources and activities to prepare personnel to comply with the mandates of the law. Dr. Vergara obtained a 3-year grant from the state of Florida to design and establish a statewide training program to prepare neonatal and early intervention physical and occupational therapists. To accomplish this task, she created a series of self-study materials that the American Occupational Therapy Association published in 1993 as a two-volume set titled *Foundations for Practice in the Neonatal Intensive Care Unit and Early Intervention: A Self-Guided Manual.* In 1993, Dr. Vergara was inducted into the American Occupational Therapy Association's Roster of Fellows for her contributions to the enhancement of the profession through the development and promotion of educational programs in early intervention.

Dr. Vergara's interest in infusing a family-centered, developmentally supportive perspective into the training and service delivery of neonatal personnel has challenged her to conduct similar training programs in countries such as Mexico and Honduras. She plans to establish two training centers in Mexico to provide ongoing preparation of neonatal personnel.

Rosemarie Bigsby, Sc.D., OTR, FAOTA, Clinical Assistant Professor of Pediatrics, Brown University, Providence, Rhode Island; Coordinator of NICU Services, Infant Development Center, Department of Pediatrics, Women & Infants' Hospital, 101 Dudley Street, Providence, Rhode Island 02905

Dr. Bigsby earned a bachelor of science degree in occupational therapy from Western Michigan University in 1974, an advanced master of science degree in occupational therapy from Boston University in 1980, and a doctor of science degree from Boston University in 1994. She holds a Board Certification in Pediatrics from the American Occupational Therapy Association and in 1993 was named a Fellow of the American Occupational Therapy Association for her contributions to the practice of occupational therapy with infants and children.

Dr. Bigsby's experience as a pediatric occupational therapist spans three decades, during which she has worked in a variety of settings as a clinician, supervisor, and consultant. When she began her career, sensory integration and early intervention were emerging practice arenas. The potential for applying principles of sensory integrative theory to practice in early intervention captured her interest, prompting her to advance her education and to eventually engage in research with preterm infants and their families. In the 1980s, following her graduate studies, she became Chief Occupational Therapist at Meeting Street School (now called Meeting Street Center), a center in East Providence, Rhode Island, for school-age children with multiple disabilities. She participated on the multidisciplinary diagnostic team as well as the Parent Program for Developmental Management, one of the first early intervention programs in the country, which was founded by the late Dr. Eric Denhoff. In 1990, she began her doctoral research under the mentorship of Dr. Barry Lester, focusing on physiologic and behavioral indicators of self-regulation in preterm infants. Since that time, she has contributed to a number of grant-funded research studies as a trainer and consultant.

Dr. Bigsby has practiced in the NICU at Women & Infants' Hospital since 1992 in the combined roles of therapist, educator, and researcher. She was instrumental in translating the model for psychosocial and developmental support to NICU infants and their families—first described by Dr. Elaine C. Meyer, Dr. Lester, and colleagues—from a research protocol to a clinical service that is provided by the Infant Development Center team.

Dr. Bigsby has authored numerous journal articles and book chapters and co-authored the American Occupational Therapy Association guidelines for NICU practice and the *Posture and Fine Motor Assessment of Infants* (The Psychological Corporation, 2000). She also has served as a contributor to the *Neonatal Network Neurobehavioral Scale* (NNNS) (Lester & Tronick, forthcoming from Paul H. Brookes Publishing Co.). Dr. Bigsby's research focuses on motor development, behavioral cues, physiologic regulation, and feeding in early infancy. She has been invited to speak both nationally and internationally, and each year, she teaches several 2-day multidisciplinary workshops on assessment and intervention in the NICU.

About the Contributors

Elaine C. Meyer, Ph.D., R.N., Assistant Professor of Psychology, Harvard Medical School, Boston, Massachusetts; Clinical Psychologist, Children's Hospital Boston, 300 Longwood Avenue, Boston, Massachusetts 02115

As a registered nurse and a clinical psychologist, Dr. Meyer specializes in pediatric psychology. She is Staff Psychologist of the Medical Surgical Intensive Care Unit and Director of the Program to Enhance Relational and Communication Skills (PERCS) at Children's Hospital Boston. In addition, she is Assistant Professor of Psychology in the Department of Psychiatry at Harvard Medical School. Dr. Meyer has presented nationally and published widely on parental perspectives of neonatal and pediatric critical care illness and hospitalization and on the development and efficacy of multimodal psychosocial interventions to serve families.

Michael E. Msall, M.D., Professor of Pediatrics and Human Development, Brown Medical School, Providence, Rhode Island; Director of Research, Child Developmental Center, Hasbro Children's Hospital, 593 Eddy Street, Providence, Rhode Island 02903

Dr. Msall attended the Feinberg School of Medicine at Northwestern University in Chicago; completed pediatric residency training at Brown Medical School in Providence, Rhode Island; and completed fellowship training in developmental pediatrics, neurodevelopmental disabilities, and developmental genetics at The Johns Hopkins University and the Kennedy Krieger Institute in Baltimore. He is a fellow of the Society of Developmental Pediatrics and the American Academy of Cerebral Palsy and Developmental Medicine and is subspecialty board-certified in developmental and behavioral pediatrics and neurodevelopmental disabilities in pediatrics. Dr. Msall's research efforts include developmental aspects of measuring and enhancing functional independence and quality supports in children with prematurity, cerebral palsy, spina bifida, autism, Down syndrome, Rett syndrome, genetic disorders, and neurosensory disorders. He collaborates with colleagues in developmental psychology and demography to understand pathways of risk and resiliency in child disability.

Betty R. Vohr, M.D., Professor of Pediatrics, Brown Medical School, Providence, Rhode Island; Director of Neonatal Follow-Up, Women & Infants' Hospital, 101 Dudley Street, Providence, Rhode Island 02905

Dr. Vohr has been Director of the Neonatal Follow-Up Clinic at Women & Infants' Hospital since 1974. In addition to this and her work as Professor of Pediatrics at Brown Medical School, she has been Medical Director of the Rhode Island Hearing Assessment Program since 1990. Also since 1990, Dr. Vohr has been National Coordinator of the National Institute of Child Health and Human Development Neonatal Research Network's follow-up studies in the United States. Dr. Vohr's primary clinical and research interests continue to focus on improving the long-term outcomes of high-risk premature infants.

Acknowledgments

Families often describe the NICU experience as one that they wish never to undergo again, yet, in retrospect, hold dear. Initial feelings of loss, sadness, and fear give way to overwhelming love and pride—pride in the resilience of their tiny sons and daughters and in themselves for enduring such a difficult time. As we reflect on the 6 years during which this book evolved, we are struck by the parallels that can be drawn between our lives and the NICU experience. Soon after our first meeting, unpredictable, life-altering events occurred within our families that brought heartbreak, loss, and sorrow. These emotions were eventually replaced with joy, pride, and a great sense of satisfaction, culminating with the completion of this book.

First, we thank our families—our major source of motivation, strength, and support—for their unselfish love and understanding, without which we would not have been able to complete this work. We dedicate this book to the late Rev. Juan Vergara and to Tom Bigsby, our husbands; to Elsie's mother Elsie Rodriguez; to Elsie's daughters Esther, Debbie, and Chely; and to Rose's sons Jim and Michael. You are everything to us!

We also thank the many colleagues, students, and families who taught us what to teach and whose stories and photos enliven and enrich this book, particularly the patients and staff of Women & Infants' Hospital in Providence, Rhode Island. Special thanks to Barry M. Lester, Ph.D., and Wendy Coster, Ph.D., for their wisdom and mentorship and for doing so much to uphold and support us professionally.

1

Supporting Infant Occupations in the NICU

OVERVIEW

Infants who are born healthy after a full-term pregnancy typically possess the necessary skills to become active participants in their own development from the moment of birth. The infant's ability to suck on his or her hand for self-soothing or to signal the need for care and attention by crying are simple but purposeful activities, or occupations, of infancy. The availability of family members to understand and respond appropriately to their infant's behaviors becomes an interactive process that enhances the caregivers' capacity to meet their infants' needs.

Admission of an infant to the neonatal intensive care unit (NICU) limits the infant's opportunities to engage in activities that are typical of healthy newborns. Moreover, NICU admission drastically alters the family's opportunities to engage in typical occupational roles such as caregiving. This chapter presents a conceptual approach to neonatal intervention based on promoting the development of infant occupations, as well as family occupations related to their infant's care. It introduces a framework of childhood occupations proposed by Coster (1996) that can be used for analysis of the tasks and activities in which newborns are expected to engage from birth. Two types of infant occupations are identified: learning (exploring) and apprenticeship (procuring, socially interacting, and feeding). A multifactorial approach is used to examine internal factors (underlying capacities) and external (contextual) factors that support, limit, or prevent participation in occupations by infants, particularly those who are premature or sick (Humphry, 2002).

Infant-related caregiver occupations include parenting tasks such as providing care and necessary resources, facilitating and regulating the infant's state of arousal, modulating the infant's environment to optimize the infant's occupations, promoting social interaction appropriate to the infant's capabilities, and reciprocating the infant's engagement efforts. The interdependency between the occupations of the infant and those of the caregivers, namely the parents and NICU personnel, in fostering the infant's social engagement and participation in his or her environment is emphasized. The importance of considering cultural values and family expectations to optimize the NICU infant's ability to engage in neonatal occupations is underscored. Common roles and occupations of NICU families are described, and general strategies for supporting the family's participation in their infant's care are provided.

OBJECTIVES

- Explain Coster's conceptualization of occupations in children and how this theoretical model applies to neonatal intervention
- Explain the concepts of occupations, occupational performance, and occupational engagement as defined in this chapter
- Identify the types of occupations in which newborns are expected to participate, both at home and in the NICU, and compare the typical patterns of occupational engagement of healthy newborns and NICU infants
- Describe the underlying capacities and contextual elements that support an infant's engagement in the various types of occupations
- Identify factors that limit or prevent an infant's engagement in expected occupations
- Identify the caregiver occupations associated with infant care and factors that may enhance or interfere with the family's fulfillment of parenting roles in the NICU
- Describe typical roles and occupations of siblings and how NICU experiences affect these roles and occupations
- Describe the ways by which neonatal therapists may enhance occupational performance in infants and in their families

DEVELOPMENTALLY FOCUSED NEONATAL INTERVENTION

Medical and technological advances since the late 1960s and early 1970s have markedly enhanced the survival of infants born prematurely or with life-threatening illnesses. Unlike their counterparts who are born healthy, these infants enter this world at a disadvantage, facing many challenges when they are most fragile. One such challenge is their limited ability to engage in the typical occupations that enable healthy infants to become active participants in their own developmental process.

Although technological advances have successfully fostered the survival and medical well-being of newborns, addressing developmental aspects of their care continues to be a challenge for neonatal professionals. Developmentally focused neonatal therapies flourished during the 1970s and 1980s, with inconsistent benefits reported (see Chapter 2).

Developmentally focused neonatal intervention has historically relied on adaptation of popular theories and practice models that were originally conceptualized for older children. Until the 1990s, the majority of theoretical approaches used in delivering services to infants were based on assessment and treatment of specific factors believed to be affecting the infant's development (e.g., neuromuscular, sensorimotor, cognitive, social, emotional), specific capacities (e.g., self-regulation, attention, alertness, visual pursuit, state modulation, muscle tone, postural control, motor coordination), or skills (e.g., gross motor, social, fine-motor adaptive). Using these approaches, the therapist assesses for the presence or absence of particular factors, then makes inferences as to the potential effect that such a deficit or disorder could have on the infant's performance. Performance expectations associated with factors other than age are seldom regarded in assessments of underlying factors. Elements such as the characteristics and meaningfulness of a given task or activity—that is, the context for the activity, which can change from moment to moment—may also have an impact on the infant's overall performance (Coster, 1996). Omitting these contextual components from an infant's assessment results in intervention programs focused almost exclusively on development of underlying factors and skills at the expense of other, perhaps equally important and more practical, aspects of performance (Coster, 1996).

Neonatal intervention programs in many regions of the United States are based on the assumption that gains in underlying factors or specific skills ultimately translate into improved performance. Although the influence of other factors on the NICU infant's ability to engage in neonatal occupations or activities has been discussed in the literature since the 1980s, in reality, some neonatal therapists still neglect to consider factors such as culturally valued expectations, the effect of the environmental context on performance, or the characteristics or meaningfulness of a task (Case-Smith, 1998).

Recognition of the family as the most important and constant influence on the developmental outcome of infants and toddlers has prompted professionals to redirect and broaden the focus of early assessment and intervention. Legislation passed in 1986 and subsequently reauthorized as Part C of the Individuals with Disabilities Education Act (IDEA) Amendments of 1997 (PL 105-17) recognized the importance of the infant's environmental context, namely the family, in addressing the infant's needs (34 CFR § 303). Part C mandates consideration of the family's needs, concerns, and priorities in the development and implementation of intervention plans for infants with disabilities or at risk for disabilities (American Occupational Therapy Association, 1997). (See Chapter 2 for further details.)

Most developmental therapists agree that the goal of intervention is to optimize the infant's development of age-appropriate occupations, tasks, or activities. Focusing assessment and intervention on the family context, however, requires identification of family-valued activities for the infant, as well as factors likely to facilitate or interfere with the infant's engagement in those activities. By examining the family's expectations for the infant and the resources available to meet those expectations, the therapist can focus on the main goal for the infant's intervention—that is, to become "an increasingly full participant [in occupations] that meet one's cultural [i.e., family] expectations and one's individual needs" (Coster, 1996, p. 8).

NEONATAL OCCUPATIONS

A major focus of developmentally focused neonatal intervention in the NICU is the provision of an environment that supports the participation of infants and their families in their expected occupations (Gorga et al., 2000; Holloway, 1998). Although a number of neonatal disciplines have claimed to have an environmental intervention focus, the definitions of *occupations* and *occupational performance* proposed in this book are new to neonatal practice. To adopt an occupation framework in the NICU, a clear definition of *infant occupations* is necessary, particularly because traditional adult-based definitions of the concept are not easily applicable to infant intervention (Coster, 1998; Humphry, 2002).

Infant occupations are thus defined as appropriate tasks and activities that are valued in either the family's culture or the NICU culture, within which an infant is expected to participate (Coster, 1996, 1998). Humphry further added that occupations are "patterns of actions that emerge through transactions between the child and environment" (2002, p. 172). *Occupational performance*, or *engagement*, is the infant's participation in the tasks and activities expected by either the family or the NICU personnel.

The extent and quality of the infant's participation results from his or her transactions with the environment. Engagement in expected occupations requires a foundation of basic skills or capacities, as well as favorable contextual conditions that support the infant's participation in such tasks or activities.

Under these parameters, what can be classified as infant occupations, and how do infants develop occupations? Although there is some discrepancy in the literature regarding what should be considered infant occupations (Humphry, 2002), it can be argued that there are two basic types of activities or occupations in which children participate as they learn the adult occupations valued in their cultures:

1. *Learning occupations* (or *acquisition occupations*) are activities that help the child develop skills considered important for adults within his or her culture but that are somewhat different from the adult form of the occupation—for example, schooling activities (Coster, 1996). Exploring is an example of an infant learning or acquisition occupation.

2. *Apprenticeship occupations* are activities that help integrate the child into the routines of his or her culture. An apprenticeship occupation resembles the adult form but is simpler or less demanding. Adults use apprentice methods of teaching to progressively expose the infant to the demands of the adult forms of the occupation. The caregiver and infant engage in a "shared enterprise" (Coster, 1996) or "scaffolding" relationship (Primeau, 1998) that enables the infant to develop an age-appropriate version of the family's valued occupation. Activities of daily living and simple chores are two examples of apprenticeship occupations (Coster, 1996). Feeding and procuring (care soliciting) are examples of apprenticeship occupations.

The extent to which an infant can engage in these types of occupations depends on critical elements. These include infant factors (i.e., basic capacities and abilities) and environmental or contextual factors, both physical and social, at the particular point in time. Within this framework, the NICU therapist's main role is to design an intervention plan that fosters the infant's occupational competence to the extent of his or her abilities and tolerance and is consistent with the family and NICU contexts. This requires the therapist to have a thorough understanding of many factors:

1. Which occupations are valued in the family and NICU cultures

2. Which factors are interfering with the infant's engagement in those occupations

3. What constitutes "readiness" for engagement in the valued occupations

4. What support, individual or environmental, would facilitate the infant's participation in the valued occupations

The therapist's role also includes determining how the necessary support can be provided to facilitate the infant's engagement in tasks and activities that promote his or her health, growth, and development without compromising the integrity of the infant's systems. Such support helps the infant become a more active participant in the occupations valued and expected within his or her culture.

The proposed framework may be used to describe the types of occupations in which a NICU infant may be able to engage—that is, exploring, procuring, socially interacting, and feeding—and to identify the specific occupations valued within the infant's culture. The framework may also serve as a practical guide for assessing the individual capacities that underlie an infant's performance and the critical elements necessary for the infant to engage in the valued occupations. For example, an infant who is having difficulty engaging in social interaction with his or her caregiver may be experiencing problems with individual capacities such as lack of alertness or physiologic instability. Likewise, the social interaction difficulty could be the result of a critical element, such as a noisy or bright environment, an overstimulating caregiver who does not support the infant's social interaction efforts, or a combination of environmental and individual factors that interfere with the infant's occupational engagement. Table 1 categorizes the occupations of newborns and the elements that support occupational engagement based on this framework.

Occupational Engagement in the Neonatal Period

Shortly after birth, healthy full-term infants are able to actively engage with their environment and, to a certain degree, express to their caregivers when they need attention (see Chapter 8). They have the central nervous system maturation to do so and, typically, the necessary environmental conditions to actively engage with their caregivers. In contrast, premature infants often do not have the necessary maturity for this extent of active engagement (see Chapter 9). Similarly, infants who are sick or physiologically unstable may need to focus energy on maintaining their stability and, therefore, are frequently less available or unavailable for this type of interaction (see Chapter 8). Furthermore, the NICU environment, especially the incubator and

Table 1. Occupations of newborns and elements that support participation

Occupations	Elements of support	
	Infant factors	Contextual factors
Procuring	Self-regulation	*Physical context*
Social play	Physiologic stability	Modulated environment
Feeding	Muscle tone	Activity level
Exploratory play	Muscle strength	Temperature
Visual	Endurance	Containment
Auditory	Postural control	
Oral	Reflex development	*Social context*
Tactile	Arousal/alertness	Caregiver sensitivity
Proprioceptive	State modulation	Caregiver availability
Vestibular/kinesthetic	State transitions (asleep–awake–crying)	Caregiver engagement
		Number of caregivers
	Sensory processing	
	Sensory modulation	*Cultural context*
	Perceptual skills	Values
	Cognitive skills	Beliefs
	Visual skills	Traditions/customs
	Auditory skills	Expectations
	Motor control	
	Oral-motor control	*Temporal context*
	Physical development	Most functional periods
	Weight	Discretionary time available
		Nursing/medical care needs
		Day–night rhythm
		Family routines

life-support equipment, isolates infants and interferes with family support and engagement.

Newborns spend more than 80% of their time sleeping, and this percentage is even higher for infants who are born prematurely or who are sick (Prechtl, Fargel, Weinmann, & Bakker, 1979). Infants' opportunities for engagement are limited to their brief periods of alertness. Although an infant sleeps much of the time, sleeping does not clearly meet the criteria for consideration as an occupation under the framework presented in this chapter. The ability to regulate sleep, however, is one of the most important underlying capacities or elements of support that infants need to engage in occupations (see Table 1). For example, an infant who can habituate to disruptive stimuli in the environment will be able to achieve the deep sleep needed for body growth. Moreover, it is believed that sleep may help the infant maintain or regain the neurobehavioral stability required to achieve a quiet alert state (see Chapter 8). The infant's state of arousal, specifically quiet alertness, determines in part the extent to which he or she is able to engage in tasks or activities within the environment. Although modulating states of arousal is not an occupation, it is a critical element of support underlying occupational performance.

Common Infant Occupations

In their alert periods, infants engage in a variety of occupations, most of them interrelated. Exploring is the most common learning/acquisition occupation; procuring, socially interacting, and feeding are the most frequent apprenticeship occupations. These occupations are not mutually exclusive—performance of one may contain elements of the others. Each neonatal occupation interacts in the development of the others and of more complex occupations; however, each occupation is described individually for clarity, with references to common patterns of interrelation when appropriate.

Exploring

Exploring can be considered a learning activity that plays a crucial role in building skills important to the development of adult occupations valued in the infant's culture (see Table 1). Exploration of the environment has been regarded for many years as infants' primary mode of learning. Adults in Western societies generally value and promote children's exploration through the provision of sensory-rich environments and experiences. For decades, Western culture has recognized the importance of exploration for infant development. Piaget (1976) considered sensory exploration the basis for the development of cognitive skills.

Sensory exploration is also considered an important element in the development of sensory integration skills in infants (Ayres, 1972; Stallings-Sahler, 1998). Caregiver–infant play at this stage consists predominantly of activities involving various forms of sensory exploration: tactile, vestibular/proprioceptive, visual, or auditory (Burke, 1998). During the first few weeks of life, infants explore predominantly through observation—that is, in nonmotor ways except for eye movements. Visual exploration becomes a critical learning mechanism for infants. For example, studies have demonstrated that newborns show preference for certain visual stimuli, such as a human face, especially the mother's face (Slater & Kirby, 1998; Valenza, Simion, Cassia, &

Umilta, 1996). This type of behavior suggests that infants have the ability to scan and explore visual images and to learn through visual exploration (see Chapter 8).

Tactile, oral, postural, and vestibular exploration, although less obvious, are other important learning mechanisms of newborns. Discrimination of auditory (Ecklund-Flores & Turkewitz, 1996; Werner, 1996) and olfactory (MacFarlane, 1975; Marlier, Schaal, & Soussignan, 1997; Schaal, Marlier, & Soussignan, 1998) stimuli has also been demonstrated in newborns (see Chapter 8), suggesting that these systems may also be involved in exploratory activities.

As a learning occupation, exploring underlies and supports an infant's engagement in apprenticeship occupations. Exploration and observation may enable the infant to scan facial expressions, search for eye contact, search for and follow his or her caregiver, play on his or her mother's breast (oral and tactile exploration), and seek comfort positions and cuddling (proprioceptive exploration). Exploring behaviors such as these enable the infant to engage in more complex forms of interaction with caregivers. For example, Figure 1 shows exploratory play between an infant and her brother. The play was initiated shortly before the photograph was taken because the brother had called his sister's name. The infant grinned even before she turned around to look at her brother, but her face lit up in a big smile when she saw his face. This incident suggests that the infant was using (at least) two modalities to explore and interpret her play environment. It is possible that her initial smile was a response to using auditory processing to recognize a familiar voice but that her smile brightened after she confirmed the familiarity of the input through her more mature visual exploration abilities.

Neonatal therapists must recognize that exploring is one of the most basic but also one of the most important and valued occupations for infants. Intervention planning must provide for the development of individual and contextual elements of support that foster infants' engagement in exploration.

Procuring

Procuring activities enable the infant to interact with the environment in a proactive, care-soliciting manner rather than in a reactive, care-receiver way. The infant becomes a "procurer" (care solicitor) when he or she can exhibit behaviors that communicate his or her needs to caregivers. For example, an infant engaged in interaction with a caregiver may turn his or her face away to "procure" a break from the caregiver when

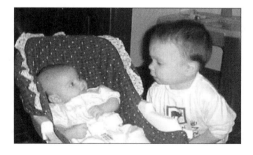

Figure 1. This 4-week-old full-term infant is demonstrating her ability to participate in social interaction with her brother. (From Vergara, E. [2002]. Enhancing occupational performance in infants in the NICU. *OT Practice, 7*[2], 8–13. Copyright © 2002 by the American Occupational Therapy Association, Inc. Reprinted with permission.)

the interaction is becoming too stressful. An infant may procure a feeding by sucking on his or her fist to indicate the need to be fed. An infant may pull away from his or her caregiver when unable to cuddle. Procuring as such becomes the first milestone toward achievement of independence, a highly valued right in many cultures. The ability to procure caregiver support decreases absolute dependence on caregivers. Although infants are by nature totally dependent on caregivers for the fulfillment of their needs, infants who can make their needs known to caregivers take an active role in securing their own care.

The seemingly simple task of procuring by communicating needs to caregivers may be complex for some newborns, particularly those who are sick or premature. Procuring is manifested through a variety of verbal (i.e., crying) or nonverbal behaviors or signals that reflect the infant's level of stress and need of support at any given moment (Als, Lester, Tronick, & Brazelton, 1982a; Bigsby, Coster, Lester, & Peucker, 1996). (This content is detailed in Chapters 8 and 9.) Procuring requires important underlying capacities, such as self-regulating states of arousal (including crying), sensory processing/sensory modulation, and cognitive skills (see Table 1). Procuring also requires an environment that supports the infant's efforts. When stressed, a stable, well-regulated, healthy infant may actively search for internal and external strategies to decrease the effect of the stressor. The ability to elicit stress-reduction behaviors depends on the infant's underlying (internal) capacities (e.g., self-regulation, postural and motor control) and contextual (external) elements of support. The infant produces behaviors that either minimize the effect of the stressor (internal elements) or signal to the caregiver that additional help is needed (external elements). For example, an infant who is sensitive to overhead lights may cover his or her face with a hand to block the light (internal element). This hand-on-face behavior also serves as a cue to the caregiver that the lights are stressful and need to be dimmed or turned off (external element). A sensitive caregiver who lowers the lights (external support) after observing the infant's procuring signals would be reinforcing the infant's use of this behavior in similar future situations. Conversely, a NICU infant with limited physiologic and motor skills who is not well organized or regulated or who has undergone a stressful procedure may not have the ability to procure either internal or external support elements. Therefore, this infant may be more dependent on the caregivers' provision of external supports. Need fulfillment and quality of life for this infant will depend almost entirely on the nurturing roles of caregivers for a longer period of time than typically needed. As NICU infants become more medically and physiologically stable, they become increasingly able to meet environmental challenges in more active ways through enhanced procuring abilities.

Engagement in procuring occupations ultimately leads to the achievement of higher levels of development and functional performance—for example, grasping a desired object rather than pointing at it. Procuring occupations, in turn, enhance the infant's ability to engage in social interaction. Specialized support from the developmental team may be necessary to enable NICU infants to gradually optimize occupational performance by taking on a more active role in procuring than they would when relying solely on their own capacities.

Socially Interacting

The ability to socially interact with caregivers is another important culturally valued and expected occupation of newborns in many cultures. Early social interaction activities are believed to form the basis for the acquisition of adult social interaction patterns.

Although families differ in their expectations regarding their infant's participation in social interaction, all children are expected to develop socially appropriate patterns of behavior. They learn these behaviors explicitly and implicitly through an apprenticeship process or a "shared enterprise" (Coster, 1996; Rogoff, 1990) or a skill-building scaffolding (Primeau, 1998) apprenticeship process with their caregivers. Emerging appropriate social interaction behaviors are reinforced implicitly through caregiver modeling and graded demands as children grow.

From the moment of birth, parents in many cultures dedicate much effort to engaging in social interaction with their infants. Most healthy newborns are able to initiate or participate in social interaction soon after birth. Caregiver availability and contingent responsiveness facilitate the infants' participation in interactive tasks. For example, the infant in Figure 1 has had ample opportunities for social interaction. She has parents who value, promote, and are frequently available for social interaction; a brother who enjoys interacting with his sister; and a small number of relatives and friends who interact with her during frequent visits. In contrast, infants in the NICU who are sick and premature may not have the readiness or the contextual elements of support for this type of engagement. Because of medical or physiologic instability, some may remain unavailable for social interaction for a long time (see Chapters 8 and 9).

Caregiver availability may affect social interaction in the NICU in a number of ways. First, caregivers may not be available to provide positive social interaction. Second, caregivers may change constantly, requiring the infant to adapt to different social interaction styles. Third, contingency of the interaction may be limited if the caregiver is not available when needed. Furthermore, NICU infants may require considerably more external support to engage in social interaction (e.g., decreased environmental stimulation, postural containment, timing of visual contact), which may not be available when needed (see Figure 2). These issues make participation in social interaction occupations more difficult for NICU infants.

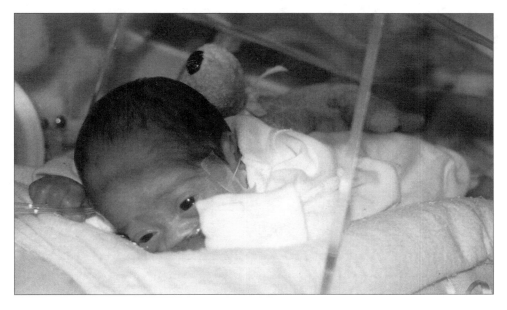

Figure 2. Limited alertness may affect this premature infant's ability to engage in social interaction.

Quality of social interaction is another factor that affects the infant's participation. Social interaction opportunities of healthy newborns are generally associated with pleasurable sensory experiences, which are offered by a limited number of close relatives or friends in a supportive environment. The quality of an infant's experiences positively reinforces his or her social engagement efforts. When this happens, the infant may respond adaptively by increasing and enriching his or her participation in these activities. For example, positive social interaction opportunities with a limited number of caregivers have enabled the infant in Figure 3 to develop a rather sophisticated, synchronized, mutually enjoyable social interaction style. Mutual reinforcement has enabled both mother and infant to "learn" to interpret each other's social signals and to take turns during the interaction based on each other's responses or needs. In contrast, social interactions within the NICU context are frequently associated with medical or nursing care, which is provided by many individuals with potentially different interactive styles. Interactions often expose infants to disruptive, aversive, intrusive, and painful sensory experiences. Under these circumstances, any efforts at social interaction may be negatively reinforced unless appropriate external support and positive experiences are offered.

Unlike other aspects of bedside care, social visits with parents and siblings in the NICU bear a greater resemblance to the normal experiences of healthy infants and their families. Moreover, infants' participation in social interaction activities with their families strengthens the bonds of attachment and offers family members opportunities to engage in caregiver occupations with their infant.

Neonatal therapists should foster opportunities for positive social interactions between an infant and his or her family. The goals of intervention in this area are to

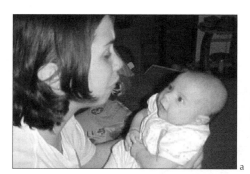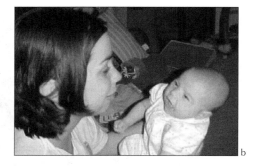

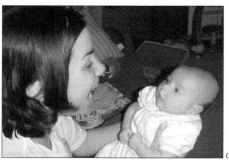

Figure 3.   This mother is engaged in a reciprocal social interaction process with her full-term infant. The process begins when the mother talks to the baby (a). The mother pauses momentarily (b) (i.e., turn taking) until the baby is able to organize a response manifested by smiling and cooing (c). Finally, the mother reinforces the infant's response as the interaction begins to dwindle. (From Vergara, E. [2002]. Enhancing occupational performance in infants in the NICU. *OT Practice, 7*[2], 8–13. Copyright © 2002 by the American Occupational Therapy Association, Inc. Reprinted with permission.)

enable the infant to engage in pleasurable social interactions and to give families the necessary skills to facilitate their infant's apprenticeship development of social interaction. This may require working directly with the infant to maximize his or her internal capacities, as well as optimizing external support through consultation with NICU staff, the parents, and other family members. Facilitating social engagement requires learning to modify the environment in response to the infant's procuring efforts. The therapist can assist caregivers by guiding their observations of the infant, helping them gain sensitivity and responsiveness to their infant's social cues, and assisting them in providing the infant with critical elements of individual and contextual support to promote interaction (Hanzlik, 1998).

Feeding

Feeding is a basic need and one of the most natural occupations of newborns. It is considered the infant's "primary work" (Glass & Wolff, 1998). The infant who is learning to feed is also engaged in a shared enterprise or scaffolding relationship with the family, as he or she learns the family's values and expectations associated with feeding. These values and expectations determine many aspects of the family's approach to feeding their infant.

Taking nourishment is a dependent task for the newborn. Although infants depend entirely on caregivers to provide the source of nourishment, infants play an active and important role in the feeding process. An infant's capacity to solicit a feeding depends on his or her procuring abilities. Shortly after birth, most healthy newborns cry when they need to eat, and to a certain extent, infants are expected to solicit food by waking up, fussing, or crying. Soliciting food becomes a specialized form of procuring. Some parents choose to feed their infants on demand—whenever the infant wakes up or cries for food. Infants fed on demand usually gain weight efficiently, indicating that they are capable of procuring from caregivers the needed nourishment and of getting the necessary oral intake to subsist and grow. Infants who have problems engaging in feeding tasks—those who do not cry for a feeding, have difficulty becoming sufficiently alert to feed, cannot regulate their respirations during feedings, present specific feeding or social interaction difficulties, or react to environmental sensory stimulation in ways that interfere with feeding—are more likely to experience difficulty obtaining nourishment and gaining weight (Glass & Wolff, 1998). These infants may be at greater risk for developing failure to thrive unless adequate external support is given (Gaining & Growing, 2000).

Although receiving nourishment is a dependent process for the infant, aspects of feeding that involve more active participation on the part of the infant may be considered apprenticeship occupations. Feeding activities carry strong cultural implications. Factors such as when, what, how, and where to eat or to be fed are passed on from parents to children as apprenticeship occupations. The decision to feed on demand versus on a schedule is often determined on the basis of the family's particular culture and individual preferences or expectations. Within the NICU context in particular, the majority of the infants are fed on a schedule. An infant's ability to solicit his or her own food is less essential when feedings occur on a schedule. Infants who do not need to solicit food may experience delay in learning that crying or fussing is an effective strategy for obtaining food and other needs. In contrast, the type of feeding schedule used in the home will depend on the family's preference, particular culture, and, perhaps, the cultural patterns of their community. One could speculate that in cultures that are less structured or that highly value independence, parents may feed infants more on demand, whereas in cultures that are more structured or that emphasize parental control, parents may schedule feedings more rigidly. From an occupation's perspective, on-schedule feeding conceptually may appear to be more conducive to the development of habits and ultimately feeding regularity; however, there is no empirical evidence to support this assumption.

Feeding method—breast versus bottle—is another factor with powerful cultural implications for infants. For many years breast feeding was discouraged in some Western cultures, but a return to breast feeding has occurred since the 1980s. Education about the benefits of breast feeding has raised awareness and given cultural value to this feeding method. At the beginning of the 21st century, many parents in Western culture expect their infants to engage in breast feeding. Although expressing milk from the breast may require more work than feeding from a bottle, mothers who value breast feeding are often willing to work with their infants until both the mother and the infant succeed in this feeding method (see Figure 4). Concerns may arise when an infant whose parents' culture expects breast feeding is unable to do so because of medical instability or contraindications, immaturity of the oral motor mechanisms, or other problems. The developmental team must work with the infant and the family to identify and provide support that—as medical, physiologic, and motor issues resolve—facilitates the infant's engagement, to the extent possible, in this important occupation.

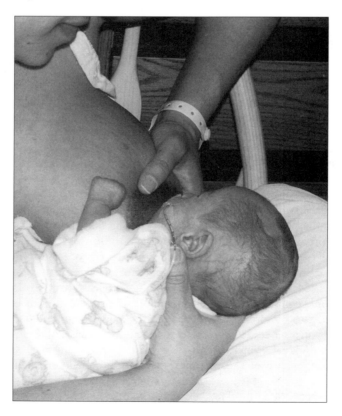

Figure 4.   This mother is introducing the breast to her premature infant while the infant is being gavage-fed by nasogastric tube.

Another issue affecting engagement of NICU infants in feeding is having to cope with feeding styles of multiple caregivers. An infant learns to feed through a dyadic interaction with the caregiver. Feeding success results from the infant's responding adaptively to the caregiver's feeding style, the caregiver's adapting to the infant's feeding style, or a combination of both. A good match between caregiver and infant is of utmost importance for engagement in feeding activities. Healthy infants who possess good adaptive skills and only have to adapt to one primary caregiver may soon achieve this dyadic interaction. This is often not the case for NICU infants, who may have poorer adaptive skills and must constantly adapt to different caregivers. In the best scenario, a NICU infant will be exposed to a minimum of two caregivers each day (one per shift). Furthermore, settings where nurse assignment is rotated limit opportunities for the caregiver and infant to get to know each other's feeding style, potentially delaying achievement of effective and efficient feeding. Under these circumstances, environmental context inconsistency makes it more difficult for infants to become increasingly active in feeding. Parental involvement in feeding in the NICU helps decrease the number of feeders to whom the infant is exposed and the issues associated with this situation. It also begins the learning process between the parent and infant prior to and in preparation for the transition home upon discharge from the NICU.

Participation in feeding is likely to improve when everyone involved in the infant's care uses a consistent feeding approach—the one that works best for that particular infant. The neonatal therapist should ensure that all people involved in feeding an infant are appropriately informed of the infant's most effective feeding method and have demonstrated competency in the use of this specific feeding technique with the infant.

ENHANCING INFANT OCCUPATIONAL PERFORMANCE

A newborn's ability to engage in age-appropriate learning and apprenticeship occupations depends to a large extent on a variety of underlying internal capacities, as well as on critical contextual elements of supports (see Table 1). The maturation of the body systems and developmental experiences result in the emergence of underlying capacities. The rapid growth and maturational changes in the infant's first year, especially during the first few months of life, bring about ongoing changes and adaptations in the development of these underlying capacities and, ultimately, in the child's occupational performance. Basic underlying capacities include functions such as self-regulation of physiologic processes (e.g., breathing, body temperature, oxygen saturation), state of arousal, reflex development, muscle tone, postural and motor control, sensory processing and modulation, oral-motor control, vocal (crying, fussing) and nonvocal communication, visual and auditory skills, and perceptual and cognitive skills (see Table 1). Impairment in these underlying capacities is believed to interfere with function and occupational engagement (see Chapters 8 and 9 for more detail).

Traditional versus Occupation-Based Approaches

Traditional intervention approaches focus on the development of underlying capacities or performance components as a mechanism to improve functional performance.

Working exclusively at the level of underlying capacities, however, may not adequately address the developmental needs of infants, which ultimately is to become increasingly active participants in activities valued within their cultures. Issues such as ongoing changes in contextual influences as children develop challenge the traditional component-based intervention approaches. Occupation-based contextual approaches, in contrast, focus intervention on an infants' engagement in expected occupations, his or her engagement patterns and capabilities, and internal and contextual factors that interfere with or support the infant's participation in such occupations. These approaches focus on enhancing the infant's participation, specifically in the family's expected and valued occupations within the constraints and support of the infant's environmental context.

Fostering occupational performance in NICU infants is an even greater challenge. For much of the time that infants are treated in the NICU, they are critically ill and dependent on life-sustaining technology. During this period, these infants appear to be internally focused and passive—that is, they are striving to achieve and maintain physiologic stability while conserving energy for healing and growth (see Chapters 8 and 9). Lack of physiologic stability hampers an infant's efforts to engage in occupations. The ability to engage in tasks and activities depends in many ways on the stage of maturity of the infant's rapidly developing body systems. The therapist needs to assess the infant's level of maturity and readiness for engagement to establish an effective occupation-based intervention plan in the NICU.

The neonatal therapist who functions as an occupation-based developmental specialist in the NICU helps enhance the infant's performance during each stage of illness and recovery in a variety of ways. Areas of intervention include the following: 1) assessing the infant's individual strengths and vulnerabilities; 2) recommending appropriate modifications to the care environment; and 3) providing external assistance as needed to optimize the infant's physiologic stability, behavioral organization, and consequently, his or her overall performance. Individualized infant assessment is an aspect of this model that can be accomplished by many neonatal therapists, depending on their expertise. Not all neonatal therapists, however, possess the educational and theoretical background or qualifications required to become the team "expert" on other aspects of occupation-based care—designing or modifying the infant's context and providing external support to optimize performance. Each institution should determine which team members are most qualified to provide this form of support to the infant and the family, based on the professional expertise of their team members.

Occupation-based care is best accomplished in collaboration among the various members of the infant's NICU team, including the family and medical professionals (VandenBerg, 1997). Each member of the team contributes his or her unique perspective on the infant's performance, and each plays a significant role in accommodating the care plan to the infant's needs.

Framework for Intervention

An occupation-based infant intervention framework must contemplate the intricate multidimensional or multifactorial processes involved in the development of occupations. Factors such as refinement and maturation of nervous system structures, physical relations of body parts, practice of emerging skills, refinement of specific abilities (i.e., sensorimotor, cognitive, perceptual, emotional, and social), and the environmental context are intimately interrelated and in constant interaction (Thelen, 1995). All of these factors enrich the infant's tasks and activities. Other factors, such as increased alertness and arousal, foster the infant's engagement in occupations and decrease the amount of time spent sleeping or in less active tasks (Colombo, 2001). Figure 5 depicts the major factors that influence an infant's participation in procuring, exploring, feeding, or socially interacting within a NICU setting, as well as the complex interrelation that exists among the various factors. In this model, infant capacities are central to the infant's occupational engagement but form just one of numerous factors that may affect participation and performance. As seen in Figure 5, the infant's capacities are strongly influenced by characteristics of the NICU environment such as sound, light, activity, the infant's positioning arrangement, and medical and nursing procedures. In addition to the NICU environment, the infant's ability to engage in occupations is heavily dependent on the caregivers' availability, sensitivity, and involvement. This model further suggests that infant, environment, and caregiver factors are constantly changing; therefore, from a systems perspective, the infant's ability to participate and opportunities for participating in occupations within the NICU setting result from the ongoing interaction among the various factors. Furthermore, infant

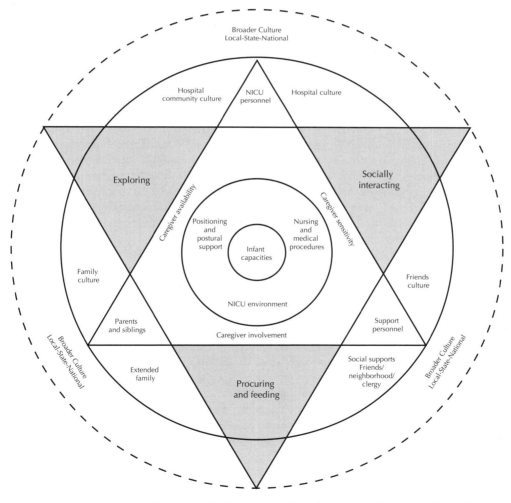

Figure 5. A systems perspective of occupational performance in NICU infants showing the array of elements that may influence an infant's participation in occupations in the NICU.

participation is embedded within the cultures of influence: the hospital culture (e.g., staff, other NICU parents, visitors), the family culture (e.g., expectations, values, beliefs), and the prevailing culture of the family's community. The extent and quality of an infant's ability to engage in such occupations are the result of interaction within the entire system.

Occupation-Based Assessment

Neonatal therapists must keep in mind the complexities of the developmental process when analyzing occupational performance in infants. A common mistake is to develop intervention plans based on speculation about the functional implications of the observed underlying factors or performance components' deficits. Although formal instruments to assess occupational performance in infants are not available, when planning intervention programs for infants, therapists are strongly urged to observe each infant's engagement patterns during routine care and other elements intimately associated with occupational performance. These elements include family values, concerns, needs, and priorities, as well as the physical and social environments of the infant. A comprehensive assessment of the infant's performance should indicate not only the status of underlying factors or the age level at which the infant is functioning but also the specific areas that limit the infant's participation and the factors that enhance participation.

Lack of adequate assessment instruments for infant occupations makes it necessary to conduct an individualized, in-depth analysis of the activities that an infant is expected to perform—prior to assessing the infant directly. This analysis must identify which tasks and abilities or underlying capacities the infant must master for effective participation in the family's expected activities or occupations. Other factors that may influence participation, such as the intrinsic characteristics of the activity and contextual elements, should also be analyzed. An analysis of this type generates an informal but structured criterion-referenced assessment against which to compare the infant's performance. Table 2 presents a breakdown analysis of three sample tasks under the procurer occupation. This example is included as a template for the analysis of other infant occupations.

Beyond the neonatal period, an infant's participation in occupations becomes more active and more complex, involving other performance areas and a broader environment. Emergence of mobility promotes exploring. Procuring activities become less crucial once the infant is able to explore and actively bring the environment closer to him or her through enhanced mobility, relying somewhat less on the caregivers. Social interaction activities become more salient as cognitive, language, and social skills improve, provided that the environment reinforces the infant's emerging social behaviors. With minimal reinforcement, the infant begins to occupy his or her time with other culturally relevant activities such as performing or entertaining play. Learning occupations also begin to blossom at this age in the form of active sensorimotor learning. Educational activities are particularly important and strongly reinforced in cultures where literacy is highly valued.

Working with infants, however, is further complicated by their continued, albeit decreasing, dependency on caregiver support for optimal performance. An occupational performance difficulty in an infant could stem from caregiver inability to recognize, respond to, or support the infant's performance efforts and needs, rather than from the infant's own inability to perform. The role of the caregivers—in this case,

Table 2.　Sample analysis of a newborn's procuring (care soliciting) occupation

Tasks	Activities	Underlying capacities
Making nourishment needs known to caregiver	Searching for breast Squirming Fussing/crying Sucking on fists	Arousal Reflex development Sensory processing Motor control Social/emotional regulation State modulation
Seeking comfort	Eye-to-eye contact Smiling or crying Cuddling Adopting flexed postures	Arousal/alertness Self-regulation Sensory processing Motor control Social/emotional regulation State modulation
Seeking opportunities for exploration	Arm flinging/kicking Visually fixating Visually scanning Reaching Stretching	Arousal/alertness Cognitive skills Perceptual skills Visual skills Sensory processing Motor control

the family—becomes instrumental for eliciting the infant's optimal occupational performance and engagement.

OCCUPATIONAL ROLE OF THE FAMILY

Parental Occupations and Role Fulfillment

One of the greatest frustrations for parents whose infant is admitted to the NICU is having to relinquish their parenting roles to strangers who are considered the "experts" on their infant's care. Although there is no real critical period for the development of attachment (Bruer, 2001), the separation and fear that results from NICU admission may delay the attachment that begins to form between an infant and his or her parents shortly after birth. Even experienced parents suddenly find themselves unable to fulfill the parenting role they had been anticipating. Parents often experience fear, anxiety, depression, and decreased self-confidence after the birth of a high-risk infant, especially when the infant's life depends on frightening life-saving equipment and procedures. Parental apprehension about handling or even touching the infant is aggravated by the limitations imposed by the wires, tubes, and alarming equipment to which the infant may be connected. The few parenting opportunities that family members may find are further hampered by the restrictive NICU environmental context.

Depending on the length of hospitalization, self-efficacy—typically associated with successful role fulfillment (Trombly, 1995)—may be detained for NICU parents unless opportunities are created to foster their engagement in their preferred parenting occupations during their infant's NICU stay. Inability to fulfill basic parenting roles during this very important period for the family could lead to poor self-concept and self-esteem that, if prolonged, could potentially interfere with parental abilities beyond NICU discharge.

Typically, the birth of an infant and the infant's subsequent procurement behaviors entice parents to interact with their infant, offering parents the opportunity to practice a variety of caregiving and child-rearing occupations. Parenting a newborn generally requires adoption of the following occupations or roles:

- *Provider* of the necessary resources to satisfy the infant's needs (e.g., handling, feeding, dressing, bathing, toileting)

- *Facilitator/regulator* of the infant's state and social interaction (e.g., calming, consoling, cuddling, helping the infant go to sleep, arousing)

- *Environmental modulator* to ensure the infant's comfort and exposure to the most optimal child-rearing environment (e.g., controlling temperature, lights, and noise; providing developmentally appropriate toys and activities)

- *Reciprocator/social interactor* to promote social exchanges between the caregiver and the infant (e.g., interpreting and appropriately responding to the infant's nonverbal—and later verbal—communication; timely and contingent social play, "taking turns")

For as long as the infant remains in the NICU, these roles are largely fulfilled by nursing personnel. However, parents should be offered opportunities to begin to perform their caregiving occupations to the extent possible.

A process similar to Table 2's analysis of infant occupations may be employed to analyze parental occupations, tasks, and activities that are necessary to perform a particular caregiving role, especially for NICU infants. Table 3 presents an example of this process for analyzing the parent's role as the infant's facilitator/regulator. Three of the most important areas for which NICU infants need regulation support

Table 3. Sample breakdown analysis of three performance areas under the facilitator/regulator (care provider) occupation of the caregiver

Performance areas	Tasks/activities	Components/capacities
Assisting the infant in falling asleep	Observing the infant for signs of fatigue, drowsiness, or restlessness	Cognitive skills
		Perceptual skills
	Offering assistance as needed (nesting, singing/playing music, positioning the infant for hand-to-mouth soothing, making rhythmic movements)	Social/emotional regulation
Consoling/enhancing the infant's self-calming abilities	Modulating one's face, voice, and touch and the environment	Social/emotional regulation
	Cuddling	State regulation
	Positioning the infant optimally for hand-to-mouth soothing	Sensorimotor processing
Providing opportunities for the infant's exploration	Arousing the infant to a quiet-alert state	State regulation
	Offering the infant appropriately modulated face-to-face interaction and visual, auditory, tactile, and movement stimuli	Social/emotional regulation
		Sensorimotor processing
	Watching for signs of fatigue or the need for a change of activity	Perceptual skills
		Cognitive skills

from their parents are analyzed: facilitating sleep, consoling/self-calming, and exploring the environment. The tasks and activities listed would enhance parental performance of the occupations required to support the infant's performance efforts. The components and capacities listed are the underlying capacities that parents need for engaging in the tasks and activities necessary to perform their caregiving role in these areas.

Parenting in the NICU

Although performing facilitator/regulator occupations becomes spontaneous and easy for most parents, parents of sick or fragile newborns may encounter considerable difficulty in fulfilling such basic tasks during their initial parenting experiences. Self-efficacy in parenting is best achieved when there is a "goodness of fit" between the parent and infant (Thomas & Chess, 1989). Goodness of fit presupposes that parental resources (e.g., physical, financial, social/emotional) are adequate to meet the needs of the infant and the parents. The greater the infant's needs (e.g., for an infant in the NICU), the more resources the parents may need to fulfill those increased needs. Parents and infants who experience a poor fit are likely more vulnerable to ineffective parental role fulfillment. Thus, a major component of neonatal intervention should be to decrease the family's vulnerability and increase their resiliency by enhancing goodness of fit between the infant's needs and parental resources. (See Chapters 3 and 11 for more details.)

Sibling Occupations

Siblings also may be affected by the special circumstances resulting from NICU admission. Although siblings of healthy, full-term infants are often allowed to perform basic caregiving activities for their new brother or sister (e.g., offering a toy, washing the infant's face), this type of involvement generally is not possible in the NICU. Anecdotal evidence suggests that siblings may resent a new brother or sister more than usual when they are not allowed to socially engage with the infant. If persistent, sibling resentfulness or rejection may become an additional source of stress for the family unless sibling opportunities for social role participation are nurtured.

Promoting Parental Occupations in the NICU

Family-centered intervention in the NICU fosters family involvement in all aspects of an infant's care to the extent the family is willing and able to become involved. Parents are given the opportunity and knowledge necessary to begin fulfilling their own occupational roles as parents—that is, as providers, protectors, caregivers, educators, and facilitators of their child's development. Through participation in developmentally supportive, occupation-based care, parents learn to identify and respond appropriately to their infant's particular capacities and needs. Involvement in the infant's care reinforces parents' role identification and performance, as they gain awareness of the complexity of their infant's condition. Moreover, parents who are involved in their infant's care have a more realistic view of their infant's health status, have more appropriate expectations for their child's developmental outcome, and are better prepared to optimize their child's potential. These parents have been shown to experience less stress and to have a better quality of feeding interaction with their infants than parents who have not received family-based intervention (Meyer et al., 1994). They may have learned ways to optimize their resources and to deal with stress and risks associated with their infant's care, thereby enhancing their resiliency and minimizing their vulnerability (McCubbin & McCubbin, 1996). Finally, and perhaps most important, these parents are better prepared for the difficult transition from hospital to home, which is a major component of the continuum of care for high-risk infants (Meyer, Lester, Boukydis, & Bigsby, 1998) and an important practice arena for neonatal therapists. This topic is covered at length in Chapters 3 and 11.

CONCLUSION

It is imperative that developmentally focused NICU therapists recognize all of the elements involved in the delivery of best practice neonatal care, the foremost element being the family. Only through family collaboration can neonatal therapists support occupational engagement of infants and their families.

2

Historical Evolution of the Neonatal Therapist's Role

OVERVIEW

This chapter discusses the roles of the neonatal therapist and the factors that have influenced these roles since the 1970s. Content focuses on the factors and philosophies of care that led to the establishment and evolution of developmental services for newborns, particularly the regionalization of perinatal services, outcome studies, and the creation of legislation that became Part C of the Individuals with Disabilities Education Act (IDEA) Amendments of 1997 (hereafter called "IDEA Part C"). The chapter emphasizes the prevailing philosophies of care and the roles of neonatal therapists in the different levels of care of newborns.

OBJECTIVES

- Describe the elements that promoted the evolution of developmental services for newborns and their families since the 1970s
- Compare the theoretical frameworks that underlie two major developmental care approaches used with newborns: supplemental sensory stimulation and individualized developmentally supportive care
- Describe neonatal approaches that have gained in popularity since the 1990s: infant massage, kangaroo care, and complementary/alternative care
- Describe the levels of nurseries established through the regionalization of perinatal services
- Explain the roles of neonatal therapists in each of the levels of newborn care, particularly their role as members of the developmental team
- Identify the knowledge base that neonatal therapists must possess and the importance of being adequately and appropriately trained to provide neonatal intervention services
- Identify the parameters of IDEA Part C—its purpose, its applicability in the NICU, and which of its various services apply to neonatal intervention
- Recognize the importance and the rights given to the family under IDEA Part C

EVOLUTION OF NEONATAL DEVELOPMENTAL SERVICES

Since the 1970s, a variety of professions have been providing developmental services to newborns. Initially, only infants with obvious chromosomal or congenital anomalies or with established conditions (e.g., Erb's palsy, spina bifida, hypoxic ischemia, progressive neuromuscular diseases, other severe motor problems or congenital conditions) were referred for developmental or therapeutic services during the newborn period. Infants generally had to be medically stable and usually spent some time either in the NICU or at home before they were referred for therapy. At that time, intervention consisted predominantly of traditional developmental stimulation, neurodevelopmental treatment, and, when necessary, splinting. Other areas included interventions based on underlying factors such as muscle strengthening, gross and fine motor coordination, and range of motion. Referrals for neonatal intervention with medically fragile infants were rare.

Prior to the 1970s, the mortality rate of medically complex/fragile infants was very high. From the time when the incubator was invented in the early 1900s and Dr. Julian Hess established the first special care unit for preterm infants in 1923 until the 1960s, the focus of neonatal care was on providing warmth, protection from infection, and feeding (Plaas, 1994). Many infants with severe respiratory or cardiovascular conditions or who were extremely premature died during the neonatal period (Merenstein, 1994). Few survived long enough to be referred for therapy. Advances in clinical and life-support technology dramatically improved infant survival. As the number of surviving small and sick infants increased, so did the need to develop specialized nursing facilities to provide the complex, technologically advanced care that these infants required. Regionalized NICUs were established in the 1970s to address this need.

Initially, the survival of very low birth weight (VLBW) infants (those weighing less than 1,500 grams [g]) came at a high cost of morbidity: the same technology that was saving their lives was contributing to the development of serious secondary complications. Survival often meant having to face the life-long challenges imposed by conditions such as chronic respiratory disorders, cerebral palsy, blindness, or cognitive and hearing impairments. Early intervention programs emerged in the mid-1970s to address these developmental issues (Hack, Fanaroff, & Merkatz, 1979; Meisels & Shonkoff, 2000; Sweeney & Swanson, 1990). Since then, developmental professionals—including occupational therapists, physical therapists, speech-language pathologists, psychologists, and others—have played an important role in the provision of neonatal intervention for fragile infants.

The most striking benefit of technological advances has been the increased survival of VLBW infants and extremely low birth weight (ELBW) infants (those weighing less than 1,000 g). Infants born as early as 23 weeks after gestation, some weighing less than 500 g, may survive. Factors associated with higher survival in the literature include higher gestational age, higher birth weight, and female gender. Although long-term neurological and developmental involvement continues to be more prevalent among infants born extremely premature or sick, many of these infants surprisingly develop within normal limits, exceeding most odds and expectations (Allen & Capute, 1989; Cohen, 1987; Epstein, 1987; Hack et al., 1979; Hack, Friedman, & Fanaroff, 1996; Hack et al., 2002; Miller et al., 1995; Msall, Buck, et al., 1994; Ounsted, Moar, & Scott, 1988; Sweeney, Heriza, Reilly, Smith, & VanSant, 1999; Sweeney & Swanson, 1990).

Traditional Supplemental Stimulation

Survival of ELBW infants has prolonged the length of their neonatal intensive care period and added new and more complex developmental concerns for neonatal health care professionals. As more of these infants survived, it became obvious that the developmental issues they were presenting were as critical as many of their medical issues.

Initially, the philosophy of care for low birth weight (LBW) and premature infants was strictly developmental—that is, to stimulate and, to the greatest extent possible, normalize the infants' development. Developmental personnel who were novices to neonatal intervention began to notice that these infants, especially VLBW infants, presented very different behavioral patterns compared with full-term infants at birth. These unique issues raised the urgency to explore new intervention theories and strategies to address the intricate needs of this growing population of infants, thereby enabling them to develop in ways more similar to those of full-term infants.

In the early 1970s, this difference in development was explained as the result of the infants' shorter exposure to the intrauterine environment (Linn, Horowitz, & Fox, 1985). Moreover, it was also believed that preterm infants experienced sensory deprivation postnatally and that the differences in development may have been a consequence of deprivation. These beliefs led to the development of supplemental sensory stimulation programs, which were designed to simulate the intrauterine conditions and accompanying sensory experiences that these infants were believed to have missed (Field, 1980; Heriza & Sweeney, 1990). Traditional supplemental sensory stimulation programs focused on enhancing primarily tactile, vestibular, proprioceptive, and auditory stimulation. Stimulation was presented either unimodally (one sensory modality at a time) or multimodally (more than one sensory modality combined). Enriched sensory stimulation was offered as a strategy to bridge or decrease the gap between normal intrauterine development and the postnatal extrauterine development of premature infants. The following effects were originally associated with supplemental sensory stimulation (Field, 1980; Heriza & Sweeney, 1990):

- Increased weight gain
- More optimal scores on certain developmental tests
- Decreased crying
- More quiet sleep
- Improved interaction
- Greater attentiveness

Several research studies later, in the 1980s, neonatal researchers concluded that supplemental sensory stimulation programs failed to close the differences and developmental gap between preterm infants approaching term age and their full-term counterparts. Although some developmental gains were associated with supplemental sensory stimulation, these programs did not achieve the clinical developmental benefits anticipated. Many infants, in particular the most fragile ones, could not tolerate the extra stimulation inherent in these programs. Supplemental stimulation programs seemed to be effective only with the older, larger, more stable preterm infants.

In the process of seeking potential explanations for the differential development of preterm infants, an alternate conceptualization of neonatal environmental influences on development began to emerge (Gottfried, Wallace-Lande, Sherman-Brown,

King, & Coen, 1981). The new view proposed that instead of being deprived of stimuli, infants receiving neonatal intensive care were exposed to excessive, mostly aversive sensory stimulation (Field, 1980; Gottfried et al., 1981; Heriza & Sweeney, 1990). The developmental differences of NICU infants were explained in part as being the consequence of sensory stress or overload resulting from such stimuli as constant lighting, elevated noise levels, and frequent intrusive medical and nursing procedures. Sensory overloading was considered to be even more dangerous for the younger premature infants who, because of immaturity of their nervous systems, were more susceptible or unable to tolerate or habituate to sensory stimuli (Gorski, Hole, Leonard, & Martin, 1983). Based on the new philosophy, a change in focus of developmental intervention from supplemental stimulation to environmental modulation emerged. The latter philosophy proposed designing or modifying the environment according to the infant's individualized needs, capabilities, and vulnerabilities to minimize potentially stressful stimuli while allowing some exposure to organizing sensory experiences (Als et al., 1986; Gottfried et al., 1981; Heriza & Sweeney, 1990; Lawhon & Melzan, 1988). Without negating the potential benefits of simulating the intrauterine environment, proponents of this theory emphasized the importance of modulating the infant's environmental context prior to, or in preparation for, exposure to stimuli that could consequently tax his or her functional abilities (Als et al., 1986; Lawhon & Melzan, 1988).

Developmentally Supportive Care

The individualized developmentally supportive care programs evolved from environmental modulation principles. Although some findings remain inconclusive (Symington & Pinelli, 2001), a few studies suggest that fragile infants cared for under individualized developmental care principles exhibit improved developmental outcomes in comparison with infants treated in traditional settings (Als & Duffy, 1989; Als et al., 1986, 1994). Most neonatal therapy services offered at the beginning of the 21st century in developed countries have an individualized developmental care perspective. The potential benefits of individualized developmental care over traditional nursing care are detailed in Chapter 3.

Individualized developmentally supportive care is the prevailing philosophy in most NICUs throughout the United States. In a study by Shannon and Gorski (1994) involving 530 NICU multidisciplinary team members, this type of care was rated as the most important among the following six categories of developmental services in the NICU:

1. Individualized developmentally supportive care
2. Direct caregiving procedures
3. Parent participation
4. Environmental modification
5. Sensory stimulation
6. Positioning

In contrast, sensory stimulation was rated as the least useful of the six developmental service categories (Shannon & Gorski, 1994). These findings further support the philosophical and clinical transformation that has occurred in the management and care of the NICU infants.

Individualized Supplemental Sensory Intervention

The focus on supplemental sensory intervention resurfaces periodically. A few such programs have gained much acceptance and popularity. Infant massage involving tactile and proprioceptive stimulation has been the most popular form of supplemental sensory stimulation used with newborns since the mid-1980s (Ottenbacher et al., 1987; Scafidi, Field, & Schanberg, 1993). It has been the subject of extensive research since the 1990s. Much of the research comes from the Touch Research Institutes at the University of Miami's Mailman Center for Child Development.

Massage and gentle human touch are safe for most preterm infants once they are medically stable (Browne, 2000; White-Traut & Nelson, 1988). Benefits associated with massage of premature or LBW infants include improved daily weight gain and reduced length of NICU stay. Other benefits include enhanced mother-infant communication and interaction (Barratt, Roach, & Leavitt, 1992; Onozawa, Glover, Adams, Modi, & Kumar, 2001). Small benefits of increased weight and decreased complications at 4–6 months corrected age have also been reported. No significant benefits have been associated with gentle, still touch (Vickers, Ohlsson, Lacy, & Horsley, 2002). The methodology of studies reporting other benefits in the literature was challenged in an extensive meta-analysis evidence-based review conducted by the Cochrane Collaboration (Vickers et al., 2002). These authors concluded that "the evidence that massage for preterm infants is of benefit for developmental outcomes is weak" and "consideration should be given as to whether this is a cost-effective use of [therapists' or nurses'] time" (pp. 1–2). Therapists must keep in mind that this area is still in great need of research. Therapists must consider which infants are likely to benefit most from massage (Scafidi et al., 1993) and must consider the cost to the family when recommending its use. Having the family provide the massage may enable an infant (and his or her family) to receive its benefits at no increased cost.

Skin-to-skin contact, also termed *kangaroo care,* is a popular means of providing warmth, sleep, and tactile comfort, as well as an opportunity for more intimate parent–infant interaction for preterm infants in the NICU (Affonso, Bosque, Wahlberg, & Brady, 1993; Feldman, Weller, Sirota, & Eidelman, 2002; Gale & VandenBerg, 1998; Ludington-Hoe & Swinth, 1996). Some of these supplemental stimulation programs are being used in combination with individualized developmental care principles. In some developing countries, particularly in South America, skin-to-skin or kangaroo care is used as an alternative to the incubator with striking results. Compared with infants who were cared for in incubators, infants provided with continuous (24-hour) skin-to-skin care had a lower risk of death, spent less time in the hospital, had similar developmental outcomes at 1 year of age, and had less severe infections than the infants in the comparison group (Charpak, Ruiz-Pelaez, & Charpak, 2001). These findings are consistent with those of other countries reported in the literature. Skin-to-skin care was once considered a form of alternative care, but with its increasing popularity, it has become part of the routine care in many NICUs.

Research evidence suggests that using supplemental sensory intervention programs with healthy, stable infants is safe. Readers are cautioned, however, that the safe use of some of these programs with the more fragile, younger, or sick infants has not been well documented. Supplemental sensory stimulation, even in its mildest forms, may be contraindicated for many NICU infants. Regarding skin-to-skin care, Gale and VandenBerg (1998) pointed out that each NICU infant must be evaluated individually for physiologic and behavioral stability before this and other forms of intervention are implemented. Neonatal therapists must exercise extreme caution and critical judgment when considering the use of supplementary stimulation approaches with infants in the NICU. The final decision should be made in cooperation with the family and other members of the medical team. See Chapter 11 for greater detail on this topic.

Complementary or Alternative Care

A variety of "alternative experiences" have been gaining popularity in NICUs in some parts of the United States, many without clear evidence to support their use with infants. These forms of care are promoted by the holistic medical movement (Jones & Kassity, 2001). Some complementary alternative therapies attempt to replicate intra-uterine experience within the NICU environment. Examples of complementary alternative NICU therapies include light therapy, music therapy, aromatherapy, reflexology, osteopathy, and chiropractic care (Jones & Kassity, 2001). Infant massage is also categorized as a complementary alternative form of therapy (Jones & Kassity, 2001). Until more research is available, neonatal therapists must exercise extreme care in using these approaches, particularly with the smaller infants with more serious medical problems.

REGIONALIZATION OF PERINATAL SERVICES

One of the factors that promoted the initiation and expansion of developmental services for newborns was the regionalization of perinatal services (Pettett, Bonnabel, & Bird, 1989). In the days before regionalization, it was not uncommon to find several hospitals within the same community providing services to infants requiring all levels of care, ranging from healthy newborns to those in need of the most critical care. As medical and technological advances in neonatology unfolded in the 1960s, neonatal care became increasingly specialized and costly, equipment and procedures needed for sustaining the infants' lives became more and more complex, and services other than nursing and medical became essential. It became practically impossible for the smaller hospitals to offer the technological and personnel support required to provide neonatal care of adequate quality to reduce mortality and morbidity. In search of a potential solution to this situation, the medical community engaged in an exhaustive evaluation of the existing systems. Alternative service delivery models that would be cost-effective and efficient while securing the highest quality of perinatal services possible were explored. In the early 1970s, following the recommendation of the American Medical Association (AMA; 1974), the Committee on Perinatal Health was formed to draft guidelines for regional perinatal services. This committee included representatives from the American Academy of Family Physicians, American Academy of Pediatrics, American College of Obstetricians and Gynecologists, AMA, and National Foundation-March of Dimes. The resulting guidelines were published in 1975, paving the way for the establishment of regional perinatal centers around the country, with private and public funding.

Passage of the National Health Planning and Resources Development Act of 1974 (PL 93-641) made it possible for individual states to develop regional perinatal centers. By 1979, there were more than 200 perinatal centers across the United States (Pettet et al., 1989). As of 2003, most communities have convenient access to a regional perinatal center. These centers are usually housed in teaching hospitals affiliated with a medical school, are staffed by qualified attending neonatologists, and offer the latest technology for saving and supporting the lives of infants who are sick and fragile. Guidelines for establishment of regional perinatal centers are included in the *Action Guide for Maternal and Child Care Committees* report (AMA, 1974). Regionalization of perinatal services pursues the following objectives (Fanaroff & Merkatz, 1993, p. 2):

1. Identification of high-risk pregnancies early in the perinatal period
2. Further identification of high-risk factors within the intrapartum period
3. Development of interhospital agreements on criteria for transfer of mothers and infants within the network
4. Development of support systems of consultation, laboratory services, education, and transportation within a region
5. Development of a record-keeping system that adequately monitors the performance of the entire program

Levels of Neonatal Care

Regional perinatal centers generally offer three levels of neonatal care:

- Level I: normal newborn nurseries
- Level II: intermediate (continuing) care nurseries
- Level III: neonatal intensive care units

An additional level of care is available in certain specialized medical centers that provide extracorporeal membrane oxygenation (ECMO) therapy. There is compelling statistical evidence that a system in which neonatal services are offered based on the degree of expertise and the resources required improves the quality of perinatal services. For example, the risk of death among preterm infants delivered at a Level I or Level II center is 24% higher than that of infants delivered at a Level III center (Paneth, Keily, Wallenstein, & Suser, 1987). The effect of specialized neonatal services on infant morbidity and developmental outcome is less clear and has been the subject of some controversy in the literature.

Level I: Normal Newborn Nurseries

Level I centers serve infants who are healthy or require minimal observation and/or care. Infants who require short periods of warming in an enclosed Isolette (incubator), brief courses of phototherapy for jaundice, or limited diagnostic workups may also receive care in a Level I nursery. Supplemental oxygen and intravenous (IV) feedings usually are not provided in this setting. Minor surgical procedures, such as circumcision, are provided at this level of care. This is often the only level of nursery available in smaller, community-based hospitals.

Level II: Intermediate (Continuing) Care Nurseries

Level II centers serve infants who need more specialized care than available in the normal newborn nursery but less specialized care than available in Level III nurseries. Level II nurseries can be found in regional hospitals as well as in many community hospitals. The Level II nursery often functions as a "step-down" unit for the NICU, caring for preterm infants who are no longer critically ill but need to grow and gain sufficient weight before being discharged. Infants who require IV antibiotic therapy or alimentation, feedings by oral or nasal gavage, phototherapy for hyperbilirubinemia, or oxygen supplementation administered by nasal cannula or oxyhood are appropriately served at the secondary level of care. The Level II nursery is a vital component of service delivery in neonatal care because it allows infants who need a certain degree of specialized care to remain in or close to their community. Level II care also makes it possible for infants who are recovering from a critical illness or from extreme prematurity to be transferred closer to their home for the remainder of their hospital stay, which greatly facilitates family visitation and participation in the infant's care. Level II nurseries are staffed by neonatologists and neonatal nurses with specialized training.

Level III: Neonatal Intensive Care Units

Level III centers are also called special care nurseries or tertiary care centers. These centers house the sickest and most fragile newborns. Level III nurseries provide highly specialized services to infants who require close observation or who are critically ill and thereby require life support and complex medical and nursing intervention. Level III nurseries are usually affiliated with major medical schools and are staffed by qualified attending neonatologists and neonatology fellows, providing the greatest expertise and specialized care. Level III nurseries serve preterm or term infants who are technologically dependent or medically fragile, requiring mechanical ventilatory support, specialized nursing, advanced diagnostic services, or surgical care. In addition, Level III centers serve infants with conditions such as respiratory distress, sepsis, neonatal seizures, and congenital anomalies or genetic disorders. Critically ill infants requiring specialized care often need to be transported to Level III nurseries that are far from their community. Those requiring a higher level of care, such as ECMO, need to be transported to specialized nurseries, often found in larger medical centers.

Summary

Most major medical centers housing Level III nurseries also provide Level II and Level I care. Both Level III and Level II nurseries require highly specialized medical, nursing, and developmental staff, as well as a long list of support personnel, including neonatal therapists. Level I and sometimes Level II nurseries may be located in smaller, community-based hospitals. The availability of support services in community hospitals varies.

Maternal Transport

Infants born in local community hospitals who need more complex services than can be safely provided in the Level I nursery are frequently transferred shortly after birth to a nearby hospital able to provide the necessary level of care (Pettett et al., 1989). When the need for specialized services is known or suspected before birth, arrangements are often made to transport the mother to a regional perinatal center for the anticipated high-risk delivery. Maternal transport has the following advantages: 1) initiation of treatments such as tocolysis to forestall the premature birth for as long as possible; 2) administration of antenatal steroids to hasten the maturation of the fetal heart and lungs; 3) close monitoring of the mother and fetus by medical personnel who are experienced with high-risk pregnancies; and 4) access to specialized services and resources, should these be necessary, immediately after delivery. Medical specialists from neonatology, genetics, cardiology, neurology, endocrinology, and other areas are also available after maternal transfer to improve expectant families' understanding of the risks and benefits of treatment or available care alternatives. Maternal transport also avoids the risks involved in transporting a perhaps unstable newborn, either by ambulance or by helicopter, to the nearest available perinatal center. When neonatal transport is compared with maternal transport, percentages of severe morbidity decrease sharply (e.g., 11.8% versus 4.9%) (Hohlagschwandtner et al., 2001). The major disadvantage of maternal transport is that the infant often is not in the family's community, thus limiting the family's visits and participation in infant care (Page & Lunyk-Child, 1995).

ROLE OF THE NEONATAL THERAPIST

The role of neonatal therapists in the NICU is multifaceted. They must function as consultants, diagnosticians, interventionists, and family support providers within a highly stressful environment. Neonatal therapists must have appropriate advanced-level training on which to base clinical decisions, a working knowledge of a broad range of neonatal conditions and their potential course of treatment and action, and the confidence that comes with experience. In the best settings, neonatal therapists are part of a team of professionals that can provide comprehensive services for the developmental, behavioral, and mental health needs of infants and families. For obvious reasons, the NICU is not considered an appropriate setting for entry-level practitioners or therapy assistants (Anzalone, 1994; Gorga et al., 2000; Hunter, Mullen, & Dallas, 1994; Sweeney et al., 1999). Neonatal practice demands appropriately trained and experienced professionals who understand the complete course of infant development and can speculate on future expectations. These professionals should have the necessary credibility to assure the families that their infants are "in good hands."

Within the Level III setting, the critical illness status and extreme fragility of the infants and the emotional vulnerability of their families must be added to the previously mentioned considerations. Gorga et al. (2000), Hunter et al. (1994), Sweeney et al. (1999), and VandenBerg (1993, 1996) outlined the specialized knowledge base required to function as a developmental specialist in the NICU. VandenBerg spoke to the necessity of going beyond knowledge of normal infant development, atypical infant development, and family dynamics. Other areas of essential knowledge required for working in the NICU include the following (VandenBerg, 1996):

- Fetal and newborn brain development
- Medical conditions of premature and full-term neonates
- Neonatal preterm and full-term infant behaviors and development
- Ecology of the NICU
- Staffing and cultural patterns in the NICU
- Parenting in the NICU

The NICU is characterized by fast-paced delivery of medical care with limited time to accommodate new learning. In this environment, seemingly simple interventions such as alterations in feeding, positioning, or handling can result in dramatic changes in physiologic stability. Interventions that appear quite benign may have far-reaching positive *and* negative consequences because infants in the NICU experience life-threatening conditions at the same time as enormous growth and development of the cardiorespiratory, gastrointestinal, and central nervous systems. Thus, the principle of "less is more" applies in the NICU as in no other setting. To emphasize this point, Garbarino (1990) quoted Hardin's First Law of Ecology. In essence, this law states that a person can never do just one thing; any action taken will have a number of reverberating consequences, many of which will be unforeseen and/or unknown. The NICU therapist must be a keen observer and have the knowledge and acumen to immediately assess not only the apparent short-term consequences and benefits but also the potential liabilities and long-term effects of interventions.

Levels of Neonatal Intervention

Neonatal intervention is most commonly provided in Level II and Level III NICUs. Because infants in Level III nurseries are often too fragile or too sick to receive direct developmental intervention, therapists at this level of care primarily provide consultation services, especially in the areas of positioning, energy conservation, and environmental design. The infant's developmental needs are met indirectly through modification of the environmental context. The main focus of intervention at this level is to decrease the infant's exposure to stress and optimize his or her neurobehavioral organization, especially during periods of medical and physiologic instability. At this level, infants are evaluated predominantly through observation to avoid unnecessary handling that may aggravate their often compromised physiologic stability. Assessment must be ongoing because the medical instability of these infants means that their support needs may change from minute to minute. Intervention in Level III nurseries also focuses on the family members, helping them to identify, interpret, and appropriately respond to their infant's signals and to recognize and respect the infant's limited readiness for interaction. Parents are also assisted in identifying ways to engage in simple but important parental tasks such as wiping their infant's skin or tucking their infant's extremities, as tolerated.

In the Level II nursery, intervention focuses on areas similar to those addressed in the Level III nursery but may be more aggressive. Infants in the Level II nursery, although still somewhat fragile, may tolerate lengthier and more intrusive evaluations and interventions. Intervention may involve more handling, and infants' developmental needs may be addressed more directly. For example, a therapist may work hands-on with an infant to enhance self-regulation through development of hand-to-mouth behaviors or to improve the infant's feeding skills. To the extent desired by and feasible for the family, family members are encouraged to participate in their infant's assessments and intervention processes for as long as the infant stays in the Level II nursery. Closer to discharge, the therapist prepares the family for the infant's transition to the home (see Chapter 11).

Therapy services in Level I nurseries are infrequent because infants at this level are typically healthy. Occasionally, therapists may receive referrals for consultation regarding feeding, self-regulation, or other developmental issues of otherwise healthy Level I infants. Assessment results may indicate the need for extended therapy. If the infant is otherwise healthy, this form of intervention is usually of short duration. Infants who require more prolonged or complex intervention usually have more serious problems than those commonly handled in Level I nurseries. These infants may be transferred to a Level II nursery for at least a short period of time, until they overcome the problem or other recommendations are made. Less frequently, an infant with a non–life threatening condition who is otherwise healthy (e.g., has Erb's palsy or minor congenital anomalies) may be cared for entirely in the Level I nursery until he or she is ready for discharge. To prevent discontinuation of services, when an infant is likely to require ongoing therapy, a referral for early intervention is recommended and arranged prior to discharge.

Intervention Approaches and Perspectives

Neonatal therapists use advanced theoretical frameworks that are reflected in their approach to practice. Also reflected in successful practice is the recognition that there is no single approach to practice that will be effective with all patients. The most effective approach is the one that best meets the infant's needs within the performance context formed by the infant's individual strengths and vulnerabilities; the opportunities and constraints inherent in that particular NICU environment; and the influences of the medical team, the developmental team, and the family (see Chapter 3).

The neonatal therapist must gain the trust of the medical team and of the family that all interventions will be carefully evaluated and implemented only with team involvement. This requires finesse in dealing with all levels of the medical hierarchy—from nurses, respiratory therapists, nutritionists, and social workers to pediatric interns, nurse practitioners, neonatology fellows, and attending neonatologists. A wide variety of medical specialists may become part of an individual infant's treatment team, including physicians from radiology, neurology, cardiology, infectious diseases, endocrinology, hematology, urology, nephrology, gastroenterology, genetics, orthopedics, otolaryngology, pediatric surgery, plastic surgery, developmental and behavioral pediatrics, and psychiatry. Neonatal intervention services must also be orchestrated with other health care services such as respiratory therapy, nutrition, and social work. Input from a variety of sources and services must be considered before cautiously embarking on a particular course of intervention.

Therapy services in neonatal intensive care settings can be summarized into the following categories:

- Consultation to care providers
- Developmental diagnosis
- Direct intervention
- Facilitation of parent roles
- Facilitation of transition home from a developmental perspective
- Follow-up monitoring
- Early intervention

Therapists may need to offer all of these services to perform effectively in neonatal care settings.

NEONATAL INTERVENTION SERVICES AND IDEA PART C

One other factor that fostered the delivery of neonatal intervention services was the creation of Part H of the Education of the Handicapped Act Amendments of 1986

(PL 99-457). This piece of legislation was originally established as a nationwide strategy to accomplish the following goals:

- Enhance the development of infants and toddlers with or at risk for disabilities and minimize their potential for developmental delay.

- Reduce the cost of education by minimizing the need for special education and related services when infants and toddlers with or at risk for disabilities reach school age.

- Minimize the likelihood of institutionalization of individuals with disabilities and maximize their potential for living independently in society.

- Enhance the capacity of families of infants and toddlers with or at risk for disabilities to meet the special needs of their children.

Part H was subsequently reauthorized as Part C of the Individuals with Disabilities Education Act (IDEA) (34 CFR § 303).[1] Amendments to the original legislation have been inconsequential to the delivery of neonatal services.

Grant monies were made available in the late 1980s to states willing "to develop and implement a statewide comprehensive, coordinated, multidisciplinary, interagency program of early intervention services for infants and toddlers with disabilities and their families" (34 CFR § 303). States were also required to provide the necessary training to ensure that early intervention personnel were appropriately and adequately trained to provide services in compliance with the law.

Part C requires that services must be available, as necessary, to meet the developmental needs of each eligible child and the needs of the family related to the child's development (34 CFR § 303.12). All of the major disciplines that fall under the rubric of neonatal therapists (i.e., occupational therapy, physical therapy, speech-language pathology, psychology) are included among the early intervention services listed under Part C. Although the law provides specific definitions for each service, it stipulates the following general roles for service providers (34 CFR § 303.12):

1. Consult with parents, other service providers, and representatives of appropriate community agencies to ensure the effective provision of services in that area.

2. Train parents and others regarding the provision of those services.

3. Participate in the multidisciplinary team's assessment of the child and the child's family.

These roles are consistent with those typically carried out by neonatal therapists.

Part C stipulates that early intervention programs must address all of the following developmental areas, as necessary: physical, cognitive, language and social, psychosocial, and self-help skills. It also defines the overall scope of practice for each of the disciplines, giving leeway to the programs regarding how the various team members will collaboratively address the developmental needs of each eligible child. Table 4 includes the definitions of Part C for the most common neonatal services (§ 303.12).

The major intent of Part C is to minimize the incidence of developmental delays in infants and toddlers with disabilities. It highlights the importance of recognizing

---

[1]Readers are encouraged to review IDEA Partnership's web site (http://www.ideapractices.org) for the most current information.

Table 4. Definition of early intervention services under the Individuals with Disabilities Education Act (IDEA) Amendments of 1997 (PL 105-17), Part C (34 CFR § 303)

Discipline	Definition	Services
Occupational therapy	Services to address the functional needs of a child related to adaptive development; adaptive behavior and play; and sensory, motor, and postural development. Designed to improve the child's functional ability to perform tasks at home, at school, and in the community.	Identification, assessment, and intervention Adaptation of the environment and selection, design, and fabrication of assistive and orthotic devices to facilitate development and promote the acquisition of functional skills Prevention or minimization of the impact of initial or future impairment, delay in development, or loss of functional ability
Physical therapy	Services to address the promotion of sensorimotor function through enhancement of musculoskeletal status, neurobehavioral organization, perceptual and motor development, cardiopulmonary status, and effective environmental adaptation.	Screening, evaluation, and assessment of infants and toddlers to identify motor dysfunction Obtaining, interpreting, and integrating information appropriate to program planning to prevent, alleviate, or compensate for movement dysfunction and related functional problems Providing individual and group services or treatment to prevent, alleviate, or compensate for movement dysfunction and related functional problems
Psychology	(No definition provided in IDEA Part C)	Administering psychological and developmental tests and other assessment procedures Interpreting assessment results Obtaining, integrating, and interpreting information about child behavior and about child and family conditions related to learning, mental health, and development Planning and managing a program of psychological services, including psychological counseling for children and parents, family counseling, consultation on child development, parent training, and education programs
Speech-language pathology	(No definition provided in IDEA Part C)	Identification of children with communicative or oropharyngeal disorders and delays in development of communication skills Referrals for medical or other professional services necessary for the habilitation or rehabilitation of children with communicative oropharyngeal disorders and delays in development of communication skills Provision of services for the habilitation or rehabilitation of children with communicative oropharyngeal disorders and delays in development of communication skills

the role and importance of the family in meeting a child's developmental needs and optimizing his or her developmental potential (Hanft, 1988). It has given the family an active (although voluntary) role in the development of the individualized family service plan (IFSP) to guide the delivery of services. The IFSP identifies the child's strengths and needs; the family's priorities, resources, and concerns related to their child's development; and the services that must be provided to address the identified needs (§ 303.344).

Although not all states mandate development of an official IFSP in the NICU, most regional perinatal centers will not discharge an infant until a needs and strengths assessment of the infant and the family is performed and documented and a plan to address those needs is identified. The degree to which family members participate in the establishment of the plan varies across NICUs, but participation is ultimately up to the individual family because it is strictly voluntary (§ 303.405). Most institutions offer families their rightful opportunity to participate in this process at their will and convenience.

CONCLUSION

Including the family in intervention planning and implementation has been a natural outflow of regionalization of services. The neonatal intensive care system provides all of the elements necessary to implement the principles of IDEA Part C with families from the moment of their child's birth. It is the most ideal setting for early identification of infants with or at risk for developing disabilities who would be likely to benefit from the provisions of Part C. Simply mandating the NICU as the first environment for implementation of IDEA, however, does not automatically imply that neonatal therapy personnel, although certified and licensed, are adequately trained to provide services in compliance with Part C. Neonatal therapists must become well acquainted with the scope and intent of the law, particularly with the definition and extent of practice for their specific discipline. This ensures that their services are delivered in accordance with the legislative guidelines.

3

Perspectives on Developmental Theories Applicable to NICU Intervention

OVERVIEW

When asked to identify their personal theoretical framework for intervention, developmental therapists (e.g., occupational and physical therapists) often give examples of preferred theoretical approaches, such as neurodevelopmental therapy or sensory integration treatment. These treatment approaches are only two of many that may fit into broader frameworks for intervention in a particular setting.

The personal theoretical framework for any developmental therapist should be consistent with the philosophical base of his or her profession. Within the NICU, however, this framework must also be grounded on the belief that the family has a strong influence on the infant's developmental outcome and vice versa. Therefore, both the infant and family are recipients of neonatal services. From this perspective, the ultimate goal of neonatal intervention should be to optimize the infant's and the family's ability to perform their required tasks and occupations throughout the infant's NICU stay and after the infant goes home. The personal framework of therapists who work with infants and their families must be sufficiently adaptable and flexible to incorporate new models and approaches in developmental care as more is learned about human development throughout the life span. This chapter presents an overview of the major theoretical approaches or models applicable to developmental neonatal intervention. Emphasis is given to approaches that focus on the interaction among the infant, the family, the occupation (or task), and the environment.

OBJECTIVES

- Explain how biological and environmental influences interact in an infant's developmental process
- Recognize the importance of considering biological and environmental factors when working to optimize the development of infants
- Identify the developmental theories that are founded on the interaction between an infant and the environment

- Describe the principal tenets of the major theories and approaches followed by therapists in the delivery of services to infants in the NICU and their families

- Explain the relevance of each theory discussed, areas of congruity between the theories, and compatibility of the various theories with family-centered care

- Explain "goodness of fit" as it relates to intervention with infants and their families

- Identify resiliency or protective factors that have been found to mediate risk factors in development

- Recognize the importance of keeping abreast of emerging theories in behavior and development to provide quality early intervention services

DEVELOPMENTAL MECHANISMS: CHANGING VIEWS

Decades of debate have surrounded the question of whether nature (biologic constitution) or nurture (environment) exerts the primary influence on developmental outcome. Wachs noted that three types of questions have surfaced from this debate: 1) "Is the environment influencing development?" 2) "What are the specific components of environment that relate to development?" and 3) "How do various components of the environment interrelate and 'translate' into variation in developmental outcome?" (1992, p. 8). Studies of the effects of sensory deprivation and stimulation (Harlow, 1958; Skeels, Updegraff, Wellman, & Williams, 1938) and of neuronal plasticity within the central nervous system (Rakic, 1991) demonstrate that environment and experience can play as important a part in the developmental process as genetic endowment (Horton, 2001; Lichtman, 2001). The notion that normal development occurs in a predictable sequence of steps that are directly related to changes in central nervous system development prevailed for decades after Gesell (1928) proposed it. This early *hierarchical neuromotor development theory* failed to explain the variability and flexibility seen in motor and cognitive behavior among typically developing children. This model also left the profound influence of the environment unexplained.

Several theories evolved later to address what the previous theories had left unanswered. Piaget (1952) was one of the first theorists to address the question of how developmental changes occur. He proposed a *theory of adaptation*: assimilation of new experiences with previous ones, accommodation in response to changing experiences, and eventual adaptation to a more mature level of functioning. Pediatric therapists embraced the adaptation theory, as it incorporates principles important in intervention such as adjustment to challenge or change, as well as individual motivation and purpose in coping with stress and challenge (Gilfoyle, Grady, & Moore, 1981; King, 1978; Llorens, 1969). However, the adaptation model also fails to provide an explanation for those periods in normal development when infants and young children not only exhibit variability in their behavior but also appear to lose previously acquired skills (Trevarthen, 1982). These periodic regressions, often observed just before achievement of a higher level of performance, have been the source of further speculation and inquiry about additional influences on development.

Later models conceptualized development as a complex process with a number of interrelated and interactive components influencing developmental progression (Bateson, 1996; Lichtman, 2001; Siegel, 1999). For example, in their *transactional theory*, Sameroff and Chandler (1975) moved beyond biological risk and genetic endowment to examine not only the environment, but also the combined contributions of infant and caregiver to early development. The infant, the caregiver, and the social and physical environment are viewed in this theory as contributing substantially and interdependently to developmental outcome. Potential effects of factors such as socioeconomic status, social support, infant–caregiver reciprocity, and individual behavioral characteristics of infants and caregivers may affect infant development. Since the mid-1970s, neonatal therapists and other medical and health-related professionals who wish to assist families in optimizing infant outcomes have been encouraged to incorporate principles of transactional theory in their approach to intervention, thus considering the family as a contextual unit within their infant's environment. Transactional theory has had a significant impact on clinical practice with infants and families. For example, since the 1980s, *family-centered care* (Dunst, Trivette, & Deal, 1988; Simeonsson & Bailey, 1990) has been widely adopted in early intervention programs as an approach to service provision. In this approach, the family participates in a collaborative relationship with early interventionists in identifying needs and priorities for service, recognizing the many factors that may ultimately contribute to an infant's developmental outcome.

Dynamical systems models are more comprehensive, acknowledging the numerous interrelated components that influence the progression of development (Bateson, 1996; Siegel, 1999). According to Thelen, *dynamical systems theory* proposes that human development is "a product of not only the central nervous system, but also of the biomechanical and energetic properties of the body, the environmental support, and the specific (and sometimes changing) demands of the particular task" (1995, p. 81). These properties are dynamic in the sense that they are constantly changing; they also are unique to each individual. Elements within these properties reflect both nature and nurture, as well as stability and flexibility within the infant and the environment (Thelen & Fogel, 1989). According to the dynamical systems theory, any loss of stability offers an opportunity for organization of a new response and, thus, for change. Variability in performance is welcomed as it provides for increased flexibility in the individual's responses. Somatic changes in size and weight that occur with growth provide additional challenges, which, in combination with changes in the environment, result in unstable performance and further opportunity for the individual to work toward alternative behavioral solutions. As each emerging strategy is applied under a variety of conditions and constraints, it is modified through internal feedback and self-regulatory processes and is reinforced through practice (Sporns & Edelman, 1993). The greater the number of options for action (i.e., "affordances"; Gibson, 1979) offered by the caregiving environment, the greater the possibilities for developmental progress.

To summarize, the following elements are incorporated into intervention based on the dynamical systems theory: individual physical and behavioral characteristics, environmental affordances and context, task characteristics, adaptation, and self-regulation. Each element is incorporated into the therapist's assessment and into the plan for family-focused intervention. For example, application of the dynamical systems' approach to the development of feeding skills in premature infants involves considering a variety of factors. Some of the factors include an infant's alertness, physiologic stability, responsiveness, posture, and motor control; the size of the infants' intraoral cavity; control of oral motor structures; environmental stimuli present; the feeding mode (e.g., breast or bottle); the type of nipple (e.g., size, pliability); the amount of the feeding; and caregiver responsiveness. Affordances may involve changing the feeding mode, nipple type, feeding schedule, feeding posture, environmental stimuli, or a combination of any of these factors.

Thelen (1995) added the elements of purposefulness (goal direction) and motivation inherent in a task into her synthesis of the dynamical systems model. In doing so, she reinforced the importance of psychosocial factors, including the interaction between the child and the caregiver and the child's interest in the task, to the dynamics of development. In the previous discussion of feeding, another affordance could be changing the caregiver–infant interaction style to elicit improved responses from the infant, even refraining from interacting with an extremely sensitive infant during feeding. These additions render the dynamical systems model even more consistent with the objectives of the therapist providing services in the NICU.

THEORETICAL MODELS AND APPROACHES RELEVANT TO PRACTICE IN THE NICU

Neurobehavioral Development

The trend in NICU settings toward individualized, developmentally supportive care is the consummation of years of study by investigators interested in the effect of the NICU environment (including caregiving) on preterm infants. Through these investigations, it became clear that the NICU environment, although providing necessary life-sustaining care, can be aversive and, at times, detrimental to the infant's physiologic stability and psychosocial development. Several models have been constructed to describe the behavioral organization of preterm infants in the NICU and the developmental processes that support preterm infant behavior. Gorski, Davison, and Brazelton (1979) proposed a hierarchical model of neurobehavioral development to explain the developmental progression of a preterm infant's interactions with the environment. In their model, the first stage is observed early in the gestational period. Infants in this stage are initially "in-turning"—that is, responding to environmental stimuli exclusively on a physiologic level. The infant is predominantly in a sleep state, without the ability to regulate states of arousal. Movements are involuntary and jerky. Infants at this stage are not likely to respond to caregiver efforts to engage them in interactions with the environment. This stage is followed by a "coming-out" phase in which the infant has more frequent periods of physiologic stability and is therefore able to respond actively to the environment. The infant who is "coming out" may maintain an alert state for brief periods during caregiving and also maintains color, oxygen saturation, respirations, and heart rate in acceptable, predictable ranges during some interactions. These improved abilities afford caregivers the opportunity to elicit short-duration visual, auditory, and social responses. An infant at this stage is still susceptible to becoming overstressed. Attempts to engage the infant must be kept brief. Finally, Gorski and colleagues described "active reciprocity" as the stage in which a preterm infant has the capacity for self-arousal and self-soothing, actively seeks stimuli, and tolerates some stressful interactions without a loss of physiologic stability.

The stage manifested is indicative of the infant's neurobehavioral development. Although in the first two stages the infant focuses internally (i.e., maintaining a stable physiologic state), at the active reciprocity stage the infant is capable of actively contributing to social interactions with caregivers, thereby providing mutually satisfying experiences. This model has been applied clinically in helping parents understand their infants' social interaction abilities and readiness.

Synactive Theory

Synactive theory is a related model, applicable to preterm infants in the NICU (Als, Lester, & Brazelton, 1979). Like Gorski and colleagues (1979), Als and her collaborators also focused their attention on the behavioral organization of preterm infants. Close observation of individual preterm infants in the NICU revealed common behaviors that signal vulnerabilities and capacities to cope with the intrusive nature of the NICU setting. In the synactive theory (Als et al., 1979), as in other later developmental theories, a preterm infant is conceptualized within a dynamic system formed by the interaction among the infant, the caregiver, and the environment. In this case, the preterm infant is viewed as a developing organism, coping with an environment for which he or she is neither physiologically nor neurodevelopmentally prepared. This theory posits the development of the preterm infant as an ever-expanding process of differentiation of specific subsystems (autonomic, motor, state of arousal, attentional/interactive, and self-regulatory). *Self-regulation* can be defined as the ability to actively cope with environmental demands and to interact with the environment. Synactive theory also has a hierarchical component such that the physiologic functions (e.g., breathing, autonomic regulation of heart rate) must gradually be stabilized to provide a foundation for motor development (e.g., postural adjustments and active efforts to self-soothe by sucking the hand). Physiologic and motor functions, individually and

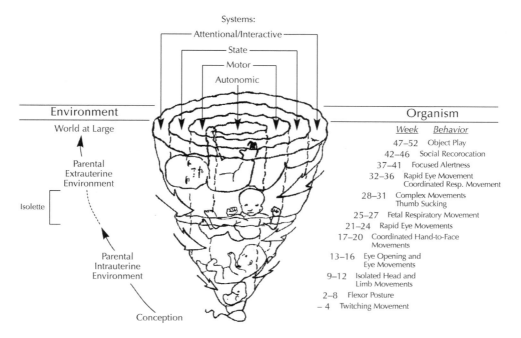

Figure 6. Model of the synactive organization of behavioral development. (From Als, H. [1982]. Toward a synactive theory of development: Promise for the assessment and support of infant individuality. *Infant Mental Health Journal, 3,* 229–243; reprinted by permission.)

together, contribute to regulation of states of arousal (i.e., maintaining a quiet alert state), enabling the infant to attend to the environment and to engage in social interaction without experiencing undue distress. Ultimately, when the subsystems are functioning well, the infant is able to self-regulate, relying less on environmental supports and more on his or her internal mechanisms for recovery of physiologic homeostasis and behavioral organization when faced with stressful events. The subsystems are not only seen as building on each other, but they also are considered to be continually interactive and mutually supportive—thus, the term *synaction*. Figure 6 illustrates Als's (1982) conceptualization of the interrelation between subsystems in development.

Infants vary to the extent that they are able to rely on the individual subsystems. An infant who may have strengths in the physiologic subsystem may display immature motor organization, resulting in poorly regulated states of arousal (Als, 1986). For example, when faced with a stressful event such as a rapid position change, the infant may initially startle and display appropriate autonomic reactivity (increased heart rate) and physiologic recovery (a vagal response, which brings the heart rate back within the infant's resting range). However, the infant's motor subsystem may not have developed sufficiently to support the infant's efforts to actively tuck his or her limbs for self-soothing and to regain a calm state of arousal. In this case, the infant may require external assistance from a caregiver to recover—for example, modifying the infant's position to enhance flexion of the limbs, thus inhibiting the tendency to startle and assisting the infant's efforts to bring his or her hand toward the face for self-soothing (see Figure 7). Without the benefit of this external support, the infant may become increasingly aroused with each startle and movement, expending precious energy on futile attempts to self-regulate; eventually, he or she may experience physiologic distress, such as apnea, bradycardia, and oxygen desaturation. The economic cost of providing external supports is minute when compared with the cost to the infant (namely, unnecessary energy expenditure and hypoxia) when support is withheld.

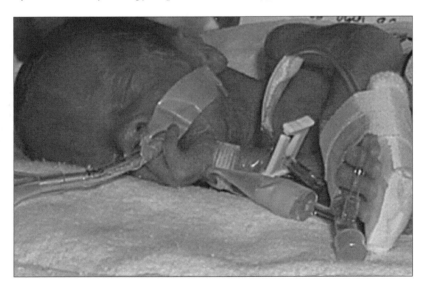

Figure 7.   This extremely premature infant is able to self-soothe and self-regulate by bringing his hand to his mouth.

Another infant may demonstrate good regulation of physiologic and motor functions but may not be able to tolerate sustained social interaction when it involves the combination of visual and auditory stimuli. This infant may initially respond to such social approaches with motor behavioral cues signaling mounting distress (e.g., gaze aversion, arm extensions, finger splaying). Faced with a continuing demand for interaction perceived as aversive, the infant may eventually begin to show signs of autonomic instability (e.g., color change, decreased oxygen saturation, decreased heart rate). A caregiver who is attentive to the infant's behavioral cues and cognizant of the infant's strengths and vulnerabilities will be more likely to recognize signs of stress and modify the interaction before the physiologic subsystem becomes unstable. For example, by continuing to engage the infant visually but ceasing the auditory stimulation, the caregiver can reduce the complexity of the stimulation, providing an opportunity for the infant to reorganize his or her response and to regain a calm, alert state. Hallmarks of synactive theory as a model for developmental intervention in the NICU are 1) determining the unique behavioral profile of each preterm infant and 2) providing an environment that is individually responsive to that infant's behavioral cues and allows opportunities for "balanced behavioral function" (VandenBerg, 1993).

Implications of the Synactive Theory for Neonatal Intervention

The synactive theory, a model borrowed from the field of developmental psychology, is totally congruent with intervention models that focus on optimizing an infant's performance abilities. The ability to self-regulate is the most important underlying capacity that enables infants to engage in their expected tasks or occupations. An infant who is able to self-regulate displays behaviors that signal to caregivers how he or she is tolerating the stimuli from the environment. This can be interpreted as procuring attention from the caregiver. Self-regulation, as an underlying capacity, enables the infant to act on the environment to interrupt or decrease the effect of an aversive stimulus. For instance, this infant may avert his or her gaze or cover his or her eyes with a hand if a visual stimulus exceeds his or her tolerance. Conversely, an infant who lacks stability of the subsystems and has poor self-regulation abilities is less able to procure or engage in social interaction. An infant with poor regulation abilities is only able to interact with the environment in a more dependent, passive, or reactive mode; thus, he or she is more susceptible to environmental influences. In turn, caregivers have to modulate the environment by providing external support to optimize this infant's performance on the basis of the cues that the infant may display through his or her procuring efforts. In this case, the infant's engagement in tasks or activities expected by the family is limited and dependent on the contextual elements of support—that is, the caregivers' ability to interpret and appropriately respond to the infant's cues or signals. Neonatal therapists may apply principles of the synactive theory to interpret and facilitate newborns' efforts to procure and engage in interaction with their caregivers. This content is detailed in Chapters 8, 9, and 11.

Among preterm infants in the NICU, maintaining a calm state translates to conservation of precious energy for healing and growth. In this setting, where physiologic dysregulation can have drastic consequences, simply watching and waiting, attending to an infant's behavioral cues, and modifying caregiving accordingly can produce impressive results. Early work on this concept focused on neonatal nurses as the primary caregivers. Procedural modifications were recommended to reduce stress and/or help infants to manage the stress that inevitably accompanies care in the NICU (Lawhon, 2002; White, 2002). Als and two groups of colleagues (1986, 1994) have since demonstrated improved weight gain, earlier nipple feeding, and earlier hospital discharges among preterm infants provided with assessment and individualized developmentally supportive care following principles of synactive theory. Related studies at other centers have reported similar findings (Becker, Grunwald, Moorman, & Stuhr, 1991, 1993). Other—and perhaps more remarkable—benefits reported by Als et al. (1994) included lower incidence of intraventricular hemorrhage (IVH) and decreased duration of mechanical ventilation and supplemental oxygen among a group of infants cared for using individualized developmental support as compared with randomly assigned control groups given traditional care. Moreover, developmental outcomes of the intervention group were improved at 3 years of age. These studies give encouraging evidence for the benefits of the developmentally supportive approach to the care of newborns. However, readers must be aware that the effectiveness of developmental care interventions has been challenged in the literature. Although sound evidence of its benefits to preterm infants exists in terms of improved short-term growth, decreased respiratory effort, decreased length and cost of hospital stay, and improved neurodevelopmental outcomes at 24 months, most other benefits are based on small studies, some having methodological flaws (Symington & Pinelli, 2001).

Applying principles of the synactive theory to developmental assessment and intervention in the NICU may enhance an infant's physiologic and behavioral regulation and, therefore, his or her capacity to function within a challenging environment. Several formal assessment instruments and programs can be used to guide care planning based on this theory: the Newborn Individualized Developmental Care and Assessment Program (NIDCAP) and the Assessment of Preterm Infant Behavior (APIB), both of which were developed by Als and colleagues (1979, 1982a, 1982b); the NICU Network Neurobehavioral Scale (NNNS) (Lester & Tronick, 2001, in press; Tronick & Lester, 1996); and the Neonatal Behavioral Assessment Scale (NBAS) (Brazelton & Nugent, 1995). All of these assessments require formal training and certification for appropriate administration and interpretation. Involving the family in these types of assessments and in informal behavioral observations can be especially rewarding. Through their participation in the assessment process, family members become more knowledgeable about their infant's communicative style and individual thresholds for stimulation (Als, 1995; Nugent, 1985). See Chapter 10 for further information on the assessments and for principles of infant assessment.

The neural and behavioral mechanisms underlying the synactive approach to developmentally supportive care remain unclear. Certain assumptions of the theory are being tested. For example, Becker et al. (1993) reported less time in active sleep and more time in quiet sleep among infants provided individualized developmentally supportive care by trained nurses, based on NIDCAP observations. They also reported less quiet alert time among the infants receiving developmentally supportive care. Because optimizing quiet alert periods in support of the infants' active involvement with their environment is a primary goal of developmentally supportive care, particularly for older infants, Becker et al. were unable to explain these findings. It may be that the intervention strategies based on the synactive theory are more effective in modulating environmental stimuli to assist the infants in protecting their sleep and reducing arousal than in enhancing arousal for the desired brief periods of quiet alert time. An alternative explanation is that the meaning ascribed to certain behaviors within the NIDCAP assessment protocol may not accurately represent the infants' individual state of arousal or level of stress and/or availability for caregiving. To demonstrate the validity of specific behavioral cues as accurate indicators of periods of stress or availability among preterm infants at various gestational ages, these behavioral cues must correspond to some other measure of arousal, such as changes in physiologic measures (i.e., heart rate, respiration rate, and oxygen saturation). Bigsby and colleagues (1994, 1996) demonstrated such relationships in preterm and full-term infants at 3 months corrected age. Bigsby and Lester conducted a pilot study to investigate the relationship between behavioral and physiologic measures among preterm infants in the NICU (Bigsby, 1994; R. Bigsby & B. Lester, personal communication, June 1997).

Until more studies are completed, the assumptions that underlie developmentally supportive care may be questioned. Nonetheless, the positive results that have been documented suggest that this approach should be a part of every NICU-based therapist's assessment and intervention repertoire. Therapy should emphasize careful observation and individualized program planning that incorporates principles of synactive theory along with other congruent family-based approaches appropriate to the NICU setting. Doing so will enhance the performance abilities of individual infants *and* their caregivers (Holloway, 1994).

Sensory Integration

Therapists in the NICU have adopted sensory integration (SI) approaches widely in their roles as developmental specialists (Hunter, 1997; Vergara, 1993). As described previously, synactive theory is a form of dynamical systems theory that is congruent with current best practice in pediatric physical and occupational therapy. Specifically, there are parallels between synactive theory and sensory integration theory (Ayres, 1972; Holloway, 1990). According to sensory integration theory, a child's ability to process sensory input and integrate it with other sensory information for adaptive use enhances his or her performance abilities. Provided that the environment offers the appropriate type(s) and amount(s) of sensory experiences—the "just-right" challenge—the child, theoretically, will begin to have increasingly complex adaptive responses (Ayres, 1972). For example, when working with an older infant in the NICU, the environment must be designed to foster exploration. Toys graded to the infant's developing capacity must be readily available to promote the visual, oral, and manual exploration needed for the development of more complex perceptual, motor, and cognitive skills. Conversely, if the child's sensory "diet" is impoverished or provides stimuli that the child perceives as noxious, his or her behavior may become disorganized. If developmentally appropriate objects or toys are not provided, the infant may experience delay in the development of exploratory play. In contrast, an overabundance of toys or overly arousing stimuli in the immediate environment may overwhelm the infant's sensory system and potentially disorganize his or her performance.

Older infants may exhibit signs of stress or of over- or underarousal similar to behaviors identified by Als (1986) among neonates in the intensive care unit (Stallings-Sahler, 1998). The synactive and sensory integration theories both posit that the experiences offered within the environment and the task demands need to "match" the individual capacity of the child to process and make use of experiences and, in turn, develop adaptive skills or behaviors. Therapists experienced in assessment and intervention based on sensory integration theory may find the parallels between sensory integration and synactive theories useful in constructing their individual theoretical frameworks for intervention in the NICU.

Neurodevelopmental Approaches

Neurodevelopmental approaches are also used with considerable frequency in the NICU. The most common is the neurodevelopmental therapy (NDT) theory originally proposed by Bobath and Bobath (1984). This approach focuses on providing the infant with sensorimotor experiences to promote development of normal movement and postural patterns. Since the 1990s (approximately), the focus of NDT has been gradually evolving to incorporate dynamical systems principles; thus, traditional NDT, as proposed by the Bobath, is seldom encountered. Infant positioning is the primary area to which NDT principles are effectively applied in the NICU (see Chapter 12). Proper NDT-based positioning is believed to promote optimal postural development in infants in the NICU. More invasive NDT intervention strategies, however, may be too taxing for small and sick infants and, therefore, should be reserved for more physiologically stable, older infants.

"Goodness of Fit": A Relevant Concept for Pediatric Occupational Therapists

Although Thomas and Chess originally proposed their "goodness of fit" model more than two decades ago, their concept of achieving a match between characteristics of the infant or child and the caregiving environment remains as relevant as ever:

> Simply defined, goodness of fit results when the child's capacities, motivations, and temperament are adequate to master the demands, expectations, and opportunities of the environment. Such consonance between child and environment promotes optimal positive development. Poorness of fit, on the other hand, results when the child's characteristics are inadequate to master the challenges of the environment, and this leads to maladaptive functioning and distorted development. Goodness or poorness of fit are never abstractions. They have meaning only in terms of the values and demands of a given socioeconomic group or culture. (1989, p. 380)

The role of the NICU therapist incorporates adapting the developmental milieu to accommodate infant preferences and sensory thresholds. This role is consistent with the previous definition of goodness of fit, as well as with the current emphasis on family-centered care (see Chapter 11). A NICU therapist who incorporates the needs, priorities, concerns, and abilities of the family into the plan of care while considering sociocultural aspects of the caregiving environment is more likely to arrive at goodness of fit.

Allowing the family's priorities to drive the direction of intervention may be a novel and, in some cases, threatening notion, particularly in an acute care setting (McGrath & Conliffe-Torres, 1996). For example, when making decisions about an infant's care, a therapist may fail to involve or ignore input from parents with a low level of education, assuming that their understanding is limited and that they are not capable of providing appropriate input for decision making. The parents' participation in their infant's care may be restricted on the basis of such biases, whereas the appropriate manner to handle the situation is to promote goodness of fit by adapting the information and type of parental participation to their level of understanding. This may be somewhat challenging for therapists who are new to family-centered care. Still, the rewards of embracing the latter approach to practice far outweigh any perceived pitfalls.

Meyer, Lester, and colleagues (1998) gave three examples in which family-based intervention emphasizing goodness of fit resulted in positive outcomes for high-risk infants and their families. They also offered strategies for family-based intervention, organized by the following domains: infant behavior and characteristics, family organization and functioning, caregiving environment, and home discharge/community resources. These strategies are summarized in Table 5 and covered in depth in Chapter 11.

To be effective in the NICU setting, therapists must be prepared to collaborate with other team members as necessary. They must incorporate each theoretical model and approach relevant to the NICU into their practice with infants and families.

RISK, PROTECTION, AND INDIVIDUAL RESILIENCY

The concepts of risk or protective factors within the environment and individual resiliency have received increasing attention because a number of studies have shown positive outcomes among infants raised in stressful or impoverished environments (Werner, 1990, 2000). These studies identified certain characteristics of infants who could be described as resilient in the face of adverse conditions such as biological risk, maternal depression or mental illness, and poverty. Resilient infants were active and cuddly, did not have problems eating or sleeping, and were able to elicit warmth and affection from their caregivers (Werner, 2000). In short, these infants had good self-regulation, were socially responsive and interactive, and were able to actively procure from the environment the care that they needed. They were somehow able to invoke from their caregivers the necessary attention to survive and thrive. Such findings underscore the importance of behavioral organization, self-regulation, and an infant's ability to procure not only within the NICU but also during the transition home and throughout infancy.

One could surmise that the importance of these resilience-building capacities would be magnified among infants with multiple biological and/or environmental risks. A longitudinal study of premature infants with varying degrees of illness and/or neurologic injury found that infants with relatively high levels of protection (high resiliency) indeed outperformed those with few protective factors (low resiliency) on developmental assessment at 4 years, regardless of the degree of biologic risk (Lester et al., 1994). These results suggest that stress and adversity need not be removed from an infant's life to obtain a positive outcome, something Werner (2000) emphasized. Werner instead suggested that protective factors may be strengthened through a number of avenues, including alternative caregivers who can provide loving care and build competence and confidence in the child. Moreover, assessment must be aimed not only at identifying vulnerabilities and risk factors, but also at the equally important protective factors in the lives of the infants and families served. Family resiliency is such a protective factor (see Chapter 11). Resilient families are able to face the overwhelming challenges of the NICU experience. However, they need not come to the experience with all of the resources necessary to activate their resiliency. Resiliency resources are expanded when team members assist families in recognizing and using their existing strengths, as well as in identifying their needs and priorities.

Just as neonatal therapists can provide external support to an infant to enhance behavioral and physiologic regulation, family resiliency can be bolstered by the appropriate amount of external support from the team. To accomplish this, the team must build a mutually trusting relationship with the family. This process is not unlike that of intervening with an infant who requires a "just right" challenge. Both processes

Table 5. Intervention domains and strategies

Domain of intervention	Common intervention strategies
Infant behavior and characteristics	In the context of NBAS[a] assessments, help the parents to learn about infant's capacity for adaptation to the environment, unique behavioral cues and signals, consolability, ability to regulate state, likes and dislikes
	Help parents to recognize the infant's signs of overstimulation and how to address these through environmental and interactional modifications
	Relieve parental anxiety about the infant's appearance and behavior through shared behavioral observations, education, and support
	Explain the concept and utility of corrected age for preterm infants
	Explain the wide range of variation and individual differences in preterm infant development
	Demonstrate infant behavioral and developmental gains using serial NBAS examinations
Family organization and functioning	Review how the birth of an infant impacts upon structure and function to accommodate roles as spouses and parents of a high-risk infant
	Discuss emotional issues and adjustment to the high-risk birth and hospitalization
	Provide the opportunity to discuss marital issues and identification of the birth as a stressor that may contribute to marital tension
	Address the educational, supportive and visitation needs of siblings and extended family members
	Discuss ways to balance hospital and home responsibilities
	Provide family counseling and appropriate referral, if needed
Caregiving environment	Demonstrate infant caregiving and handling techniques (e.g., feeding, consoling, bathing, social interaction)
	Foster a graduated caregiving role for parents in the nursery setting, in preparation for home discharge
	Support parent efforts at caregiving, learning to pace feeds, and observing for signs of behavioral disorganization
	Provide privacy for parents to get to know their infant
	Modify environmental stimulation appropriate to infant's level of sensitivity in hospital and home settings
	Support and reinforce positive parenting behavior and caregiving skills
	Encourage regular visitation
Home discharge/ community resources	Discuss parental concerns and readiness for home discharge
	Help identify and mobilize available informal and formal social support
	Facilitate multidisciplinary discharge planning meeting to review infant and family's special needs and to target discharge date
	Arrange overnight hospital visitation prior to discharge
	Make referrals to community resources (e.g., WIC,[b] VNA,[c] parent support group, local transportation services)
	Empower parents in their role as advocate for the infant to access appropriate community resources
	Foster parents' relationship with community pediatrician
	Provide access to family resource library (written material and videotapes)

Domain of intervention	Common intervention strategies
	Foster family's receptiveness to changes in therapeutic service providers by demonstrating knowledge of and confidence in other programs
	Facilitate an enriched home environment with appropriate infant supplies, equipment and toys

From Meyer, E.C., Lester, B.M., Boukydis, C.F.Z., & Bigsby, R. (1998). Family-based intervention with high-risk infants and their families. *Journal of Clinical Psychology in Medical Settings, 5*(1), 58; reprinted by permission.
[a]NBAS = Neonatal Behavioral Assessment Scale (Brazelton, 1973, 1984; Brazelton & Nugent, 1995)
[b]WIC = Special Supplemental Nutrition Program for Women, Infants and Children
[c]VNA = Visiting Nurses Association

are enhanced by taking a dynamical systems approach in which challenges provoke temporary instability that facilitates or induces a self-regulating response and subsequent adaptation to a higher level of functioning. Therapists and other members of the NICU team must take a similar approach to infant and family resiliency and adaptation. That is, they need to facilitate a dynamic system (with self-regulating capacities that may require intermittent external support) to achieve the ultimate goal of strong and flexible children and families.

CONCLUSION

Neonatal therapists need to draw from a number of current developmental models to construct principles for intervention in the NICU. Ongoing modification of treatment principles will be necessary as factors that influence development continue to emerge from research. Ultimately, the most effective therapeutic approach is one that recognizes and incorporates the needs and capacities of the infant and family within their environmental context.

4

Personnel and Teamwork in the NICU

OVERVIEW

Chapter 4 is the first of three chapters describing the NICU environmental context. It begins by listing and describing the preparation and major roles of relevant NICU personnel. Emphasis is given to members of the developmental team. The importance of teamwork for promoting the well-being of infants and their families is discussed. Practical suggestions for appropriately interacting with and gaining respect from nursing and medical personnel are provided.

This chapter concludes with a short case illustration in which an occupational therapist is following through with a request to initiate feeding intervention with an infant. The therapist begins by consulting with other team members prior to initiating the intervention. Based on the therapist's input and observations, the team decides to postpone intervention. This case example emphasizes the value of teamwork and highlights the cautious approach that must be taken when working in the NICU.

OBJECTIVES

- Identify the various professions that provide services in the NICU
- Describe the roles of the various members of the NICU team, particularly the developmental team
- Compare the level of professional preparation required of the various team members
- Recognize that role delineation may vary across NICU settings depending on factors such as the facility's philosophy and policies, as well as the team members' type of professional preparation
- Explain the importance of teamwork, recognizing the professional limits and roles of the various members of the team, clearly delineating those limits and roles when working with infants in the NICU, and recognizing areas in which overlapping roles may be inevitable
- Identify factors that promote and factors that challenge effective teamwork in the NICU
- Identify the elements of the teamwork process illustrated in the case example provided

NICU PERSONNEL

Personnel delivering services in the NICU encompass a wide range of individuals with very different professional preparations and roles. Developmental therapists working in the NICU must become familiar with the major responsibilities, functions, and authority levels of key NICU personnel as well as with role delineation and potential areas of overlap. Although the basic preparation of professionals is generally uniform across NICUs, role definition for some personnel may vary depending on the institution's philosophy and policies and the specialized training and orientation that individuals may have received previously (McCanless, 1994). In particular, areas of expertise among developmental team members may overlap. Preparation and roles of technical personnel may vary even more than those of the professional team.

To facilitate role assignment while avoiding service duplication, institutions may occasionally assign roles on the basis of the training that the team members have received. Disciplines with roles that tend to overlap in the NICU include nurses, occupational therapists, physical therapists, speech-language pathologists, early childhood educators, child life or other developmental specialists, and psychologists. Role definition may become a source of friction when someone feels entitled to a given role that has been assigned to a professional in a different discipline. To avoid such issues, therapists should examine their personal philosophy about neonatal intervention and their perceived roles and responsibilities in the NICU prior to accepting a new job. This self-assessment should serve as the basis to determine compatibility between the therapist's and the NICU's views on role delineation. The following sections summarize the major responsibilities typically assigned to members of the developmental team.

Medical Team

The medical team is composed of physicians, nurses, and other ancillary personnel responsible for the infant's primary care. Representatives from the medical team (e.g., neonatologist, nurse) *must* be available *in* the NICU at all hours of the day and night.

Attending Neonatologists

Attending neonatologists are physicians who have completed their residency training in pediatrics and an additional fellowship in neonatal medicine. They are ultimately responsible for the care provided in the NICU, as they provide guidance and training to the neonatology fellows, residents, and medical students. In addition to patient care and teaching responsibilities, many attending neonatologists are engaged in clinical research and academic and administrative pursuits. They rotate on and off service, usually on a monthly basis.

Neonatology Fellows

Neonatology fellows are physicians who have completed their residency in pediatrics and are engaged in fellowship training in neonatology. Under the attending neonatologist's supervision, neonatology fellows are responsible for the care provided in the NICU and for ongoing teaching of residents and medical students. Generally, fellows also are expected to complete at least one clinical research project and to give several scholarly presentations throughout their 3-year fellowship. They usually serve on a rotating (monthly) basis.

Pediatric Residents

Pediatric residents are physicians who have completed medical school and are engaged in residency training to become a pediatrician. Typically, they rotate on and off service (monthly) in the nursery. The NICU experience usually offers pediatric residents many specialty rotation options. Residents may also be responsible for consultation in the NICU as part of another specialty rotation. In this way, they receive their supervision and training from neonatology fellows and attending neonatologists, as well as the large number of specialists who consult in the NICU. Residents are often responsible for particular infants' plans of care and, under the neonatal fellow's supervision, for procedures such as intubation and placing catheters and percutaneous lines. They also assist during infant deliveries and provide pediatric care for patients in the Level I newborn nursery (Karlowicz & McMurray, 2000).

Medical Students

Medical students are baccalaureate program graduates who are in the process of completing medical school. The NICU rotation is usually offered to medical students as an opportunity for exposure to critical care medicine. Medical students participate in patient rounds, during which they can absorb a large volume of information. They are often responsible for tracking a particular infant's progress and reporting changes that occur or do not occur. The students' patient care responsibilities generally are limited and closely supervised.

Physician Assistants

Physician assistants provide services in some NICUs. These professionals have completed a certification program that prepares them to assess patient symptoms, formulate a preliminary diagnosis and a suggested course of treatment, and then consult with the attending physician before implementing a change in treatment. They are usually not licensed to prescribe medication and must work under the supervision of a physician at all times.

Nurse Practitioners

Registered nurses who have a baccalaureate degree in nursing and a master's degree in a specialized area of practice are qualified to become certified nurse specialists (CNSs) or nurse practitioners. Some nurse practitioners have made neonatal care their specialty and have completed the NICU experience and examination requirements for certification as neonatal nurse practitioners (NNPs). Although desirable, this credential is not required for practice in many NICUs. Nurse practitioners without the NNP credential usually spend the necessary time under supervision to demonstrate that they have the advanced knowledge and experience for assisting with deliveries, resuscitating newborns, and performing procedures such as intubation and catheterization (Karlowicz & McMurray, 2000). They are also licensed to prescribe and administer medications with the approval of an attending physician. In many nurseries, they are their patients' primary care providers and are important sources of information, consultation, and referral for neonatal therapy (Beal & Quinn, 2002). Experienced nurse practitioners may work in collaboration with the pediatric residents and may assist as "first-line teachers" for incoming first-year residents (Frank, Mullanery, Darnall, & Stashwick, 2000).

Neonatal Nurses

Neonatal nurses are registered nurses (and sometimes licensed practical nurses) who are graduates of accredited nursing training programs at the associate's degree level or higher and have completed all requirements for licensure and certification. They usually have completed additional training in neonatal intensive care, which includes closely supervised on-the-job proctoring by an experienced neonatal nurse, advanced coursework, and, in some cases, they have earned the advanced certification credential of the National Association of Neonatal Nurses (NANN). Neonatal nurses implement infants' care plans and, in many cases, become primary care providers for specific infants. Neonatal nurses usually become the experts on these infants' individual needs. They are the custodians of their fragile patients and are justifiably protective of them in the face of large numbers of specialists and consultants who may examine the infants each day. In addition, a neonatal nurse often is the team member most familiar with an infant's family members and with issues that need to be addressed to achieve a family-centered approach to care.

Nurse Managers

Nurse managers are registered, licensed nurses who have advanced knowledge and extensive experience in neonatal nursing. They are responsible for the smooth operation of the NICU. Typically, nurse managers attend rounds to become familiar with the severity and care needs of each infant, and assign infants to nurses accordingly. At the first report that the nursery will receive a new patient, whether by transport from another hospital or via the delivery or operating rooms, the nurse manager ensures that adequate space is available for the incoming neonate, along with appropriate equipment and support personnel standing by to perform all necessary procedures. When there are problems interpreting care plans for family members or involving family members in the care of their sick infant, nurse managers are often an important source of guidance and consultation for neonatal therapists.

Respiratory Therapists

Respiratory therapists are graduates of an accredited program in respiratory therapy at the associate's degree level or higher. They are responsible for the careful monitoring of each patient's respiratory status and for provision, adjustment, and maintenance of the various ventilatory supports in use in the NICU. They also provide hands-on treatment in the form of chest physical therapy, which involves vibration and percussion to clear the lungs of mucus and improve air exchange and administration of bronchodilation medications. Respiratory therapists can be extremely helpful to the neonatal therapist seeking to understand how an infant's respiratory status may affect his or her efforts to self-regulate, feed, or interact with caregivers.

Nutritionists

Nutritionists are registered dietitians, often with master's degrees, who have additional experience and training in pediatric and neonatal nutrition. NICU infants require a careful balance of nutrients in parenteral and oral feedings to maintain physiologic stability and provide adequate nutrition for healing and growth. The neonatal nutritionist tracks weight gain and physical growth and recommends changes to maintain nutritional intake during the hospital stay and neonatal follow-up (Fenton, Geggie, Warners, & Tough, 2000). The neonatal therapist and the nutritionist often work side-by-side in discharge planning and during follow-up visits to optimize nutritional intake when feeding difficulties arise.

Discharge Planners/Case Managers

Discharge planners/case managers are usually registered nurses with extensive experience in neonatal and early intervention. They follow the progress of individual infants, anticipate the need for parent education, and set up specific training for family members as infants draw closer to discharge. They also work closely with third-party payors to ensure availability and coverage for needed services and equipment during the hospitalization and after discharge. They also work with the developmental team to generate a carefully detailed discharge plan that can be used by the infant's family and/or visiting nursing personnel to facilitate continuity of care at home (Robison, Pirak, & Morrell, 2000).

Developmental and Psychosocial Care Team

The developmental and psychosocial care team consists of ancillary service providers who may become involved in the infant's care on a referral basis.

Developmental Specialists

Developmental specialists are pediatric health care professionals who typically have completed the entry-level requirements in their particular field and have also obtained advanced training and education in areas such as neonatal assessment, infant development, family-centered care, and infant–caregiver interaction (Ashbaugh, Leick-Rude, & Kilbride, 1999; Ward, 1999). Occupational and physical therapists often function as the developmental specialists on the NICU team, but speech-language pathologists, psychologists, nurses, and special educators may also serve as the developmental specialist. Regardless of the specialist's professional discipline, a primary responsibility of this role is fostering infant–caregiver interaction. This is accomplished by 1) assisting family members and caregivers in recognizing and responding appropriately to the strengths and vulnerabilities of their infant and 2) supporting their relationship with the infant. The developmental specialist may also assist in modifying the caregiving procedures and environment to optimize infant physiologic stability and energy conservation for healing and growth. Ideally, the role of a developmental specialist in the NICU also includes provision of psychosocial support and interactive guidance for caregivers within a framework that recognizes the primacy of the family's needs and wishes in developing an effective plan of care. To ensure continuity of care and smooth home transitions for infants and families, some NICU-based developmental specialists follow their patients after discharge through home visits or at a follow-up clinic.

Occupational Therapists

An occupational therapist in the NICU should have completed the requirements for registry and licensure as an occupational therapist and also should have extensive clinical experience in pediatrics with children of all ages and supervised experience in the NICU. The occupational therapist in the NICU may serve as the developmental specialist as well as provide traditional occupational therapy services that focus on feeding, positioning or handling, or modification of the infant's sensory experiences to optimize energy conservation and developmental progress.

Physical Therapists

In addition to completing the requirements for registration and certification in their field, physical therapists who work in the NICU should have extensive clinical experience in pediatrics with children of all ages and supervised experience in the NICU. Like occupational therapists, physical therapists may function as the developmental specialist in the NICU. This may include providing traditional physical therapy services that focus on positioning or handling and aspects of the infant's motor development. In some settings, physical therapists also provide "chest physical therapy" procedures to improve pulmonary functioning, including percussion, vibration, and, with larger infants, postural drainage followed by suctioning, if needed. However, most NICUs in the United States rely on the respiratory therapists to perform these procedures.

Speech-Language Pathologists

Speech-language pathologists working in the NICU generally have completed the entry-level master's degree requirements for practice in their field as well as the advanced competency credentials (Certificate of Clinical Competence, or CCC, designation), considerable clinical experience in pediatrics, and supervised experience in the NICU. Like occupational and physical therapists, speech-language pathologists may be the developmental specialist in the NICU, depending on their clinical background and experience. Their work may include speech-language pathology's traditional focus on evaluation of feeding and swallowing and interventions to enhance prelanguage development and feeding.

Occupational therapists, physical therapists, and speech-language pathologists may work side by side in some NICUs, but the cost of this form of collaboration precludes its use in others. More often, these practitioners have a transdisciplinary role.

Social Workers

Social workers in the NICU have completed the necessary graduate-level training and internships for certification and licensure in clinical social work. They often have additional experience working with families in prenatal clinics, labor and delivery areas, and outpatient programs that assist women with postpartum depression or provide grief counseling to families. Social workers play one of the most important roles in implementing family-centered care in the NICU. They are often the first to learn a family's circumstances, strengths and vulnerabilities, and wishes and desires for their infant. As such, social workers are a valuable resource in individualizing the team's approach with the family. Social workers also provide ongoing psychosocial support to families in distress, offer guidance for obtaining necessary resources, and may offer social-skill–building activities for parents and siblings.

Developmental/Clinical Psychologists

Developmental/clinical psychologists who provide services to families in the NICU have doctoral degrees and often have extensive experience working with families in crisis. These psychologists typically provide assistance to families in recognizing strengths and vulnerabilities of, as well as establishing a loving attachment with, their fragile infants. They may also provide individual and family counseling to assist family members in adjusting to their altered parental and sibling roles while the infant is in the NICU and during the transition home.

Child Psychiatrists

Child psychiatrists are physicians who have completed residency training in adult and child psychiatry. They provide special assistance to families in crisis, including assessment and individual or family counseling sessions. These psychiatrists also prescribe treatment, including medication, as needed. They can be particularly helpful when mental illness or drug abuse among family members exacerbates the difficult situation of having an infant in the NICU.

Related Personnel

Related personnel include a wide variety of individuals, some who provide services in the NICU in an advisory capacity and others whose work supports smooth functioning in the NICU.

Pharmacists

Pharmacists are graduates of accredited baccalaureate degree programs in pharmacy. Those servicing NICUs usually have advanced training and experience, as the medications and parenteral nutrition utilized in neonatal intensive care require complex preparation and strict administration guidelines. Although pharmacists are not routine members of the medical and developmental teams, they may be asked to attend rounds when specific concerns need to be addressed. They also are available around the clock to answer questions from physicians and nurses regarding appropriate dosages and administration schedules for medications.

Utilization Review Personnel

Utilization review personnel typically consist of registered nurses but may also include qualified physicians from the hospital's quality improvement department, who regularly review patient records for appropriateness of services and length of stay. Similar people from third-party payment sources may be visible in the NICU, routinely reviewing records. To comply with current standards and ensure reimbursement for all eligible services, it is important for neonatal therapists to acquaint themselves with these individuals and their expectations for documentation of services.

Secretarial and Clerical Staff

Secretarial and clerical staff are often the first to greet all visitors and personnel arriving in the NICU. They are important gatekeepers who ensure that anyone entering the NICU follows rules for visitation and for scrubbing. In addition, these staff members answer telephone calls, including inquiries by family members and referrals of new patients (whether in house or by transport). They may schedule emergency or routine laboratory and radiologic procedures as well as consultations by physicians and other specialists, as ordered. These staff also may be responsible for reporting an emergency in the labor and delivery or operating room. Thus, they must be familiar with medical terminology and the myriad services needed by infants receiving intensive care; must be able to act quickly while remaining calm during a crisis; and must project a friendly, helpful demeanor to visitors and staff.

Housekeeping Personnel

Housekeeping personnel are a constant presence in the NICU and are responsible for continuously maintaining very high standards of cleanliness. They must learn when it is most appropriate to work around staff when critical care is being provided and in what manner to do so. It is helpful to have certain housekeepers designated to work in the NICU. This enables them to become accustomed to conducting their work in a way that causes little interference with caregiving, is unobtrusive to patients and families, reduces noise, respects privacy, and keeps noxious odors to a minimum.

Research Assistants

Research assistants are also a constant presence in any NICU that is affiliated with a teaching hospital, as studies are continually being conducted in this setting. They may or may not be paid and are often students from medical, psychology, or other health care disciplines. The neonatal therapist needs to become familiar with the research protocols underway in the NICU to avoid inadvertently interfering with a study protocol when intervening with an infant or family. The best way to ensure this is to always ask the infant's nurse or the research assistant or check the infant's medical record before initiating any handling or care.

Volunteers

Volunteers may also have a central role in greeting visitors and personnel, assisting visitors in checking in and scrubbing, and assisting with sibling visitation. In addition, they may assist family members in locating services throughout the hospital and may be responsible for providing informative pamphlets and brochures. Like all other members of the NICU team, they must be friendly and professional and scrupulously maintain patient/family confidentiality.

Family Members

Family members, particularly parents, play a central role in an infant's care team. Their participation in the team, however, is strictly voluntary and should be maintained within their level of comfort. Parents are encouraged to assist with their infant's routine care in the NICU to the extent of their availability, willingness, and skills, as well as their infant's medical and physiologic stability. Family input is especially important in the decision-making process regarding the infant's care.

TEAMWORK IN THE NICU

All of the previously described personnel contribute to an infant's and family's NICU experience. Families expect and deserve to be included as members of a cohesive team. They expect team members to work well together while being sensitive to the stress experienced by the family during the time that the infant is in the NICU. How well NICU personnel relate to one another as team members also has a significant impact on their ability to fulfill their own professional roles. No one functions independently in the NICU!

Hunter et al. (1994) emphasized the importance, in this environment, of engendering trust and acceptance over a period of time. The process of becoming a true partner in the care of these fragile children is slow and arduous. It requires a considerable investment of time and careful attention to one's work, the infant's and the family's needs, and the needs of other team members. For example, it is important to recognize a nurse's ultimate responsibility for the well-being of his or her patients and, thus, his or her need to retain ultimate control of these infants' schedules and activities. The wise neonatal therapist *always* checks with nursing staff before planning an assessment or intervention. A therapist who calls the nurse or stops by the nursery to discuss the feasibility of a particular developmental plan within an infant's NICU routine communicates that the therapist's concern for the infant outweighs the need to complete an evaluation. In doing so, the therapist also conveys that the nurse is a respected member of the team whose opinion is valued. Moreover, the therapist will likely learn important information about the infant's condition that may influence the decision regarding what, if anything, should be done on that particular day. The following case example portrays the vital importance of team collaboration and communication in the NICU.

A preterm infant born at 24 weeks of gestation, now 33 weeks chronological age, displayed poor nipple feeding, potentially causing a delay in his impending discharge from the NICU. The occupational therapist who received the referral to conduct a feeding assessment read the infant's medical record, then stopped at the infant's bedside to review his condition with the nursing staff. The therapist learned that during the past 48 hours, the team had discontinued Aldactone and Diuril (medications that assist the infant in clearing fluid from the lungs) in preparation for discharge. Although the infant initially nipple-fed well, his respiratory rate increased to 70 breaths or greater per minute since this medication was discontinued. Based on the nurse's report, the therapist could determine, without attempting to feed the infant by nipple, that the increased work of breathing was probably interfering with his attempts to nipple-feed. The therapist discussed this possibility with the medical team, who agreed that the change in respiratory status could be the problem. The therapist recommended waiting to assess the infant until his respiratory status improved, explaining that the infant's inability to coordinate such rapid breathing with sucking and swallowing could cause him to aspirate some liquid during nipple feeding. It was agreed that the feeding evaluation would be suspended until the infant's respiratory condition improved. The bedside care plan was modified to include the precaution that nipple feeding should be deferred until the infant's tachypnea resolved. The team appreciated the occupational therapist's interpretation of the problem and the appropriateness of her recommendation to delay further action.

In his commentary on the Vermont Oxford Network's Neonatal Intensive Care Quality Improvement Collaborative 2000, Bloom described and critiqued four "key habits" adopted by NICU teams: 1) the habit for change, 2) the habit of understanding the processes of care, 3) the habit of collaborative learning, and 4) the habit of using evidence-based medicine. Bloom recommended expanding the first habit beyond mere change to "a willingness to test new ideas in a structured way" (2001, p. 2). He suggested that NICUs that embrace these habits have the potential to improve NICU care substantially. The common thread among these four habits is communication: the commitment to sharing information, communicating not only *what* is to be done but *how* and, perhaps most important, *why* it should be done. Incorporating these four habits of communication will enhance the NICU therapist's participation as a team member.

The previous case example illustrates the importance of communicating information to the entire team. The NICU therapist noted that the infant's rapid breathing likely would have interfered with his ability to pause long enough to take a breath; in turn, he would be at a high risk of aspiration if nipple feeding occurred before his breathing was stabilized. Because the recommendation was based on concern for the infant's safety, it was particularly important to incorporate the recommendation into the bedside plan of care. Thus, communication with every member of the team involved in deciding on the infant's feeding method was required.

As with any NICU consultant, there are times when it is appropriate for the neonatal therapist to provide research evidence that supports his or her recommendations. Making such information available to the team educates team members about important benefits or precautions of treatment. It also enhances the therapist's credibility as a practitioner who provides care that is carefully considered and as a professional who is as informed by the available research as possible.

CONCLUSION

Hippocrates' rule "First, do no harm" applies in this critical care environment as in no other. The medical team members will enthusiastically support therapy services in the NICU once they trust that the neonatal therapist follows that principal rule and will proceed with assessment and intervention only when it can be done safely and comfortably for the infants in the team's care.

5

Physical Context, Equipment, Environmental Stressors, and Sources of Support in the NICU

OVERVIEW

A health care professional seeking work in a NICU must clearly understand the influence of the NICU's physical environment on an infant's functional performance and long-term outcome. The first part of this chapter describes the NICU's physical environment as highly stimulating and stressful. Environmental factors that may stress the infants, such as light and noise, and recommended guidelines for reducing stress in the NICU are discussed. A description of the equipment most commonly found in NICUs is presented. The importance of learning the purpose and basic operating procedures of equipment commonly used with NICU infants is emphasized. The risks and potential consequences of changing equipment settings are underscored. Equipment that must be operated or adjusted strictly by specialized personnel is identified.

The content on NICU equipment is followed by a discussion of the NICU environmental context. Factors likely to stress families of newborns who require neonatal intensive care are discussed. A family's reactions to the NICU, and the interactions among situational and environmental stressors as the family copes with this experience, are highlighted through a case example. This chapter concludes with a description of support groups available to assist families in coping with having an infant in the NICU.

OBJECTIVES

- Describe the most common sources of environmental stress in the NICU, with particular emphasis on noise and light levels
- Identify the most common pieces of equipment found in NICUs and describe the purposes of each type of equipment
- Recognize basic operation procedures for equipment that therapists must know for working with their patients
- Identify which equipment therapists may operate or alter (e.g., change the settings) and which are off-limits for most therapists

- Recognize the precautions and potential risks associated with disengaging an alarm or changing the settings of each piece of equipment discussed
- Identify the major stressors—situational and environmental—experienced by families when coping with having an infant in the NICU and relate this information to the case presented
- Identify the sources of support that NICU personnel made available to the family discussed in the case example to assist them in coping with the stress they were experiencing
- Give examples of support services available to families to cope with the NICU experience

THE PHYSICAL ENVIRONMENT OF THE NICU

Although there have been tremendous advances in the care provided in NICUs over the past few decades, the physical environment of NICUs continues to be a source of stress for all inhabitants. Environmental factors are discussed in the following subsections.

Sound

Each bedside is equipped with numerous pieces of equipment, some of which generate significant sound levels during their operation. For example, bubbling in ventilator tubing is in the noise range of 60–80 dBA[2] (American Academy of Pediatrics Committee on Environmental Health, 1997). Alarms sound loudly when an infant's temperature, heart rate, respiration, oxygen and carbon dioxide exchange, or IV feeding volumes reach unacceptably high or low levels. When added to the continuous sounds of respiratory equipment and the intermittent sounds of ultrasound equipment—as well as an overhead paging system, ringing telephones, and the opening and closing of Isolette and cabinet doors—the result is a steady din that staff and visitors must speak above to be heard. In one study, 86% of the peak noises were in the 65–74 dBA range, and 90% of these noises were related to human activity (Chang, Lin, & Lin, 2001). It should be noted that most adults consider noise levels between 50 and 55 dB moderately annoying (American Academy of Pediatrics Committee on Environmental Health, 1997). Peak sound levels greater than 100 dB (decibels) have been recorded with such common activities as the closing of cabinet doors (Lasky, 1995). This sound level equates roughly with the sound of a pneumatic drill (Thomas,

---

[2]Sound pressure is measured in decibels (dB). Humans perceive sound signals of similar pressure levels depending on their pitch: low- and high-pitch sounds are perceived lower than medium-pitch sounds. An "A" filter is often used to correct the values of low- and high-pitch sounds to represent what a person qualitatively hears as sound or noise. "A"-filtered sound pressure levels are expressed as *dBA*. Both scales are used in the literature, but because the dB scale is logarithmic, comparisons across scales are difficult. In general, the sound pressure of normal conversation is within 40–45 dB, whereas the sound pressure produced by a power drill is close to 90 dB. Noise levels above 55 dBA are considered annoying, and noise between 80 and 90 dBA is considered loud. Noise higher than 120 dBA causes pain and distress in adults. Prolonged exposure to noise between 85 and 90 dBA causes hearing loss. It is strongly recommended that noise in the NICU be maintained at levels below 60 dB to prevent cochlear damage (American Academy of Pediatrics Committee on Environmental Health, 1997).

1989) or a power mower (American Academy of Pediatrics Committee on Environmental Health, 1997). Because decibels increase in a logarithmic fashion, even small increases in the decibel levels of sounds can be significant. This issue has raised concern among physicians and developmental specialists, who wonder how elevated noise levels may affect the developing hearing mechanisms of preterm and full-term infants (Blackburn, 1996). Although hearing loss has not been demonstrated to result from exposure to sounds in the NICU, studies have shown effects of such exposures on auditory frequency discrimination and pattern recognition in developing animals and in humans (Graven, 1997).

The literature review conducted by the *Physical and Developmental Environment of the High-Risk Infant Center, Study Group on Neonatal Intensive Care Unit (NICU) Sound, and the Expert Review Panel,* a multidisciplinary group concerned with effects of sound on the developing fetus (Graven, 2000), resulted in recommendations that can be summarized as follows:

- The voice of an infant's mother and the sounds produced by her body during her everyday activities is sufficient for normal auditory development.
- Sound should be regularly assessed and controlled in NICUs.
- Earphones should not be used with infants.
- There is little evidence that recorded music or speech is beneficial for preterm infants; therefore, infants should not be left unattended with such devices.

It is recommended that the combination of continuous background sound and transient sound in any bed space should not exceed an hourly average of 55 dB (the perceived level of annoyance). Transient sounds (produced by voices or equipment) should not exceed 70 dB. Intensity of the sound, however, is only one of several factors that should be considered. According to Morris, Philbin, and Bose (2000), a preterm infant's maturity, birth history, and state of arousal may influence his or her response to sound. Moreover, concern about the effects of sound exposure go beyond the hearing apparatus to include effects on physiologic regulation, thus presenting a need for careful and ongoing monitoring of neonates who are exposed to noise above the recommended levels (Zahr & Balian, 1995).

Light

Lighting levels in the NICU are equally concerning. Overhead fluorescent lighting is not uncommon in NICUs. In addition, procedure lights, phototherapy lamps, and nearby windows produce added illumination. Light is measured in lux or foot-candles, with 10.76 lux being equivalent to 1 foot-candle. Daytime light levels in NICUs range from 192 to 1,488 lux (Blackburn, 1996). In a National Institute of Child Health and Human Development survey of eight NICUs, mean phototherapy light levels from within the Isolettes ranged from 7,600–19,000 lux. The mean ambient light in the eight NICUs was 731.68 lux ± 33 (Landry, Scheidt, & Hammond, 1985). In comparison, the Occupational Safety and Health Act of 1970 (PL 91-596) recommends a 430–538 lux maximum for office workers. Light levels have been shown to influence the development of circadian rhythms among preterm infants (Mirmiran & Ariagno, 2000). Despite growing evidence that NICU characteristics such as intrusive light and sound levels and the overwhelming presence of technology may contribute to behavioral disorganization and stress among infants and caregivers, few changes have been made in the physical environment of many NICUs.

There have been a number of investigations of the potentially harmful effects of light and sound on preterm infant development, state regulation, visual development, and hearing (Blackburn, 1996; Graven, 1997; Mirmiran & Ariagno, 2000). The benefits of altering the NICU environment to achieve quiet periods with decreased light, noise, and activity have also been investigated. One such study reported reductions in median diastolic blood pressure, mean arterial pressure, and infant activity (Slevin, Farrington, Duffy, Daly, & Murphy, 2000). Although some results are inconclusive, the consensus seems to be that reducing light and sound levels should be a goal, if for no other reason than providing a more restful, soothing atmosphere for the infants. The Consensus Committee to Establish Recommended Standards for Newborn ICU Design (2002) produced guidelines for the NICU environment, including the following:

- Have adjustable ambient lighting from 10 to 600 lux, as measured at bedside
- Provide controls for immediate darkening of artificial and natural lighting that are sufficient to allow transillumination when necessary
- Create a procedure for lighting that is framed to reduce illumination on adjacent beds
- Have at least one source of natural lighting (i.e., a window or skylight), equipped with shading, that is visible from patient care areas; however, to prevent heat loss, the source of natural light should be no closer than 2 feet from any infant's bedside

Bed and Family Space

Other Consensus Committee (2002) recommendations focus on the need to reduce stress among caregivers. Increased space between beds provides for more privacy at the bedside and enhances family comfort and participation in their infant's care. In addition, recommended strategies to decrease stress through family-centered care may include providing private, cozy areas for families to spend time with their infant, waiting areas for families to rest between visits and to meet other families, information areas, and places to meet privately with the medical team.

NICU Equipment

Before they can effectively assist in modifying the NICU environment to optimize infant–caregiver engagement, neonatal therapists must become familiar with the equipment commonly found in the NICU and the purposes of each piece of equipment. Equipment settings are the primary responsibility of the medical and nursing personnel, and therapists should refrain from changing settings unless authorized by medical or nursing personnel. Nonetheless, therapists must at least learn basic operation procedures for the various types of equipment required by the infants with whom they work. Therapists must know the basic precautions for working around certain pieces of equipment and, most important, know what to do in case of an emergency while working with their patients. Styles of equipment vary by NICU, so it is important for therapists to become acquainted with the operation of the equipment in their particular environment. This includes learning how to identify the sound of various alarms, appropriately respond in the event of a true alarm, and silence an alarm if it is false or the problem has been corrected. Whenever it is necessary to respond to a true alarm, therapists should know to notify the nurse in charge and document the event on the infant's medical chart as appropriate. The following subsections describe the equipment commonly found in NICUs.

Incubators

Thermal regulation is one of the most vital capacities for the survival of newborns. Cold stress is a serious, potentially life-threatening problem for sick or premature infants. Incubators provide a regulated thermal environment for infants who cannot maintain their body temperature within a safe range. This invention revolutionized the care of medically fragile newborns, particularly LBW infants. In addition to having immature central nervous systems, these fragile patients lack the ability to produce and retain heat because they lack both subcutaneous and "brown" fat (fat that is produced in the last trimester of gestation and used to metabolize heat). Infants may lose heat in four ways:

1. *Conduction* is the transfer of heat directly to another object through physical contact. For instance, when an infant is placed on a cold surface, heat from the infant's skin transfers to the supporting surface and the infant runs the risk of getting cold.

2. *Convection* is the loss of heat into the surrounding air. For example, when the incubator door is left open, the temperature decreases because the heat disperses to the surrounding environment.

3. *Evaporation* is the loss of heat into the air through conversion of moisture from an infant's skin and mucous membranes into a vapor. This is the main indication for using plastic wrap covers or for humidifying the air in incubators.

4. *Radiation* is the loss of heat from an infant's body to a nearby surface. This form of heat loss needs to be considered when toys and care supplies are kept inside the incubator.

Incubators are designed to prevent heat loss by regulating the thermal environment. Incubators primarily minimize heat loss through radiation and convection. Some incubators warm and humidify the air, reducing heat loss by evaporation. There are two types of incubators: open (radiant warmers) and closed (Isolettes).

Radiant Warmer

An open incubator, or radiant warmer, is used most often when an infant is under close observation—for example, during the first few hours of life or for immediate access to infants who require frequent or complicated medical procedures. It consists of an open bed with low Plexiglas rails (see Figure 8). The angle and height of the bed can be adjusted. A heating unit, temperature monitor, and procedure lights are located overhead. The infant's temperature is monitored by means of a heat probe that is attached to his or her skin. The reflective probe is attached to the unit by means of a thin wire. An alarm sounds when the infant's temperature is outside the range set by the caregiver. The probe must not be covered by clothing or bedding; doing so will make it function inefficiently and the infant may become overheated or too cool. The open design of this warmer allows unobstructed visual inspection and easy access to the infant for care. An infant in an open warmer need not be dressed, as there is minimal heat lost by way of radiation or conduction. However, an infant in an open warmer is more likely to lose heat by convection and evaporation. The

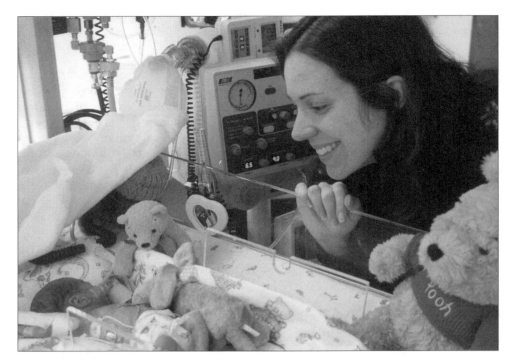

Figure 8.   An open warmer is used to enable this infant to receive the frequent and potentially life-saving medical and nursing care that she needs. Although this baby cannot yet be held, the openness allows the mother to get close to her daughter.

warmer bed may be covered with plastic wrap to prevent convection and evaporation heat loss.

Isolette

Closed incubators, or Isolettes, are used for infants who need assistance with thermal regulation but do not require frequent nursing intervention. The Isolette consists of a heated clear plastic box or cylinder that houses a flat, reclinable surface on which the infant is placed (Figure 9). Most Isolettes have ports with plastic sleeves and/or small porthole doors that open and close to reduce unnecessary cooling when reaching inside. Some sides of box-type Isolettes also drop down for positioning and handling. Cylindrical Isolettes do not have doors and tend to lose more heat when the hood is left open during infant handling. Heating elements and an air circulation fan are located underneath the infant compartment. An alarm sounds when the Isolette's temperature is outside the range set by the caregiver, which can occur when the side door, hood, or ports have been left open too long. A U-shaped plastic heat shield may be placed over the infant's trunk to retain heat around his or her body.

Weaning an infant from an incubator usually takes place over a period of several days, during which the temperature of the Isolette is lowered and eventually turned off. Then, the ports are opened to allow the infant a chance to gradually regulate his or her own temperature. Until that time, the NICU therapist must be careful to minimize heat loss when examining and caring for the infant. Infrared lights or other heating devices may be used to maintain a regulated thermal environment when

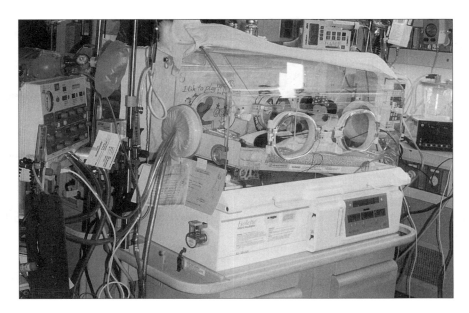

Figure 9. Isolettes are commonly used in the NICU to provide thermal regulation and protection for infants who are relatively stable.

personnel must handle infants who are unable to regulate their temperature outside the incubator for prolonged periods of time.

Isolettes are also used when infants require additional protection from the environment to regulate their states of arousal. Newer units have quieter fans and an increased capacity to muffle environmental noise. Enclosed Isolettes now dampen outside noise by approximately 10 dB but maintain an internal noise level of approximately 58 dBA. Incubator coverings attenuate the noise even more (Saunders, 1995).

Infant Cribs

There are two basic types of infant cribs in NICUs. The regular open crib is generally used with larger and older infants who no longer need thermal regulation assistance. This type of crib provides no close boundaries and may not be the most appropriate for infants who require tactile containment. Boundaries may be formed through other sources, such as rolled blankets, stuffed animals, or commercial positioning devices such as the SnuggleUp or the Bendy Bumper (available from Children's Medical Ventures, http://www.childmed.com/products). Positioning recommendations for this type of crib are detailed in Chapter 12.

Bassinet-type cribs are smaller than open cribs and are found in most Level I newborn nurseries. They consist of a basket or bucket-type clear plastic "bin" in which the infant lies dressed and swaddled. They are used with infants who may still benefit from close boundaries, no longer require thermal support, and are small enough to safely fit inside.

Both types of cribs may be used with infants in need of continued physiologic monitoring and/or oxygen administration by nasal cannula. However, the larger crib is required for infants receiving oxygen by oxyhood or ventilatory support.

Heart and Respiration Rate (Apnea) Monitors

Heart and respiration rate monitors give a warning signal should either the heart rate (HR) or the respiration rate (RR) reach unsafe limits. Alarms are commonly set to sound when HR or RR readings are outside the following recommended safe limits:

- HR between 100 and 200 beats per minute (BPM); the ideal rate is 120–160 BPM
- RR between 20 and 60 breaths per minute

Alarms also are set to sound after a respiratory pause longer than 20 seconds. When an alarm begins to sound, the infant must be visually inspected immediately to determine whether the alarm signals a true emergency. Many false alarms are set off when the infant moves. If the infant is moving and breathing and has good color, then the alarm should be disengaged and intervention continued. If the infant is not breathing or becomes cyanotic, pale, or limp, then the nurse in charge must be notified immediately. The infant's HR must be noted, and appropriate stimulation (tactile or vestibular) must be given until the infant reinitiates breathing.

Oxygen Saturation Monitor (Pulse Oximeter)

Oxygen saturation (sats) monitors measure the concentration of oxygen in an infant's peripheral circulation. Normal oxygen concentration ranges between 90% and 100%. The alarm usually is set to sound if the concentration falls below 90%. The sensor for this monitor is generally attached to one of the infant's feet or hands. It is extremely sensitive to movement, so false signals are common. One important consideration in interpreting this monitor's signals is to compare the pulse reading on the sat monitor with the reading on the HR monitor. These readings must correspond within approximately 5–10 beats. When readings do not match, they are false signals that can be ignored. The infant must *always* be checked before the alarm is disengaged.

Transcutaneous Peripheral Oxygen and Carbon Dioxide Monitors

Transcutaneous peripheral oxygen and carbon dioxide monitors measure the concentration of oxygen ($TcPO_2$) or carbon dioxide ($TcPCO_2$) through the skin. Electrodes are placed on the infant's skin to heat the area, causing oxygen and carbon dioxide to diffuse through the skin where their concentration can be measured. Transcutaneous monitors are more reliable than pulse oximetry but less accurate than blood chemistry. Neonatal therapists should not alter the settings on these monitors. The nurse in charge or the respiratory therapist should be asked to check the infant if the $TcPO_2$ or $TcPCO_2$ alarm sounds.

Ventilatory Support

The goal of ventilatory support is to optimize the clinical status of the infant by improving gas exchange using the least amount of fraction inspired oxygen (FiO_2) at minimum pressures. The strategy employed to ventilate each infant depends on that infant's condition (Eichenwald, 1997).

Bag and Mask

This type of ventilation is accomplished by hand, with a mask that fits over the infant's nose and mouth and a bag that can be squeezed to deliver oxygen or room air. It is used for resuscitation, as an interim means of ventilation prior to intubation, or when an infant is removed temporarily from a mechanical ventilator.

Continuous Positive Airway Pressure

Continuous positive airway pressure (CPAP) is used for infants who are able to breathe spontaneously but require assistance maintaining their end-expiratory lung volume. A continuous flow of warmed, humidified gas is circulated past the infant's airway at a set pressure. This is accomplished by using a set of flexible nasal prongs; a small, tightly fitted mask over the nose; or, less commonly, an endotracheal tube. CPAP is administered by a mechanical ventilator with positive pressure settings (Eichenwald, 1997).

Mechanical Ventilation

Mechanical ventilation is more invasive, administered by endotracheal tube. It has the greatest potential to cause barotrauma. Mechanical ventilation is used for infants with the following clinical conditions: severe hypoxemia (decreased peripheral oxygen, or PaO$_2$), severe hypercapnia (increased peripheral carbon dioxide, or PaCO$_2$); apnea and bradycardia unresponsive to CPAP; inefficient respiratory effort due to asphyxia, narcosis, or primary cardiopulmonary disease; or shock with hypoperfusion and hypotension. Mechanical ventilation is also used for ELBW infants who are unable to maintain ventilation secondary to immaturity (Hagedorn, Gardner, & Abman, 1989). There are several types of mechanical ventilators: intermittent mandatory, synchronized intermittent mandatory, and high frequency.

The most commonly used type of intermittent mandatory ventilation (IMV) is pressure-limited, time-cycled, continuous flow. The IMV provides a continuous flow of mixed air and oxygen, and the rate and duration of inspiration and expiration are fixed, but the infant is able to make spontaneous efforts to breathe between ventilator breaths. This type is most often used for infants with respiratory distress.

The synchronized intermittent mandatory ventilator (SIMV) is also referred to as an assist/control or pressure support ventilator. The SIMV also provides intermittent breaths at a fixed rate but is equipped with sensors to detect the respiratory efforts made by an infant. Each time the infant breathes spontaneously, the unit delivers a synchronized positive pressure breath, reducing the phenomenon of "fighting" the ventilator. This method is thought to help infants wean from the ventilator and may also be less likely to contribute to complications such as air leak or IVH.

High-frequency ventilation (HFV) is used with infants who are not responsive to conventional ventilation or for infants with air leak syndromes. There are several types of HFV: high-frequency oscillating ventilation (HFOV), high-frequency flow interruption (HFFI), and high-frequency jet ventilation (HFJV). All of these deliver small volume breaths at extremely rapid rates to avoid lung injury (Eichenwald, 1997).

Although neonatal therapists must know how to interpret ventilator alarm signals, they are not qualified to change the settings on any ventilation equipment. When working with infants who are intubated, care must be taken to keep the ventilator tubes in the same arrangement as initially set for the entire duration of the treatment. *Extreme care must be taken not to extubate the infant while handling.*

Infusion Pumps

Electric infusion pumps control the flow and rate of IV fluids, intralipids, and transpyloric feedings. Neonatal therapists must know how to interpret infusion pump signals.

When an infusion pump alarms, the nurse should be notified immediately. Therapists should neither change the settings nor disengage an infusion pump alarm without nursing consent.

Extracorporeal Membrane Oxygenation

Extracorporeal membrane oxygenation (ECMO) is a lifesaving heart and lung bypass procedure for infants with severe neonatal cardiorespiratory failure who do not respond to intensive care. The procedure involves draining the infant's venous blood, supplementing it with oxygen, and removing carbon dioxide by means of a membrane oxygenator (artificial lung), as well as returning the blood either to the venous or arterial circulation. This process bypasses the lungs, allowing them to "rest."

Contraindications for ECMO include mechanical ventilation for more than 10 days, significant intraventricular or parenchymal hemorrhage, infant weight of less than 2,000 g, and gestational age of younger than 34 weeks. ECMO is considered a treatment of last resort, and is offered only at centers that can provide the equipment as well as the highly specialized medical management required to be classified as specialized nurseries. The advent of high-frequency oscillatory ventilation and nitric oxide therapies has diminished the need for ECMO (Levy & Fackler, 1997).

STRESSORS IN THE NICU
ENVIRONMENT: EFFECTS ON INFANTS AND CAREGIVERS

Anyone who has taken care of infants in the NICU is well aware that it can be a stressful place for infants, families, and staff. The stress partially results from the apprehension that caregivers experience when they see their infant surrounded by life-support equipment and monitors (e.g., Figure 10). Some of this stress is related to specific situations and some is related to the environment in which these situations are experienced. The following case example illustrates both situational and environmental stressors for the infant as well as the family.

Jake weighed 690 g at birth. He was born at 25 weeks of gestation by emergency cesarean section after spontaneous rupture of membranes and a footling breech presentation. After Jake was stabilized in the NICU, the attending neonatologist and the NICU social worker, Juan, visited with Jake's father at the baby's bedside, explaining the difficult course ahead for Jake. Jake's father, Bill, was still dazed by the day's events. Later, he spoke of how alone and frightened he felt being Jake's first and sole visitor in the NICU. His wife, Sarah, was still recovering from the surgery, and his parents were at home, anxiously awaiting news while watching Hayley, Jake's older sister.

Bill clearly remembered Hayley's birth 3 years ago. What a different experience that had been, helping Sarah bring a healthy full-term infant into the world! Now, Bill hesitated to call their relatives with the news of Jake's birth. What could he say? He telephoned both his and Sarah's parents, relating that Jake was born by cesarean section and was critically ill and that Sarah was still in recovery. Jake's grandparents had many questions that Bill could not answer. Bill decided to wait

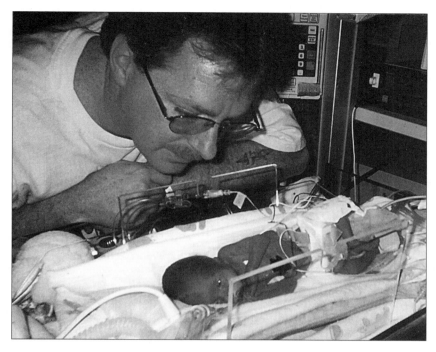

Figure 10. Observe the intensity of this father's facial expression as he looks at his premature son, who is surrounded by life support equipment.

until Sarah was awake so he could help her process what had happened and they could decide together what else to tell their families.

After making the telephone calls, Bill returned to the NICU. He felt that he needed to stay close to Jake in case the infant took a turn for the worst. Yet, Bill also felt that he should stay close to his wife so he could be with Sarah when she awakened to reassure her that the doctors in the NICU were doing everything to save their son. Juan encouraged Bill to stay with Sarah while the NICU team continued to make Jake as comfortable as possible and to stabilize him on the ventilator. The neonatologist, Dr. Peterson, said that she would come to Sarah's room later to talk with both of them.

In this example, situational stressors include the precipitous delivery of an infant who was expected to be delivered at term. When a pregnancy is characterized as high risk, whether because of difficulties in a previous pregnancy or because of complications with the current pregnancy, the obstetrician usually helps prepare parents for the possibility that their infant may be born prematurely. Often, when there are signs of preterm labor, the mother is admitted to the hospital for the remainder of her pregnancy in an attempt to forestall the premature birth. While she is hospitalized, the obstetrics team has time to educate both parents about the issues such as the possibility that their premature infant may require an extended stay in the NICU. Consultation by an attending neonatologist and/or neonatology fellow can be provided at this time to inform the parents of the likelihood of survival should the infant be born at that particularly early gestational age, as well as of the complications that the infant will likely experience during a NICU stay. Developmental outcomes of preterm infants born under similar circumstances are also discussed, as this is usually of paramount importance to prospective parents. Also important at this time is supportive counseling by social work or psychology staff, who assist the parents in dealing with their fears and apprehensions and in obtaining and using available social supports among family members, friends, and clergy. In the case example, anticipatory guidance and psycho-social support were not available to Jake's parents because of his unexpected early delivery. Postponing guidance until after the birth of the infant compounds the family's situational stress and limits their access to social supports who otherwise might be ready and able to assist them.

Several hours later, with Bill at her side, Sarah was still sedated for pain but alert enough to consult with Dr. Peterson and ask questions: "Will Jake be okay?" "How can he survive? He's so small!" "When will we be able to see him?" "When can we hold him?" The neonatologist explained that Jake would have a good chance of survival if he made it through the next 48 hours but that he would face a prolonged stay in the NICU, with many potential complications. Dr. Peterson also mentioned the possibility that Jake could have developmental problems related to the complications but that there was no way of telling how complicated Jake's recovery and development would be. Dr. Peterson then told Bill and Sarah that they probably would not be able to hold Jake for several days (until he became stable on the ventilator) but they were welcome at his side any time when the doctors were not conducting rounds in Jake's bay. Dr. Peterson explained that she would be meeting with Bill and Sarah regularly, giving brief updates at the bedside and more detailed summaries in private family meetings that would be scheduled at their convenience. The parents and the doctor then made arrange-ments for Sarah to visit Jake in the NICU.

In the NICU from which this fictional case example is drawn, the neonatologist visits new parents as soon as he or she can leave the infant's bedside. In this visit, the neonatologist explains the infant's current plan of care, provides information about the expected course of treatment, and begins to assist the parents in forming realistic expectations for their infant's outcome. This is done privately in the mother's hospital room to give parents the opportunity to react to the news, support each other, and ask questions. The social worker assigned to the family accompanies the neonatologist on this initial visit to hear what the parents are told, see their reaction, and assess their need for psychosocial support. The social worker often stays with the parents after the neonatologist leaves, providing support and preparing them for their first visit to the NICU as a couple.

Bill was glad he had seen Jake in the NICU first so he could put aside his initial shock and assist his wife. Their first joint visit was overwhelming, seeing their tiny infant lying on the warmer and attached to so many tubes and wires. The sounds were frightening, too. The nurse, Marie, spent time explaining Jake's equipment. She said that because Jake cannot breathe on his own yet, a ventilator helps him breathe through a tube going into his mouth and down into his lungs. The foil sticker with the blue wire attached to Jake's chest is his temperature probe, which keeps the warmer at just the right temperature for him. The thick gray wire attached to Jake's foot is the pulse oximeter, which measures the level of oxygen in his blood, and the thin wires attached by thin disks are for monitoring his heart rate and respiration. Marie noted that these last three items are attached to monitors that will beep if Jake's heart rate, respiration, or oxygen saturation were to reach unacceptable levels. She then explained that the IV line in his arm is for feeding and that Jake also has an umbilical artery catheter to check the adequacy of his gas exchange and other important blood levels without having to draw his blood repeatedly. Marie said that Jake is on an open incubator with a Plexiglas heat shield and a plastic-wrap covering to retain heat and moisture.

Bill was very interested in the equipment and asked a few questions about the monitors' readings. Sarah was too busy examining Jake to take it all in. She had seen pictures of infants in NICUs but never dreamed that she would see her child in a NICU. Sarah could not yet process the fact that this tiny person attached to all this equipment was her son. Although Dr. Peterson had cautioned them that Jake's survival was not assured, Sarah could see that he was breathing with the help of the ventilator and was resting calmly, surrounded by a "nest" of blanket rolls to keep his arms and legs flexed close to his body. She touched Jake's hand lightly and spoke to him, and he moved his fingers and squirmed in response.

Marie confirmed that it would be a few days before Jake's parents could hold him, but they were welcome to visit often and to talk to and touch Jake. Marie noted that Sarah and Bill also would learn ways to care for Jake (e.g., clean his mouth with a swab, take his temperature, change his diaper) and meet with the neonatal therapist to discover how their son likes to be touched, moved, and interacted with during his care. Marie encouraged them to bring a few things from home for Jake: a quilt to place in his warmer bed, a small stuffed animal to look at, a family photo, and perhaps a book or two to read to him.

Juan, the social worker, returned to assure Sarah and Bill that he would check in intermittently and would be available to meet with them any time. Juan shared that Bill and Sarah would meet the rest of Jake's team—the assistant nurse manager, neonatal nurse practitioner, neonatal fellow, and attending neonatologist—at their first family meeting in a few days. In the meantime, before signing out for the night, the neonatal fellow or attending neonatologist would visit them again in Sarah's room to update them on Jake's condition. Juan then explained visitation rules for other family members and friends and gave Jake's parents a copy of the NICU's parent handbook, which included these rules and listed the staff and the various programs available to families of infants in the special care nursery. Jake's parents were also invited to the parent orientation being held on the following Monday evening in the NICU conference room. In addition, they were invited to bring their daughter Hayley to "Kid's Klub," a sibling visitation group, on Tuesday evenings.

Sarah needed to rest. She was still experiencing considerable discomfort after her cesarean section. Yet, there were so many things to think about—everything had happened so fast. She gave Jake one last touch good-bye and asked to be wheeled back to her room.

NICU SUPPORT SERVICES

Experiencing the NICU for the first time can be overwhelming for anyone, whether he or she is a staff member or a visitor. The critical condition of the infant is a major source of stress (Reddick, Catlin, & Jellinek, 2001; Spear, 2002). The sights and sounds of the NICU environment are known to also induce stress and fatigue among NICU personnel (Oates & Oates, 1996). However, the experience of family members in the NICU is unique because it is intertwined with their fears and hopes for the infant. Every piece of equipment at the infant's bedside has the potential to increase the parents' environmentally induced stress and instill new fears and anxieties. Restrictions in visitation times further increase stress for many families. The NICU staff need to anticipate all sources of stress among family members and attempt to allay these fears by providing information and support in various formats throughout the NICU experience.

Keeping parents well informed, discussing care options with them, and facilitating parental visitation from the beginning are among the best ways of reducing situational stress for families (Spear, 2002). The neonatologist, as the leader of the NICU team, has a vital role in informing family members of the infant's status, recommending a course of treatment, and involving the family in decision making whenever there are several options to consider.

Nursing staff can reinforce the importance of the family as members of the caregiving team by welcoming them to their baby's bedside with sympathy and respect, postponing nonessential procedures until after family visits, and providing additional details relative to the care of their infant. Nurses are in a powerful position in the NICU, as they are constantly at the baby's side, implementing the care (Lawhon, 2002). When asked about sources of stress in the NICU, some parents voiced having a secondary role to nursing staff when it comes to nurturing and caring for their baby (Bell, 1997; Dobbins, Bohlig, & Sutphen, 1994). For example, in Bell's study, a group of teenage mothers reported that the alterations in their expected parental role, as well as the infant's appearance and behavior, were a greater source of stress than the sights and sounds of the NICU environment. Nurses who follow the tenets of family-centered care will seek to minimize this form of stress and enhance the parents' role in nurturing their infant by being receptive to parents' questions at any time, whether at the infant's bedside or by telephone. Family-centered nurses also assist parents to find ways of becoming involved in their infant's care (McGrath & Conliffe-Torres, 1996). All of these activities have been found to decrease the family's stress (Meyer et al., 1994).

Parents can be shown how to provide routine care, even for the sickest and smallest NICU infants. At a minimum, parents can be drawn into observations and discussions of their infant's behavior and responses to caregiving, and they can participate in making some accommodations for their infant's comfort. Bringing in a quilt, toys, and family photos helps personalize their baby's bedside and helps staff to relate to the infant as somebody's baby rather than "the 25-weeker on the oscillator in C-bay." Quietly talking, reading, or singing to the infant; touching and holding the infant; and providing skin-to-skin (or kangaroo) care are important ways that families can begin to build an emotional bond with their infant.

Situational stress among parents also may be caused by their fears of interacting with their sick infant and their concerns for the infant's eventual developmental outcome. Involving parents in developmental assessment and in formulating a developmental care plan early in the hospitalization (by scheduling assessments and meetings at times convenient for the family) can be tremendously reassuring and helpful to parents. These experiences allow parents to better observe and interpret their infant's behavioral cues, to interact appropriately, and to obtain optimal responses from their infant; they also help parents become more knowledgeable about their infant's developmental strengths and vulnerabilities at discharge (Meyer et al., 1994).

Environmental stress can also be reduced by explaining to family members the purposes of the NICU equipment, alarms, and procedures used with their infant and by giving them opportunities to ask questions. In this chapter's case example, nursing and social work staff had key roles in providing anticipatory guidance and reassurance to the family by offering additional information and support from a variety of sources (e.g., weekly parent orientation meetings).

Whether the stress is related to situational, environmental, technology-related, financial, or time issues (or a combination of factors), a number of programs can be provided to parents in the NICU to assist in their adjustment to this difficult experience. The special care nursery illustrated in the case example offered a variety of support services for families, such as a parent support group, a parent-to-parent support program, and a support group for siblings. Examples of other similar programs can be found in the literature (Plaas, 1994).

Parent Support Groups

Parent support groups are often run by a social worker, generally meet weekly, and are open to all NICU parents. Such groups include an informational component, with invited speakers on topics such as attachment, behavioral cues of preterms, and developmental outcomes of preterms. They also have a social support component, with time in each meeting for parents to interact, share their concerns and fears with the group, and obtain support from other group members. Often, parents who meet in the group setting continue to provide psychosocial support to each other on an informal basis as they meet elsewhere in the hospital.

Parent-to-Parent Support Programs

In some hospitals, parents who would like peer support on a formal basis without becoming involved in a parent support group can participate in parent-to-parent support programs. These programs pair parents of infants in the NICU with experienced parents of NICU "graduates" (Jarrett, 1996a, 1996b; Roman et al., 1995). The experienced parents are volunteers who have been specially trained to provide friendly support to current NICU parents. In such programs, parents are usually paired with others who previously faced similar challenges regarding their infant's medical status and care. These relationships can continue after infants are discharged from the NICU to assist parents during the transition home. The experienced parent volunteers are continually supported in their efforts by the social work staff, who assist parent volunteers in maintaining a friendly, nonclinical relationship with the NICU parents.

Sibling Visitation Groups

In the case story, "Kid's Klub" served as an example of a sibling visitation group. In some places, these groups are run by a NICU nurse, psychologist, or social worker; an art therapist; and volunteers. Before meetings, each child who plans to participate is given a standard health screening by a nurse to prevent bringing contagious illnesses

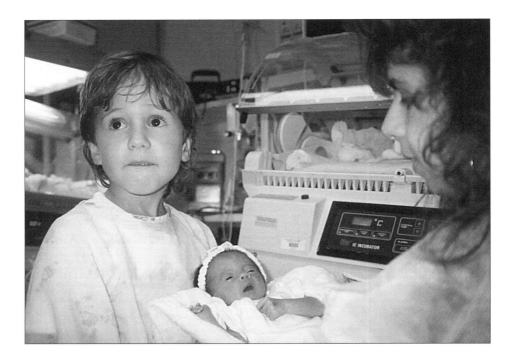

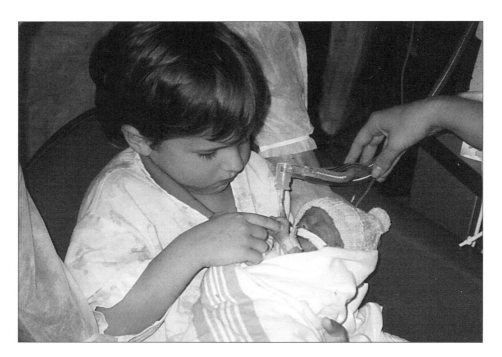

Figure 11. This boy is visiting his sister in the NICU for the first time. He initially appears apprehensive (top photo). With the support of the sibling visitation staff, he is able to warm up to his sister (bottom photo).

into the NICU. While parents visit with their NICU infants, siblings go to a conference room, where they are grouped according to age and prepared for the NICU environment by a psychologist or social worker. Explanations of what they will see and experience are tailored to the developmental level and age of the siblings and to the particular circumstances of the infants they will be visiting. For example, if an infant is extremely small and is being kept under a plastic wrap cover or has an unusual appearance because of an anomaly or surgery, these factors are explained ahead of time. Dolls and other props are used, as needed, to illustrate these explanations. The children then do an age-appropriate art project—usually making something for their sibling, such as a mobile or bright picture that can be hung at the infant's bedside. They share pizza and juice, are shown how to scrub, and then are accompanied to the baby's bedside, where their parents are waiting. A support group staff person remains with the sibling during the visit to provide guidance and supervision. Visits are usually kept to 20 minutes or less, depending on the sibling's age. This approach is successful in preparing children for the experience of seeing a fragile sibling in the NICU and begins the process of sibling attachment (Figure 11). Parents have reported that when their older children participate in such programs, they are less likely to behave in a jealous manner toward the newborn and actually become protective of their younger brother or sister (Meyer, Kennally, Zika-Beres, Cashore, & Oh, 1996). Furthermore, there is no evidence that sibling visitation increases the incidence of contagious disease in the NICU, as long as children are properly screened before each visit (Hamrick & Riley, 1992; Schwab, Tolbert, Bagnato, & Maisels, 1983).

CONCLUSION

This first glimpse into the lives of NICU parents and families and their initial responses to the NICU environment raises a number of points for the NICU therapist to consider. Infants may be referred for intervention for reasons that are infant centered, parent–infant centered, or related to specific family needs. The timing of the initial referral may vary, depending on whether it is driven by the needs of the infant, the family, or both. As described in the case story, joint observations of the infant by the therapist and the family can begin as soon as the infant is initially stabilized, providing an opportunity to forge an alliance that will continue throughout the infant's NICU stay. Although there are as many goals for developmental and therapeutic intervention as there are differences among infants, families, and NICUs, a primary objective is to work together to reduce unnecessary environmental effects on the infant while ameliorating the family's environmental and situational stress. This collaborative approach, sometimes referred to as *relationship-based intervention* (Als, 1997b; Holloway, 1994, 1998), is described in further detail in Chapter 11.

6

Medical Management
of High-Risk Infants

OVERVIEW

The purpose of this chapter is to acquaint potential neonatal therapists with prevalent medical conditions in the NICU and common medical interventions. The information contained in this chapter is basic and by no means comprehensive. Individuals seeking to become neonatal therapists must review the original sources to obtain more in-depth knowledge about the discussed conditions. A medical dictionary may be useful for unfamiliar terms, and the glossary at the end of this book serves as a resource for commonly used acronyms.

Special emphasis is given to respiratory disorders, the most prevalent neonatal conditions. Common neonatal cardiovascular and cardiopulmonary disorders are discussed. Central nervous system disorders are also discussed, with an emphasis on IVH and periventricular leukomalacia (PVL). Other disorders covered include neonatal seizures, hyperbilirubinemia, congenital anomalies and genetic disorders, metabolic disorders, and gastroesophageal reflux (GER). Retinopathy of prematurity (ROP) is discussed because of its potential implications for an infant's visual capabilities.

OBJECTIVES

- Identify the most common neonatal conditions found in NICUs
- Describe some of the respiratory disorders that are common in newborns
- Identify the common signs of apnea of prematurity and the recommended steps for helping infants to recover from apneic episodes
- Explain the potential neurologic consequences and recognize the life-threatening severity of many respiratory disorders, especially chronic lung disease (CLD) and perinatal asphyxia
- Identify the most common types of cardiovascular/cardiopulmonary disorders, recognizing the possible limitations of infants with cardiac conditions and the importance of optimizing the infants' participation while preserving energy
- Identify central nervous system disorders that are common in neonates and likely to have long-term developmental consequences

• Describe other common neonatal disorders and the implications of each for the delivery of neonatal therapy services

COMMON MEDICAL CONDITIONS OF NICU INFANTS

Infants who begin their lives in a NICU are among the most fragile of patients served by neonatal therapists and developmental specialists. Although not all of these infants have conditions that are immediately life threatening, they all need intensive medical management to prevent deterioration of or to improve their condition. Some infants require short-term observation secondary to physiologic instability at birth or possible sepsis; others require life-sustaining treatment for extreme prematurity, congenital conditions, or perinatal conditions and will remain in the NICU for months. They all share a vulnerability to medical complications that can easily become life threatening or, at the very least, affect their occupational performance and developmental outcome. Neonatal therapists seeking to become neonatal specialists must become knowledge-able about the medical conditions prevalent in NICUs and about common nursing and medical management in the NICU. Neonatal therapists are able to help optimize infants' occupational performance and participation in age- and context-appropriate activities only after recognizing the intricacies of the NICU environmental context.

Most infants in Level III NICUs have been admitted for their many medical problems associated with prematurity. Full-term neonates, however, also represent a large group in the NICU, as they may have a number of serious conditions requiring short-term or long-term NICU stays. Developmental specialists who work with high-risk newborns must be knowledgeable about the prevailing medical problems among these infants, their medical management, the ways that a medical problem may affect intervention, and the ways that intervention may affect a medical problem. Lack of adequate medical background may pose a threat to the infant's health and well-being. The following section lists the most prevalent neonatal medical problems, their causes, their potential effects on infants, and their possible effects on neonatal intervention.

Respiratory Disorders

Most NICU admissions are related to respiratory distress or hypoxemia. The causes of respiratory distress vary, including fetal distress, airway obstruction, lung immaturity, congenital heart disease, retention or aspiration of amniotic fluid or meconium, and pneumonia. Of these, severe meconium aspiration syndrome, severe perinatal pneumonia with sepsis, and respiratory distress syndrome of prematurity are classified as more serious, requiring prolonged periods of intubation with assisted ventilation, nitric oxide therapy, and, in some cases, invasive procedures such as ECMO (heart-lung bypass) (Vohr, Cashore, & Bigsby, 1999; Wolkoff & Narula, 2000).

Respiratory Distress Syndrome

Sometimes referred to as *hyaline membrane disease* (HMD), respiratory distress syndrome (RDS) is caused by inadequate pulmonary surfactant, which can lead to alveolar atelectasis, edema, and cell injury. Lung immaturity contributes to factors such as inefficient clearing of secretions and reduced surface area for gas exchange, which can exacerbate the distress. Mortality from RDS has been reduced by advances in neonatal care, including prenatal identification of infants at risk (e.g., infants likely to be delivered at extremely low birth weights), antenatal administration of steroids, surfactant replacement therapy, better management of oxygenation and fluids, and improvements in mechanical ventilation (Liley & Stark, 1997; Roberts, 1999).

Transient Tachypnea of the Newborn

Transient tachypnea of the newborn (TTN), also called "wet lung," is a transient form of pulmonary edema believed to be caused by a delay in the reabsorption of lung liquid (Lawson, 1997). Infants begin to experience respiratory distress soon after delivery, manifested by fast breathing (more than 80 breaths per minute), grunting, nasal flaring, intercostal retractions, and cyanosis. This problem is more common in full-term or near-term infants and in infants born by cesarean section because of lack of vaginal thoracic squeeze (Hagedorn et al., 1989). Oxygen is administered by oxygen hood, nasal cannula, or nasal continuous positive airway pressure (NCPAP). TTN generally resolves within 3–5 days, with no recurrence of respiratory problems (Lawson, 1997). Neonatal therapists may see infants with TNN briefly for an assessment of feeding and behavioral organization prior to NICU discharge. This can be especially helpful to parents who are anxious about their infant's condition. Parents benefit from reviewing their infant's capacities and being reassured that their infant is able to nipple-feed without distress.

Apnea of Prematurity

Apnea is the most common respiratory problem in premature infants. Stark defined *apnea* as "a cessation of respiration accompanied by bradycardia (heart rate <100 beats per minute) or cyanosis" (1997, p. 374). In most nurseries, apnea monitors are set to detect a 20-second pause in breathing because such a pause is usually sufficient to trigger an associated bradycardia. Sustained apneic spells can result in pallor, hypotonia, and unresponsiveness.

Four types of apnea have been described. *Periodic breathing* refers to a pause in breathing with or without oxygen desaturation but without a change in heart rate (Cashore, 1999). *Central apnea* refers to an interruption of breathing effort such that inspiratory muscle activity does not continue after the infant exhales. Bradycardia is associated with this event. *Obstructive apnea* refers to a lack of air flow during the inspiratory muscle activity phase that occurs secondary to a blockage in the upper pharynx. The obstruction can be a result of GER, accumulated secretions, or poor positioning of the head and neck (Cashore, 1999). *Mixed apnea* refers to episodes in which central apnea occurs either immediately before or after an obstructive event (Stark, 1997).

Incidence as well as severity of apnea tend to be inversely related to gestational age (GA) and are variable subject to lung volume. All infants born before 28 weeks of gestation have periodic breathing. Approximately 50% of infants with birth weights less than 1,500 g require treatment for prolonged respiratory pauses. By 38 weeks, most infants have outgrown their apnea, although apneic spells may persist beyond term-corrected age in some infants born before 28 weeks of gestation (Vohr et al., 1999).

Although apnea of prematurity typically results from immaturity of the respiratory control mechanisms, it also frequently occurs as a symptom of another common neonatal disorder. The following conditions can secondarily increase or aggravate the normal occurrence of apnea of prematurity: RDS, lung disease, airway obstruction, inadequate ventilation, hypoxia, premature extubation, intracranial or subarachnoid hemorrhage, hydrocephalus, perinatal asphyxia, cerebral infarct, seizures, congestive heart failure, patent ductus arteriosus (PDA), necrotizing enterocolitis (NEC), anemia, temperature fluctuation, and sepsis. Certain medications or drugs may also interfere with the respiration of infants, causing respiratory pauses. In these cases, medical attention given to correct the primary disorder usually corrects the secondary apneic disorder.

Frequent or prolonged apneic episodes affect an infant's physiologic status and may be detrimental to the infant's health and development or even life threatening. The main physiologic alterations associated with apnea are a drop in oxygen saturation followed by a sudden drop in heart rate to life-threatening levels below 100 BPM, after which the infant may require stimulation to recover. Other potential physiologic effects of apnea are as follows (Gomella, 1999):

- Decrease in arterial oxygen

- Decrease in peripheral blood flow

- Neurologic (electroencephalographic) alterations

- Increase in venous blood pressure

- Decrease in muscle tone

Heart and respiration rate (apnea) monitors are used on a regular basis with premature infants and full-term infants who are sick to detect apnea and bradycardia. The technological development of cardiorespiratory monitoring has markedly improved the survival of small and sick newborns.

The treatment of choice for the control of apnea is methylxanthine therapy, which includes aminophylline and theophylline (Gannon, 2000). Theophylline is the medicine of choice because it is thought to decrease apnea by stimulating the respiratory center and improving diaphragmatic contractility. Serum levels must be monitored to avoid theophylline toxicity and its side effects, such as tachycardia, jitteriness, irritability, feeding intolerance, vomiting, and (at very high levels) metabolic changes and seizures. Caffeine citrate is gaining popularity as an alternate choice to stimulate respiration, with fewer side effects. Caffeine serum levels must also be monitored (Stark, 1997). Mild apnea is usually closely monitored but left medically untreated. Sustained apnea may require mechanical ventilation.

Infants who have apneic spells are frequently seen by neonatal therapists—for instance, during developmental assessment and intervention or assessment of infants who are learning to nipple feed. Health professionals who work with preterm infants need to learn to identify apneic spells and what to do when an infant stops breathing. This includes reading and interpreting monitor signals, distinguishing real alarms from false alarms, and helping the infant begin breathing after a respiratory pause. The following steps are recommended for helping infants recover from an apneic spell:

- "Respond to the infant, not the monitor, checking for bradycardia, cyanosis, and airway obstruction" (Stark, 1997, p. 375).

- Allow the infant to recover spontaneously from the respiratory pause (many do).

- Apply mild tactile or vestibular stimulation if the infant does not quickly respond spontaneously; this is usually all that is needed to help the infant begin breathing again.

- Administer oxygen via nasal cannula, blow-by, or bag and mask, if required. Administration of oxygen by bag and mask should only be done by a qualified member of the medical team (i.e., a nurse, physician, or respiratory therapist).

- Administer immediate resuscitation in the presence of a serious event (indicated by pallor, cyanosis, limpness, stiffness, or unresponsiveness).

Pulmonary Air Leak Syndromes

Pulmonary air leaks result from overdistention of the air sacs, which tears the tissues and allows air to leak to adjacent areas. Infants with RDS, pneumonia, and meconium aspiration are at higher risk for air leaks because they typically require mechanical ventilation at high positive pressures. Visible signs of respiratory distress commonly seen with air leak syndromes are tachypnea, grunting, flaring, retractions, cyanosis, apnea and bradycardia, and, in some instances, asymmetric expansion of the chest (Silverman, 1997). Infants with pulmonary air leak syndromes are considered to be critically ill. Developmental intervention other than stress prevention and positioning is contraindicated in the acute stages of these diseases. Pulmonary air leak syndromes include various disorders such as pneumomediastinum, pulmonary interstitial emphysema (PIE), pneumothorax, and pneumopericardium.

Pneumomediastinum

Pneumomediastinum is a condition in which pulmonary interstitial air collects in the mediastinum. It can result from excessive pressure secondary to mechanical ventilation or from direct trauma to the airways (Silverman, 1997). Treatment consists of reducing mean airway pressures and preventing other air leaks.

Pulmonary Interstitial Emphysema

PIE is most often seen in preterm infants with RDS who require mechanical ventilation. It is the result of damage to the respiratory epithelium at the alveoli. Interstitial air interferes with pulmonary mechanics, decreasing lung compliance, and has the potential to alter lymphatic drainage and pulmonary blood flow. When the rupture extends to the pleural space, a pneumothorax can be the result (Silverman, 1997).

Pneumothorax

Pneumothorax occurs when the pleural surface ruptures and air becomes trapped in the chest cavity. The introduction of surfactant therapy has significantly reduced the incidence of pneumothorax, but pneumothorax continues to be a risk for infants treated with mechanical ventilation. Close observation may be the only treatment for infants who do not have a continuous air leak, with resolution in 24–48 hours. However, some infants may need to have air removed surgically to allow their lungs to reinflate and to prevent further lung collapse. This is accomplished by inserting one or more chest tubes into the pleural cavity or by aspirating with a needle, depending on severity. Sedation, pain medication, and induction of muscle paralysis are sometimes required.

Persistent pneumothorax can be life threatening. It may require high-frequency oscillation and, ultimately, ECMO if unresponsive to other treatments. The combined effects of hypoxia, acidosis, hypercapnia, impaired venous return, and fluctuating intracranial blood pressures that may present as consequences of pneumothorax may also result in IVH (Silverman, 1997).

Pneumopericardium

Pneumopericardium is a serious condition that occurs when peritoneal air ruptures into the pericardium—that is, the space around the heart. It occurs most often in critically ill preterm infants who are being treated with mechanical ventilation, and it can be the cause of acute changes in hemodynamics. It is the most common cause of cardiac tamponade, a condition with a mortality rate of 70%–80%; therefore, pneumopericardium is treated aggressively in symptomatic infants with continuous pericardial drainage (Silverman, 1997).

Bronchopulmonary Dysplasia

Bronchopulmonary dysplasia (BPD) is the most common name given to CLD associated with prematurity. Preterm infants who have an abnormal chest X ray and continue to require oxygen supplementation after 28 days of life are considered to have BPD. BPD can occur in preterm infants of any gestation but is most commonly seen in ELBW infants because the less mature infants are at birth, the more susceptible their lungs are to chronic lung problems. There is, however, a wide variation between perinatal centers in the incidence of BPD. Risk of BPD is reduced among infants whose mothers receive antenatal steroid treatment. Surfactant replacement therapy has also been reported to contribute to a reduction in the incidence of BPD (Parad & Berger, 1997).

BPD is the result of an initial acute lung injury caused by prolonged oxygen exposure and mechanical ventilation (Davis et al., 2002; Weingerger, Laskin, Heck, & Laskin, 2002). The inflammation and water retention within the lungs that result from the initial injury interferes with normal development of the alveoli. Poor clearing of sloughed cells and lung secretions contributes to airway obstruction, causing areas of collapse. Excessive release of growth factors results in fibrotic changes which further contribute to fluid retention and reactive airways. Poor lung compliance and inefficient exchange of oxygen and carbon dioxide result in trapping of air in the lungs (Parad & Berger, 1997).

Infants with severe BPD often require prolonged mechanical ventilation, oxygen supplementation, and close physiologic monitoring. These infants often require continued oxygen supplementation for weeks to months after discharge from the NICU and are rehospitalized at twice the rate of infants without BPD. NICU discharge instructions for infants with BPD emphasize good hand-washing practices and minimal exposure to crowds or people with symptoms of a cold or the flu to reduce the threat of contracting respiratory illnesses such as respiratory syncytial virus (RSV). For infants with BPD, such viruses can result in rehospitalization, a return to mechanical ventilation, and, in some cases, death. Therefore, the discharge plans for infants with BPD also recommend monthly injections of immunoglobulin for RSV, throughout the cold season. This immunoglobulin stimulates production of antibodies to the RSV virus, decreasing the severity of symptoms should the virus be contracted.

Neurological complications such as IVH and PVL, initially thought to be more prevalent among infants with BPD, have not been found to have a direct association with BPD. Although long-term developmental outcomes vary widely, developmental problems such as mild cognitive deficits, delays or alterations in motor coordination, and visual-perceptual motor functioning are more prevalent among infants with BPD (Hack & Fanaroff, 1989; Hack et al., 1996; Vohr et al., 2000; Volpe, 2001).

While in the NICU, infants with BPD may have periods of restlessness and irritability related to hypoxemia. Their sleep may be disrupted by their own discomfort or by frequent interventions from caregivers. Once they begin nipple feeding, they may face additional hurdles related to their increased work of breathing or the tendency toward apnea and bradycardia. The neonatal therapist in the NICU has an important role in promoting the regulation of states of arousal, preventing unnecessary stress, and enhancing nipple feeding. For infants with BPD, these intervention measures contribute to energy conservation and, subsequently, weight gain and vital lung growth. In addition, infants with BPD have limited physiologic resources to expend on social interaction. Parents and other caregivers benefit from guidance in recognizing signs of distress and of their infant's availability for social interaction. Such guidance reinforces the parental role of protecting the infant from unnecessary stress while enhancing their relationship with their infant. It also fosters the infant's development of behavioral organization. Such individualized developmentally supportive care has been associated with shorter NICU stays, decreased incidence of secondary medical complications, and improved developmental outcome of some infants with BPD (Als et al., 1986, 1994).

Perinatal Asphyxia, Hypoxemia, and Hypoxic-Ischemic Encephalopathy

Decreased concentration of oxygen in the blood is common to perinatal asphyxia, hypoxemia, and hypoxic-ischemic encephalopathy (HIE). Snyder and Cloherty defined perinatal asphyxia, or anoxia, as "an insult to the fetus or newborn due to a lack of oxygen (hypoxia) or lack of perfusion (ischemia) to various organs" (1997, p. 515). Hypercapnia, hypotension, and acidosis are primary features of hypoxemia and asphyxia. In addition, there are major effects on glucose and energy metabolism within the brain. The white matter of the neonatal brain is particularly vulnerable to the changes in glucose metabolism occurring after a hypoxic episode (Volpe, 2001). As with hypoxia, ischemia is also accompanied by changes in energy metabolism in the brain. Fortunately, compared with the adult brain, the newborn brain has fewer dendritic projections and synaptic contacts and, thus, a lower rate of utilization of cerebral energy and a lower accumulation of toxic products of injury. This is thought to contribute to the relative resistance of the newborn brain to permanent injury (Volpe, 2001).

The incidence of perinatal asphyxia is greater in high-risk pregnancies. According to Snyder and Cloherty:

> Ninety percent of asphyxial insults occur in the antepartum or intrapartum periods as a result of placental insufficiency, resulting in an inability to provide O_2 to and remove CO_2 and H+ from the fetus. The remainder are postpartum, usually secondary to pulmonary, cardiovascular, or neurologic insufficiency. During normal labor, uterine contractions and some degree of cord compression result in reduced blood flow to the placenta, and hence decreased O_2 delivery to the fetus. (1997, p. 515)

Even during a normal vaginal delivery, the newborn is exposed to some degree of hypoxia and ischemia; therefore, any additional hypoxemia that occurs is superimposed on an already stressed system. In general, as noted by Snyder and Cloherty:

Any process that (1) impairs maternal oxygenation, (2) decreases blood flow from the mother to the placenta or from the placenta to the fetus, (3) impairs gas exchange across the placenta or at the fetal tissue, or (4) increases fetal O_2 requirement will exacerbate perinatal asphyxia. (1997, p. 516)

Table 6 summarizes the major factors that may contribute to the development of perinatal asphyxia, hypoxemia, or ischemia in infants.

Hypoxic-ischemic brain injury occurs as a consequence of prolonged hypoxia and perinatal asphyxia. A sequence of events leads to ischemia and subsequent cell death (Snyder & Cloherty, 1997, p. 517, © Lippincott Williams & Wilkins):

1. Initial hypoxia impedes cerebral oxidation.
2. Lactate increases, pH drops, and phosphate compounds decrease.
3. Glucose utilization is increased.
4. Vascular dilation occurs as a regulatory response to the hypoxia.
5. Vascular dilation results in a further increase in local lactic acid production.
6. The increased acidosis results in decreased glycolysis (metabolism of sugar and water).
7. A subsequent loss of cerebrovascular autoregulation with decreased cardiac function occurs, causing a local ischemia.
8. Local glucose stores become depleted.
9. Accumulated lactic acid remains in tissues.
10. Cardiac output and cerebral blood flow further decrease.
11. Failure of energy metabolism increases, causing accumulation of ions and excitatory amino acids.
12. The osmolarity load increases, resulting in neuronal cell death.
13. Reperfusion can exacerbate cell death by releasing excessive free radicals.

Table 7 summarizes the actual stages of hypoxic-ischemic encephalopathy.

Prevention to decrease associated risk factors, early detection, and prompt resuscitation in the delivery room largely decrease the mortality and morbidity risk from prolonged neonatal hypoxia or asphyxia. Intervention consists of maintaining adequate ventilation and oxygenation, maintaining adequate cardiac output and circulation, maintaining normal temperature, preventing hypoglycemia, controlling seizures, and

Table 6.   Factors contributing to perinatal asphyxia, hypoxemia, and ischemia

Maternal	Placental/Cord	Fetal
Hypertension (chronic or preeclampsic)	Placental infarction, fibrosis or hydrops (edema)	Anemia
		Hydrops
Vascular disease	Placental abruption	Infection
Diabetes	Cord prolapse	Intrauterine growth restriction (IUGR)
Drug use	Cord entanglement; true knot	
Hypoxia[a] from pulmonary, cardiac, or neurologic disease	Cord compression	
	Abnormalities of umbilical vessels	Postmaturity
Hypotension		

Source: Snyder & Cloherty (1997).

[a]*Hypoxia* and *hypoxemia* signify different things. Hypoxia, a decrease of oxygen in inspired gases, may result in hypoxemia (among other conditions).

Table 7. Sarnat and Sarnat stages of hypoxic-ischemic encephalopathy (HIE)[a]

Stage	Stage 1 (mild)	Stage 2 (moderate)	Stage 3 (severe)
Level of consciousness	Hyperalert, irritable	Lethargic or obtunded	Stuporous, comatose
Neuromuscular control	Uninhibited, overreactive	Diminished spontaneous movement	Diminished or absent spontaneous movement
Muscle tone	Normal	Mild hypotonia	Flaccid
Posture	Mild distal flexion	Strong distal flexion	Intermittent decerebration
Stretch reflexes	Overactive	Overactive, disinhibited	Decreased or absent
Segmental myoclonus	Present or absent	Present	Absent
Complex reflexes	Normal	Suppressed	Absent
Suck	Weak	Weak or absent	Absent
Moro	Strong, low threshold	Weak, incomplete high threshold	Absent
Oculovestibular	Normal	Overactive	Weak or absent
Tonic neck	Slight	Strong	Absent
Autonomic function	Generalized sympathetic	Generalized parasympathetic	Both systems depressed
Pupils	Mydriasis	Miosis	Midposition, often unequal; poor light reflex
Respirations	Spontaneous	Spontaneous; occasional apnea	Periodic; apnea
Heart rate	Tachycardia	Bradycardia	Variable
Bronchial and salivary secretions	Sparse	Profuse	Variable
Gastrointestinal motility	Normal or decreased	Increased diarrhea	Variable
Seizures	None	Common focal or multifocal (6 to 24 hours of age)	Uncommon (excluding decerebration)
Electroencephalographic findings	Normal (awake)	*Early:* generalized low-voltage, slowing (continuous delta and theta)	*Early:* Periodic pattern with isopotential phases
		Later: periodic pattern (awake); seizures focal or multifocal; 1.0 to 1.5 Hz spike and wave	*Later:* totally isopotential
Duration of symptoms	< 24 hours	2 to 14 days	Hours to weeks
Outcome	About 100% normal	80% normal; abnormal if symptoms more than 5 to 7 days	About 50% die; remainder with severe sequelae

From "Neonatal Encephalopathy Following Fetal Distress: A Clinical and Electroencephalographic Study," by H.B. Sarnat and M.S. Sarnat, 1976, *Archives of Neurology, 33*(10), 696. Copyright © 1976 by American Medical Association. Reprinted with permission.
[a]The stages in this table are a continuum reflecting the spectrum of clinical stages of infants over 36 weeks' gestational age.

controlling brain swelling. Neurologic involvement in the form of ischemic brain lesions is common in severely asphyxiated infants. Ischemic brain lesions in full-term infants occur in the border zones between the end fields of the major cerebral arteries because these areas are the most vulnerable to a drop in cerebral perfusion. The areas most involved include the parasaggital cortex, the hippocampus, the striatum, the dentate gyrus, the amygdala, and the thalamus. The two most common sites for ischemic injury, or periventricular leukomalacia in preterm infants, are the corners of the lateral ventricles and the white matter around the foramen of Monro (Volpe, 2001). Animal studies have provided a possible explanation for the unique vulnerability of a preterm infant's brain to periventricular white matter injury. Three factors that potentially contribute to white matter lesions have been identified in the preterm infant's brain: 1) hemodynamics (i.e., limited capacity for vasodilation), 2) metabolism (i.e., poorly regulated glycolysis), and 3) specific vulnerability of oligodendroglia that are in the process of early differentiation and myelination (Volpe, 2001).

Just as the sites of ischemic injury differ between term and preterm infants, so do the neurologic sequelae. In full-term infants with parasagittal injury, there is proximal limb weakness during the neonatal period, more so in the upper than in the lower extremities, with spastic quadriparesis and intellectual impairment being the possible long-term sequelae. In preterm infants with periventricular leukomalacia, ischemia is likely to affect fibers that descend from the motor cortex past the periventricular region and into the internal capsule, controlling movement of the lower extremities. Lower limb weakness may be seen during the neonatal period, with spastic diplegia or quadriplegia and cognitive impairments occurring as possible long-term sequelae (Han, Bang, Lim, Yoon, & Kim, 2002; Volpe, 2001).

Among infants with hypoxic ischemic encephalopathy, 10%–30% develop seizure disorders related to the cortical injury. Cognitive sequelae are more difficult to predict, although they are usually related to the extent of the injury. Severely affected infants may have impaired cortical visual function with cerebral cortical atrophy noted on a computed tomography (CT) scan. During the first 2 years of life, 50% of these infants show some improvement in functional vision, possibly due to plasticity of the developing brain. Hearing impairment is less common (Volpe, 2001).

Infants recovering from episodes of asphyxia are initially quite hypotonic, may be comatose, usually require mechanical ventilation for varying periods of time, and generally tend to be extremely sick and fragile. Further physiologic stress and trauma must be avoided during the healing period. Developmental personnel need to assist family members, nursing staff, and medical personnel in adhering to strict stress modulation guidelines by designing environmental arrangements for the infant that decrease the level of aversive stimulation. Assessment of neurodevelopmental status should be ongoing throughout the recovery period, with a particular focus on regulation of states of arousal; visual, auditory, motor, and reflex responses; and oral-motor responsiveness. This information provides the medical team and the family with a consistent source of information with which to plan for intervention and discharge. Periodic follow-up evaluations after discharge from the NICU are essential to monitor developmental progress. Most infants require early intervention program services.

Cardiovascular/Cardiopulmonary Disorders

The incidence of structural heart disease in the first year of life is 4 per 1,000 live births. It is increasingly common for congenital cardiac defects to be diagnosed in utero through fetal echocardiography; however, most conditions are still diagnosed during the neonatal period. Although there are many types of heart disease, most present with one or more of the following signs and symptoms: cyanosis, congestive heart failure, heart murmur (with or without symptoms), and arrythmia (Wechsler & Wernovsky, 1997). Therefore, differential diagnosis is very complex, requiring a range of assessments including auscultation (stethoscope), transcutaneous oxygen monitoring, arterial blood gas measurement, and electrocardiography (EKG), echocardiography, and cardiac catheterization. Some of the most common cardiac disorders involve malformation or incomplete development of the heart and great vessels. Advances in ultrasound technology have made it possible to detect many structural anomalies through echocardiography; therefore, this noninvasive procedure is used extensively in fetal assessment and in the NICU to detect and monitor cardiac conditions.

Patent Ductus Arteriosus

PDA is uncommon among term infants but common in preterm infants. It occurs when the fetal ductus arteriosus fails to close shortly after birth, and its incidence in preterm infants is proportional to the degree of prematurity and low birth weight. The fetal ductus arteriosus connects the pulmonary artery to the aorta in the fetus to bypass pulmonary circulation. When the duct fails to close spontaneously at birth, much of the blood from the left side of the heart passes to the right side, resulting in hypotension and poor perfusion and potentially causing cardiovascular overload. Closure of the ductus is believed to be stimulated by increased oxygen concentration when the infant begins to breathe, as well as by metabolic factors (Gomella, 1999). The main diagnostic criterion is a characteristic murmur confirmed by echocardiogram (Heyman, Teitel, & Liebman, 1993). Respiratory difficulties are common in the more severe PDAs. PDAs that do not resolve spontaneously within a few days are treated with indomethacin or surgical ligation. Fluid intake is restricted to prevent congestive heart failure.

Atrial and Ventricular Septal Defects

Atrial septal defects (ASDs) and ventricular septal defects (VSDs) involve the septum that divides the right and left atria (ASDs) or the ventricles (VSDs). They are a common cause of congestive heart failure in neonates. ASDs are most common among infants with Down syndrome (70% of ASDs are seen in infants with Down syndrome) (Wechsler & Wernovsky, 1997). ASDs present with more symptoms than VSDs and are a cause for greater clinical concern. Early surgical closure is usually recommended for an ASD, whereas a VSD may close spontaneously over time and is usually treated with medication when necessary. Commonly prescribed medications for these conditions are digoxin and diuretics.

Tetralogy of Fallot

Tetralogy of Fallot is a combination of four specific congenital heart defects: a ventricular septal defect, an obstruction in the ouflow from the right ventricle, overriding of the aorta over the ventricular septum, and hypertrophy of the right ventricle. The severity of the obstruction dictates the symptoms, and the timing of surgical repair depends on when the infant becomes symptomatic.

Persistent Pulmonary Hypertension of the Newborn

Persistent pulmonary hypertension of the newborn (PPHN) is a potentially life-threatening disorder. It consists of an increase in vascular tension in the lungs that causes a right-to-left shunt through the ductus arteriosus and foramen ovale, often resulting in severe hypoxemia. PPHN is most common in term or postterm infants and is related to such maternal conditions as fever, diabetes, urinary tract infection, and the use of nonsteroidal anti-inflammatory drugs during the pregnancy. It is also associated with a number of neonatal conditions, including meconium aspiration syndrome, perinatal asphyxia, pneumonia, and sepsis (Van Marter, 1997). Emergency treatment is needed to interrupt the rapid progression of this disease. Respiratory management involves the initial administration of 100% oxygen, intubation, and mechanical (usually high-frequency oscillatory) ventilation, including the use of a narcotic analgesic for sedation. Correction of metabolic acidosis and management of cardiac output with pharmacologic agents are additional concerns. Inhaled nitric oxide has been added as a treatment option. For infants who do not respond to conventional management, ECMO is recommended (Van Marter, 1997).

The neonatal therapist in the NICU should be aware of cardiac conditions, as they may affect the infant's ability to engage in feeding and other activities and can contribute to cardiorespiratory distress, poor weight gain, and failure to thrive. Neonatal intervention with families of infants with cardiac conditions emphasizes careful assessment of the infant's response to various activities and recommendations for optimizing participation while conserving energy.

Central Nervous System Disorders

Intraventricular Hemorrhage

Preterm infants born before 32 weeks of gestation are most at risk for IVH. Studies in the 1980s reported a 40% incidence of IVH among infants weighing less than 1,500 g. However, rates of 12%–30% were later reported. This shift is perhaps a result of advances in preventive treatment, including the administration of antenatal steroids and of prophylactic indomethacin during the first week after birth, when the risk of occurrence is highest.

An IVH occurs in the germinal matrix tissues of the brain and may or may not extend into the ventricles and parenchyma (Figure 12). Bleeds are classified according to severity (Papile, Burstein, Burstein, & Koffler, 1978), as follows:

- Grade I: Subependymal hemorrhage, germinal matrix hemorrhage
- Grade II: Intraventricular bleeding without ventricular dilatation
- Grade III: Intraventricular bleeding with ventricular dilatation
- Grade IV: Intraventricular and intraparenchymal bleeding

Symptoms depend on severity and extent of the bleeding and may include bulging fontanelle, sudden anemia, apnea, bradycardia, acidosis, seizures, high blood pressure, hydrocephalus, and alterations in muscle tone and consciousness level. Neurologic and developmental outcomes are also related to severity of IVH, ranging from recuperation with no sequelae among infants with Grade I and II bleeds to significant neurologic injury and subsequent motor, cognitive, and language dysfunction following

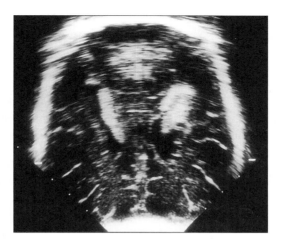

Figure 12. Ultrasound photo of the brain of a premature infant with Grade III intraventricular hemorrhage showing bilateral dilatation of the lateral ventricles.

ventricular dilatation, particularly when shunt placement is required. Clinical findings are variable and may resolve within 4 weeks in 50% of infants with ventricular dilatation. However, increasing fontanelle size, increasing ventricular size, irritability, apnea, and poor feeding are all signs of increasing intracranial pressure which, if persistent, may lead to surgical placement of a ventriculoperitoneal shunt (Vohr et al., 1999).

Periventricular Leukomalacia

PVL, an injury of the periventricular white matter, is manifested as cystic lesions at the corners of the lateral ventricles. These lesions are more commonly seen in the frontal and parietal regions on cranial ultrasound or CT scans. PVL is thought to occur secondary to changes in cerebral blood flow after IVH; however, hypotension, infections, apnea, and ischemic events are also considered risk factors for PVL. PVL occurs most often in the sickest, smallest infants. Although neurological sequelae— including vision and hearing impairments, intellectual impairments, and other developmental abnormalities may occur with PVL (Rezaie & Dean, 2002)—the most frequent clinical correlate of PVL is spastic diplegia (Vohr et al., 1999; Volpe, 2001). The extent of the cystic lesions has been shown to be correlated with the type and severity of cerebral palsy (Han et al., 2002).

Infants with IVH and/or PVL require careful developmental monitoring while in the NICU and after discharge, particularly if a shunt has been placed. These infants may begin to show atypical postures and movement while still in the nursery or may have difficulty regulating states of arousal. Positioning recommendations may be needed to avoid pressure directly on the shunt and to provide a variety of positions for comfort and normal postural development. Parents of infants with IVH and/or PVL may have additional fears about their infant's future development and usually benefit from repeated developmental assessments during the NICU stay to reinforce their infant's strengths and identify areas for developmental intervention. Because PVL is associated with long-term sequelae and the short-term sequelae may not appear until after discharge from the NICU, infants with IVH and/or PVL require careful neonatal follow-up, long-term monitoring, and early developmental intervention.

Neonatal Seizures

The neonatal therapist in the NICU should be familiar with the various manifestations of seizures, as he or she may be the first person to observe these behaviors in an infant being evaluated or treated for an associated problem. Seizures are among the most obvious and most frequently occurring signs of neurological disease in the newborn. They demand immediate attention because they are often associated with serious illness, can impede respiration and feeding, and may contribute to brain injury (Volpe, 2001). Because of the immaturity of the neonatal brain, seizures are manifested differently in newborns than in children and adults, complicating early detection. In neonates, seizures may appear in many forms (Kuban & Filiano, 1997, pp. 493–494):

- Repetitive lip smacking, chewing, sucking, or eye blinking or fluttering of the eyelids
- Abnormalities of gaze
- Generalized clonic movements (compared with the more organized focal seizures of children and adults), slow repetitive jerking (e.g., two to three per second), or posturing of the limbs
- Complex movements such as "swimming" or "bicycling"
- Rhythmic alterations in vital signs
- Apneic episodes of otherwise unknown etiology

An electroencephalogram (EEG) is usually given when seizures are suspected, although neonatal EEGs are difficult to interpret because of the immaturity of the newborn brain and increased possibility for irregularities in the tracings. Seizures may be seen in infants who have had an intracranial hemorrhage or IVH, hydrocephalus, or hypoxic ischemia, as well as in infants experiencing drug withdrawal or metabolic derangements. A variety of anticonvulsant medications can be administered, the most common ones being diazepam (Valium), lorazepam (Ativan), phenobarbital (Luminal), and phenytoin (Dilantin).

OTHER NEONATAL DISORDERS

Hyperbilirubinemia

Physiologic jaundice of infancy, or hyperbilirubinemia, does not usually require admission to the NICU; however, moderate levels of hyperbilirubinemia may require treatment to prevent increasing severity and associated neurologic sequelae. Sequelae may include transient depression of brainstem function or even permanent neurologic injury. Phototherapy treatment is used to lower the serum bilirubin levels. More severe cases require exchange transfusion. Infants usually recover quickly with no apparent long-term effects (Vohr et al., 1999). Hyperbilirubinemia is an important consideration during assessment of development and feeding, as this condition tends to decrease levels of arousal and activity. When an infant is receiving phototherapy, the neonatal therapist will need to remove the infant from under the lights briefly to assess visual responsiveness. The neonatal therapist should minimize the time that the infant is kept away from the lights and be certain to replace eye protection when returning the infant to phototherapy.

Congenital Anomalies and Genetic Disorders

Advances in prenatal testing via ultrasonography and biochemical and chromosomal analyses have made it possible to identify (prenatally, in some cases) a number of chromosome abnormalities, including trisomies 13, 18, and 21 and neural tube and other congenital defects such as cardiac, pulmonary and kidney malformations, diaphragmatic hernia, Pierre Robin sequence (a clustering of related anomalies), and cleft lip and palate. Early identification prepares the family and the obstetrical and neonatology teams for complications that may present at delivery or immediately thereafter and, in some cases, allows prenatal treatment (e.g., in the case of prenatal closure of a meningomyelocele). Neonatal therapists are frequently requested to assist in evaluating infants with congenital anomalies, particularly when they are related to the infant's functional performance—for example, oral/facial anomalies that interfere with breathing and feeding or defects that may restrict the options available for positioning and handling an infant. This can be one of the most rewarding areas of practice for the neonatal therapist in the NICU, as many problems presented by these conditions have practical solutions that can be implemented through teamwork with other professionals and the infant's family.

Metabolic Disorders

A number of rare metabolic disorders can be life threatening in the neonatal period or may result in severe developmental sequelae if left undiscovered and untreated. The American Academy of Pediatrics recommends universal screening for hypothyroidism and phenylketonuria (PKU). Some states also screen for other conditions such as maple syrup urine disease and congenital adrenal hypoplasia. Neonatal therapists encounter a few infants with metabolic disorders each year. They should be prepared to provide family-centered developmental and behavioral assessment and intervention as needed to address regulation of states of arousal, atypical posture and muscle tone, and feeding issues that may arise.

Necrotizing Enterocolitis

Necrotizing enterocolitis (NEC) is a serious disease of unknown etiology in which the immature intestine is affected, resulting in an acute intestinal necrosis. Premature infants, particularly those with extremely low birth weight, are at highest risk for the disease, although approximately 10% of infants with NEC are full term. The number of cases reported varies from year to year and from one perinatal center to another (Lee et al., 2000). Cocaine exposure, known to double the risk of NEC because of vasoconstriction, is the only maternal or fetal risk factor other than early gestation shown to have a strong association with NEC. Infants may present with respiratory distress, apnea and/or bradycardia, temperature instability, and decreased peripheral perfusion. Abdominal signs include distention, tenderness, gastric aspirates (residual amounts of the previous feeding), vomiting of bile and/or blood, and bloody stools. As NEC progresses, the infant may develop an intestinal hemorrhage; gangrene;

submucosal gas; and, in severe cases, perforation of the intestines, sepsis, and shock. The average age at onset is 12 days (McAlmon, 1997). Intestinal pneumatosis is confirmed through radiographic studies.

Kliegman, Walker, and Yolken (1994) defined three stages of NEC:

- Stage I (NEC scare or suspected NEC): The infant has mild gastrointestinal problems with nonspecific signs (increased volume of gastric aspirate, abdominal distention, feeding intolerance, apneas and bradycardias, labile temperature).

- Stage II (documented NEC): The infant may be mildly or moderately ill, and there is radiographic evidence of the disease (pneumatosis intestinalis).

- Stage III (severe NEC): The infant has unstable vital signs and signs of respiratory failure. Infants in Stage III often require mechanical ventilation. Intestinal perforation is present or likely at this stage. The infant is very sick and may die.

Surgical intervention is indicated when perforation of the intestines has occurred. Infants in the severe stage of NEC (Stage III) are too sick to receive developmental intervention. During their recovery, however, as these infants begin to tolerate feedings, neonatal therapists may reinitiate nonnutritive sucking and other types of oral stimulation as needed to counteract hypersensitivities that may have developed and to prepare for eventual nipple feeding. Helping to make feeding experiences as pleasurable as possible for the infants is an important goal when working with their families and other caregivers. Once nipple feeding is restarted, these infants usually require prolonged feeding intervention to make incremental progress.

Gastroesophageal Reflux

GER is defined as gastric acid rising to the lower third of the esophagus. GER is thought to be related to weakness of the lower esophageal sphincter. Although all babies have some degree of reflux, this condition is a concern when it interferes with feeding or causes obstructive apneic and bradycardic events during or after feeding. Signs and symptoms include excessive spitting up or vomiting, irritability 1–3 hours after feeding (or after the first half of the feeding has been taken), and breathholding/apnea with or without bradycardia. The discomfort associated with these symptoms can contribute to feeding aversion and, eventually, to failure to thrive. Infants being treated with xanthines such as theophylline are at higher risk for reflux (Cashore, 1999). Treatment may begin with reflux precautions such as positioning the infant semi-upright during feeding and keeping the infant semi-upright for 15–30 minutes after feeding (e.g., holding the infant at one's shoulder or raising the head of the bed approximately 30 degrees to allow gravity to assist in keeping feedings down). Prone positioning is also recommended for LBW infants because reflux has been demonstrated to occur less frequently in prone-lying than in side-lying. Additional measures include giving frequent feedings of smaller volume, thickening the feeding with infant cereal (a half teaspoon of cereal per ounce of formula is often recommended), and administering medication (ranitidine [Zantac] or metoclopramide [Reglan]) to relieve the esophagitis that often accompanies and can exacerbate the reflux. Antireflux medication increases motility and gastroesophageal sphincter tone but has side effects that should be considered. Metoclopramide is associated with extrapyramidal symptoms such as dystonia (Laneau et al., 1998; Sun et al., 1997). Cisapride (Propulsid) was formerly used to treat reflux, but its use has been discouraged because the drug can be deadly (Ward, Lemons, & Molteni, 1999).

GER usually resolves with maturation by 3 months corrected age because the tone of the lower esophageal sphincter improves, reducing the severity of reflux and diminishing symptoms. Until GER resolves, however, it may be a source of great discomfort for the infant and of concern to the family and physician who are trying to ensure proper nutritional intake. Neonatal therapists in NICUs and early interventionists in follow-up programs must be aware that GER can contribute to infants' feeding problems. When GER is thought to be interfering with an infant's feeding, the neonatal therapist should know the various interventions to reduce symptoms and discomfort. In addition, the neonatal therapist should always work closely with the NICU medical team, the pediatrician, and the family to identify the most appropriate medical and behavioral interventions for the infant and his or her family.

Retinopathy of Prematurity

Retinopathy of prematurity (ROP) is an eye disease that occurs in some premature infants. It is caused by an alteration in the normal development of retinal blood vessels that occurs in two stages. In the primary stage, an event such as hypoxia, hyperoxia, or hypotension causes vasoconstriction and reduced circulation to the developing retina. In the secondary stage, the ischemic retina releases growth factors that stimulate new blood vessels to grow through the retina into the vitreous. These atypical "fibrovascular" vessels are prone to hemorrhage and edema. When there is extensive growth of these vessels, they form a ring of scar tissue that pulls on the retina, potentially detaching it from its insertion (see Figures 13 and 14).

The disease process usually reaches its peak 34–40 weeks GA. Because uncorrected retinal detachment leads to blindness, early and regular retinal examinations by ophthalmology specialists are essential to track the progression of ROP and to recommend surgical intervention when necessary (Cryotherapy for Retinopathy of Prematurity Cooperative Group, 2001). Most hospitals in the United States conduct routine ophthalmoscopic examinations and follow-up exams every 2–3 weeks for infants less than 35 weeks of gestation who have received oxygen therapy, as well as for all infants less than 30 weeks of gestation (see Figure 15). Infants who are discharged from the

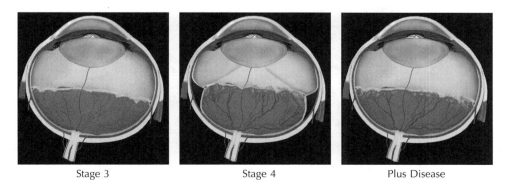

| Stage 3 | Stage 4 | Plus Disease |

Figure 13. The left image illustrates Stage 3 retinopathy of prematurity, which is characterized by abnormal vascular growth extending into the vitreous humor. Continuation of this abnormal growth may result in traction on the retina, with various degrees of retinal detachment. This is described as Stages 4A (partial detachment, not involving the macula), which is shown in the center image, and 4B (detachment involving the macula), which is not depicted in the figure. The right image shows the dilated, tortuous vasculature characteristic of Plus Disease. (Images from The Association of Retinopathy of Prematurity and Related Diseases [ROPARD]. *What is retinopathy of prematurity?* Retrieved August 5, 2003, from http://www.ropard.org/what_is.shtml; reprinted by permission.)

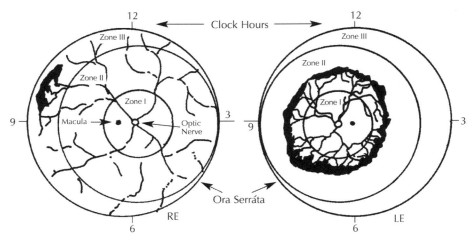

Figure 14. Schematic classification of retinopathy of prematurity. (From Phelps, D.L. [1992]. Retinopathy of prematurity. In A.A. Fanaroff & R.J. Martin [Eds.], *Neonatal-perinatal medicine: Diseases of the fetus and infant: Vol. 2* [5th ed., p. 1393]. St. Louis, MO: Mosby-Year Book; reprinted by permission.)

NICU prior to or during the peak age of ROP's progression should continue to be followed by ophthalmology specialists until their retinal vessels have fully matured.

The location and stage of ROP is reported by the ophthalmologist according to the International Classification of ROP. This classification can be summarized in terms of location, stage, and extent (Anderson & Stewart, 1997). *Location* describes the distance that the abnormally developing retinal blood vessels have travelled. The

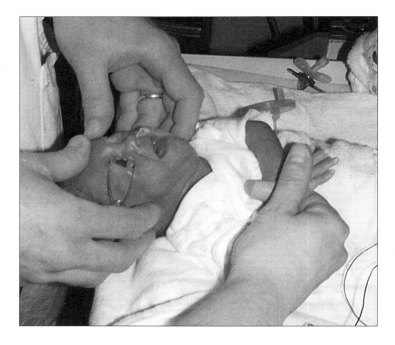

Figure 15. This premature infant is undergoing an eye examination to rule out retinopathy of prematurity.

retina is divided into three concentric circles, forming "zones," with Zone 1 surrounding the optic nerve and extending out toward the macula, Zone 2 extending toward the nasal and temporal sides, and Zone 3 extending further to the temporal sides (see Figure 14).

Stage refers to the severity of the disease. At Stage 1, a thin demarcation line appears, separating the normal retina from the undeveloped avascular areas of the retina. During Stage 2, the demarcation develops into a thick, high ridge that protrudes into the vitreous humor. At Stage 3, extraretinal fibrovascular proliferation (development of abnormal blood vessels) occurs along the edge of the ridge, extending into the vitreous humor. During Stage 4, fibrosis and scarring occurs with traction on the retina, resulting in partial retinal detachment. Stage 4 is subdivided into Stages 4A and 4B. In Stage 4A, the partial detachment does not involve the macula, and the chance for vision is good if the retina is reattached. Stage 4B is partial detachment involving the macula, and the likelihood of usable vision in the affected eye is decreased. Stage 5 is complete retinal detachment. Furthermore, *plus disease* describes the presence of vessels that have become dilated and tortuous. According to Anderson and Stewart, it is a severe form of ROP involving "iris vascular engorgement, pupillary rigidity, and vitreous haze. Plus disease that is associated with zone 1 ROP is termed *rush disease*; this type of ROP tends to progress extremely rapidly" (1997, p. 644).

Extent of the disease refers to its location. This is reported as clock hours around the circumference of the zones (see Figure 14). The additional terms *prethreshold* and *threshold* ROP refer to the preceding summary of designations (e.g., Zone 2 ROP with Stage 2 and Plus Disease). Infants with prethreshold ROP do not necessarily need surgical treatment but are monitored carefully. One in three infants with prethreshold ROP will require treatment. Anderson and Stewart noted that threshold ROP is "the level of severity at which the risk of blindness is predicted to approach 50% and thus treatment is recommended" (1997, p. 644).

Causes and Treatments

ROP is found exclusively in premature infants. It is more prevalent in preterm infants of low gestational age and low birth weight who have been exposed to high concentrations of oxygen (Askie & Henderson-Smart, 2001); however, new theories suggest that other factors may also lead to the development of ROP. Factors investigated for possible association with ROP include hypoxia or anoxia, hypocapnia, acidosis, IVH, fluctuation in blood gas tensions, sepsis, RDS, dexamethasone exposure, PDA, vitamin E deficiency, and precocious exposure to light. The term *retrolental fibroplasia* was once used when ROP was not diagnosed until extensive fibrosis and scarring had occurred, ultimately leading to blindness. This term is no longer used in the United States, as most ROPs are identified before severe fibrosis occurs.

Laser therapy is the treatment of choice to arrest the process of retinal detachment in premature infants. The purpose of laser therapy is to prevent retinal detachment by eliminating the abnormal blood vessels and preventing the build up of scar tissue. Scleral buckle and vitrectomy may be indicated in severe cases (Lee, 1999).

Neonatal therapists working in the NICU are in a unique position to evaluate functional visual performance of preterm infants who are at risk of developing ROP prior to and during its progression. The initial signs of ROP cannot be easily distinguished from a functional vision standpoint. As the disease progresses, there may be a rapid decline in an infant's responsiveness to visual stimuli. Expanding opportunities for visual experience appropriate to the infant's gestational age is always a part of neonatal therapy intervention in the NICU. Using appropriate stimuli, such as emphasizing presentation of the human face and encouraging visual exploration of the immediate surroundings, and avoiding excessive or overpowering stimuli are important guidelines when working with any preterm infant and may be helpful early interventions for ROP. In addition, helping parents become attuned to the infant's style of responding to visual stimuli will enhance the enjoyment of playful interactions and optimize visual responsiveness throughout the changes that may occur with the progression of ROP.

Nosocomial Infections

Nosocomial infections are hospital-acquired infections. They are quite common in premature and sick infants. ELBW infants are particularly susceptible to infection; therefore, preventive measures reduce but do not entirely eliminate the incidence of nosocomial infections. If the infection progresses to sepsis, an infant's survival may be at risk. Developmental services may be indicated during the active course of the infection depending on its severity. Developmental personnel must adhere to strict infection-control procedures in working with infants with an active infection.

CONCLUSION

This chapter has provided a limited overview of the most prevalent disorders and conditions presented by NICU infants. The conditions that neonatal therapists may encounter are as numerous as the variety of ways by which the conditions may be managed. Health professionals seeking to gain competence for providing therapy services to newborns must consult neonatology textbooks and many of the readings discussed in this chapter prior to initiating their practice in the NICU.

7

Embryonic Development and Neonatal Classification

OVERVIEW

This chapter begins with a review of the development of the infant from the preembryonic to the fetal stages. Emphasis is given to the embryonic periods during which the development of the various body systems occurs. The developmental anomalies that may result when the formation of the different body structures is altered or interrupted are discussed. Reference is made to the possibility that a major structural anomaly may terminate in abortion. The various types of abortion are identified.

This chapter also describes the different parameters used to classify newborns and the categories under which infants are grouped within each parameter. Classification systems described include gestational age (GA; age in weeks from last menstrual period), postconceptional age (PCA; age in weeks from fertilization), birth weight, weight-by-age relationship, and multiple births. The categories that present increased developmental risk for the infants are discussed. The risk associated with premature birth and delayed intrauterine growth is described in greater detail. The way in which the various classifications are used and the implications for the developmental management of infants in the NICU are described.

OBJECTIVES

- Identify the major stages of intrauterine development of infants: preembryonic (germinal), embryonic, and fetal

- Explain why the fourth through the eighth weeks (i.e., embryonic period) are the most critical for the structural formation of the embryo, and describe common congenital anomalies associated with malformations during the embryonic period

- Recall the most common types of abortion: spontaneous, missed, induced, and reduction

- Explain the importance of GA assessment for determining readiness for delivery and estimating neonatal risk, and identify the most common methods for calculating GA

- Explain why birth weight is one of the most important predictors of neonatal health and survival

- Explain the interrelation between weight and GA and its developmental relevance for infants
- Explain how the various newborn classification systems are used in the NICU for describing newborns and estimating developmental risk
- Identify the major risk factors associated with multiple gestations

EMBRYONIC AND FETAL DEVELOPMENT: NICU IMPLICATIONS

Prematurity, the most common condition encountered in the NICU, is an interruption in the process of intrauterine growth and development that requires the fetus to physiologically and behaviorally adapt to the extrauterine environment. The NICU therapist must be familiar with the physical and neurobehavioral characteristics of the fetus at each GA as a basis for developmental and behavioral evaluation of preterm infants. Many full-term infants who are treated in the NICU have conditions that can be attributed to a disruption or derangement in normal preembryonic, embryonic, or fetal development. Some of these conditions are responsive to therapeutic and surgical interventions, such as cleft lip and palate. Other conditions such as spina bifida, congenital heart defects, and chromosomal abnormalities may have profound implications for an infant's future growth and development. A basic knowledge of embryology and fetal development allows the therapist working in the NICU to relate these conditions to their origins (preembryonic, embryonic, or fetal) and to recognize the complex series of events in utero that may have contributed to their presentation in the NICU infant. Familiarity with the stages particularly sensitive to disruptive influences that may cause structural alterations provides a context for understanding specific conditions frequently encountered in the NICU. Although there is strong consensus about the existence of critical periods for the anatomical development of the embryo and fetus, the debate about the existence of such periods for the development of functional skills is ongoing. The presence of critical periods in the infant has also been a matter of controversy (Horton, 2001). Readers interested in a detailed presentation of the major arguments and positions on this subject are referred to Bailey, Bruer, Symons, and Lichtman (2001).

Stages of Development

During the preembryonic and embryonic stages of development, specific changes occur literally on a daily basis (Figure 16). Preembryonic development begins shortly after fertilization and lasts 2 weeks. During that time, the fertilized egg, or zygote, becomes an embryo, the multicellular organism from which all of the body systems and structures will emerge. The embryonic period begins with the formation of the embryo and lasts until the end of the eighth week after fertilization.

The changes that occur during the preembryonic and embryonic periods are often grouped for descriptive purposes into 23 stages (Carnegie Stages) (O'Rahilly & Muller, 1987). These 23 stages begin with fertilization of the egg released from the ovarian follicle and continue through the formation of the zygote, the embryo, and, ultimately, the fetus. Each numbered stage represents a significant change in the developing human. For example, Stage 8 designates the formation of the neural plate, the precursor to the nervous system. The primordial heart bulge begins to pump

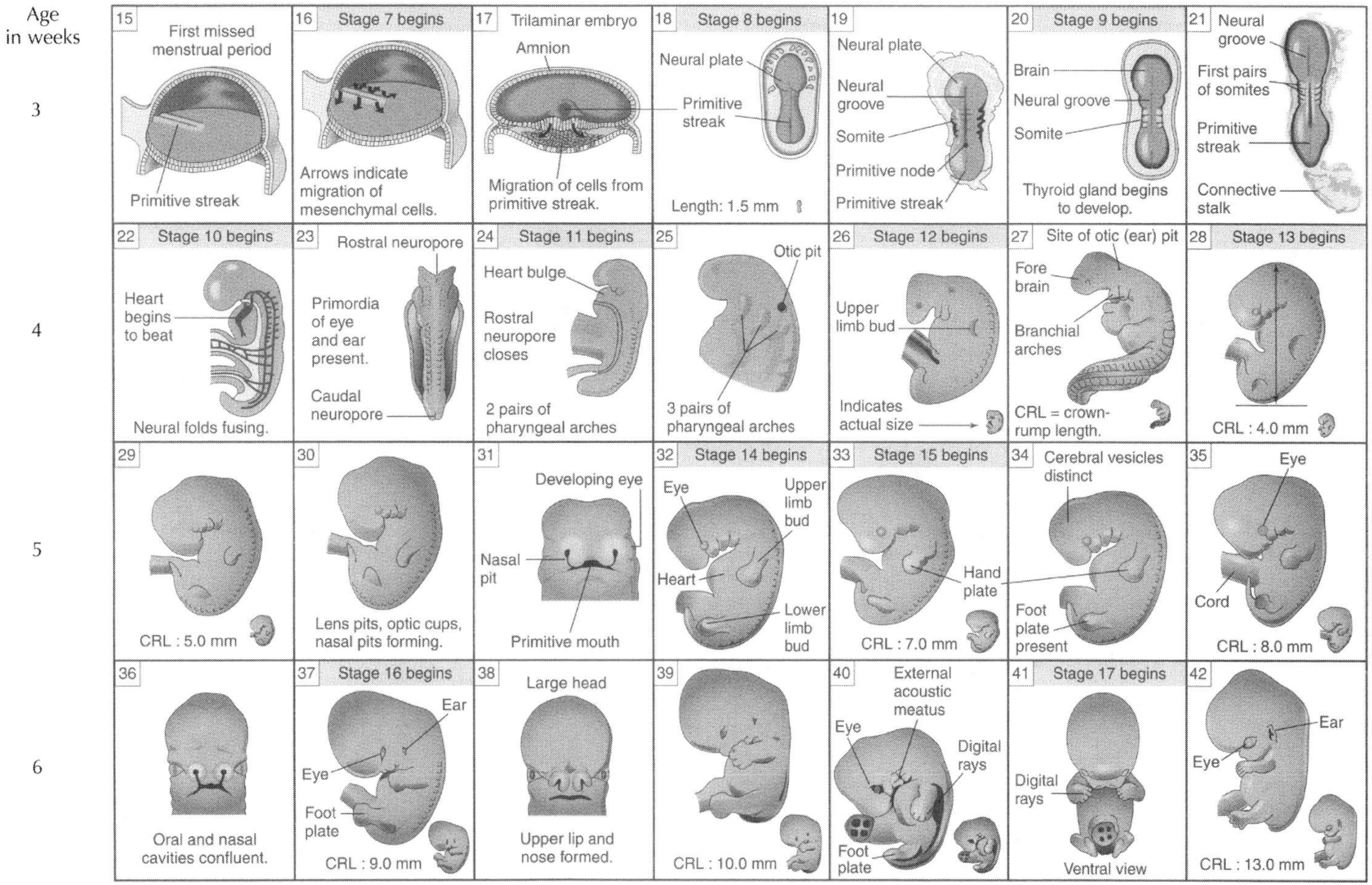

Figure 16. Developmental progression of the embryo from day 15 to day 42 after last menstrual period, showing the Carnegie Stages of development. From Moore, K.L., & Persaud, T.V.N. [1998]. *The developing human: Clinically oriented embryology* [pp. 545–546]. Philadelphia: W.B. Saunders; reprinted by permission.)

(continued)

Figure 16. *(continued)*

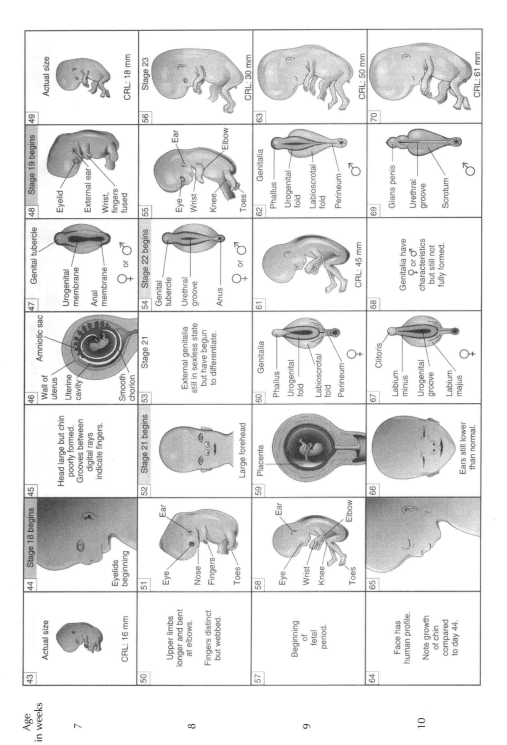

blood between Stages 11 and 12, during the third week after fertilization. Upper limb buds emerge during Stage 13. The embryonic phase of development is complete by Stage 23, the last stage, on day 56 after conception. From that day until birth, the developing human is described as a fetus.

The embryo undergoes rapid development between the fourth and eighth weeks after fertilization. During this period, all of the organs and body cavities are formed, albeit rudimentarily, and many body systems become functional. An 8-week fetus clearly has human characteristics, including facial features, a complete vertebral column, jointed extremities, fingers, and toes. By the eighth week, many important neural structures such as the forebrain, midbrain, hindbrain, cerebellum, and spinal cord can be distinguished, and the presence of all major organs can be ascertained (e.g., heart, liver, kidneys, intestines). These 4 weeks are considered to represent the most critical period of intrauterine development because a number of major congenital anomalies can be traced to them (Moore & Persaud, 1998). The following section describes the origins of some congenital anomalies that are prevalent among NICU infants.

Digestive System Anomalies

The digestive organs and many related structures emerge from specific portions of the primordial gut. The pharynx, trachea and esophagus, stomach, proximal intestine, liver, and pancreas are outgrowths of the foregut. Incomplete partitioning of these structures during development may lead to stenoses (constriction or narrowing), atresias (absence of a normal opening or cavity), and fistulas (abnormal connection or passage). The midgut is the point of origin for the lower intestines and colon; the hindgut is the point of origin for the rectum, anus, and urogenital structures. In early development, the liver and kidneys are relatively large, leaving insufficient room for growth of the intestines. Around the sixth week, the intestines begin the process of physiologic umbilical herniation, in which the contents of the midgut move into the umbilical cord to make room for organ development and to rotate around the axis of the superior mesenteric artery. By the tenth week, around the beginning of the fetal period, the abdominal cavity has enlarged sufficiently for the midgut loop to return to the abdomen and to begin to further rotate into its final position in the abdomen (Moore & Persaud, 1998). A number of congenital anomalies of the digestive system are related to this process, including abdominal wall defects such as gastroschisis (opening of the abdominal wall lateral to the umbilicus with organs protruding outside the abdominal wall) and omphalocele (incomplete closure at the base of the umbilical cord with organs protruding into the cord). Other anomalies include diaphragmatic hernia (abnormal opening in the diaphragm with abdominal organs protruding into the chest cavity) and malrotation of the intestines.

Nervous System Anomalies

During the third week, the neural plate begins to form. This structure infolds a week later to form the neural groove, with neural folds forming on either side. These folds then fuse to form the neural tube. Related cells that are not included in this fusion remain outside the neural tube to become the neural crest. The central nervous system develops from three primary areas of the neural tube: forebrain, midbrain, and hindbrain. Although the midbrain undergoes little change during embryonic development, divisions of the forebrain and hindbrain occur during the fifth week.

These divisions provide the basis for the development of the central nervous system. The peripheral nervous system emerges predominantly from the neural crest.

Some of the most common anomalies of nervous system development are neural tube defects (NTDs), such as myelomeningocele, which occur when the neural tube fails to close completely (Liptak, 2002). Other congenital nervous system anomalies occurring during the embryonic period may stem from outside influences such as exposure to teratogens (substances or agents that cause structural abnormalities in the fetus), infection, trauma, or malnutrition or from inborn errors of metabolism (e.g., congenital hypothyroidism, PKU).

Cardiac Anomalies

Moore and Persaud noted, "The critical period of heart development is from day 20 to day 50 after fertilization" (1998, p. 401). Although barely perceptible, the heart begins to beat between the end of the third week and the beginning of the fourth week of embryonic development; it is partitioned into four chambers by the seventh week. By the eighth week, the aortic arches form and further partition into the carotid, subclavian, and pulmonary arteries. Interruption in this process can result in an array of cardiac anomalies. Examples of cardiac anomalies include ASDs and VSDs, transposition of the great vessels, tetralogy of Fallot, stenoses, atresias, coarctation (compression) of the aorta, anomalies of the aortic arch, and hypoplasia of the left ventricle.

Fetal blood bypasses the lungs and is oxygenated by the placenta. During the first weeks of infancy, closure of the foramen ovale and the ductus arteriosis (structures that allow blood to bypass the lungs) enables the transition from fetal to newborn circulation. Failure of the foramen ovale to close and of the duct and umbilical arteries to constrict during the first hours and days after birth may resolve spontaneously or may be an indication for pharmacologic and/or surgical intervention.

Limb Anomalies

The limb buds first emerge from the embryonic mesoderm (intermediate germinal layer) during the fourth week, with upper limbs developing slightly faster than lower limbs. The period from the 24th to 36th days is critical for limb development. By the sixth week, the early hand and foot plates differentiate to form digital rays (i.e., the precursors to digits of the hands and feet), giving a webbed appearance to the fingers and toes. Further separation of the digits occurs through a process of programmed cell death. When these cellular changes are somehow disrupted, syndactyly (webbing) of the fingers and toes occurs.

Some limb anomalies are inherited as a dominant trait (e.g., supernumerary digits of the fingers or toes, absence of the radius, clubfoot) or caused by environmental factors (e.g., exposure to teratogenic substances). Vascular problems or disruption of circulation, such as ischemic events and embryonic bands, may also disrupt development of the limbs.

Cranio-Facial Anomalies

Development of the face begins with a single frontonasal prominence that further differentiates, giving rise to individual facial structures. The lips, tongue, and jaw arise from the maxillary and mandibular prominences. The hard and soft palates arise from the maxillary prominence and are formed between the sixth and twelfth weeks, with the most critical period for palate formation being between the sixth and ninth weeks. Cleft lip and palate, commonly seen together, actually have different etiologies. Cleft lip results from the failure of the medial nasal and maxillary prominences to merge. Cleft palate results from a failure of the palatal shelves to meet and fuse. A number of other facial anomalies may result from an interruption in the development of the pharyngeal/branchial arches. As noted in Chapter 6, Pierre Robin sequence is a clustering of related anomalies. These include a U-shaped cleft palate; retrognathia (retracted jaw); micrognathia (small jaw); and associated problems with airway maintenance, sucking, and swallowing. Apert syndrome is a skeletal anomaly involving premature fusion of the cranial and facial sutures. The cause of these errors in development is unclear, but some are related to genetic factors, environmental factors, or a combination of both.

The term *critical periods* has been used in developmental literature to refer to spans of time during which particular sensory experiences and environmental conditions are thought to exert the greatest positive or negative effects on infant development. Although the existence of critical periods in infant development continues to be debated in the literature, it could be inferred from the previous discussion that critical periods exist during embryonic and fetal development (Horton, 2001). Figure 17 depicts critical periods in development of the embryo and fetus. These are times in development when an alteration (e.g., exposure to a teratogenic substance) or a disruption (e.g., an interruption in fetal blood flow) can be traced to specific birth defects or other sequelae (e.g., mental retardation). Alcohol and a variety of drugs, both legal and illegal, are known to act as teratogens on the developing embryo, particularly in the first trimester. Maternal smoking is also known to affect the embryo and restrict intrauterine growth. Infants whose mothers smoked during pregnancy are frequently small for gestational age (SGA) (Wunsch, Conlon, & Scheidt, 2002).

Some disruptions in embryonic or fetal development, particularly the most severe ones, bring about a total cessation of development. Severe developmental anomalies or genetic conditions incompatible with life often result in spontaneous termination of a pregnancy. In other instances, a decision may be made to medically terminate a pregnancy if the mother's well-being is at risk or if the infant is known to have a terminal condition or severe congenital anomalies. *Abortion* refers to the consequences of such developmental disruptions—that is, that the embryo or fetus is expelled from the uterus, in a spontaneous or induced manner, "before it is *viable*—capable of living outside the uterus" (Moore & Persaud, 1998, p. 3). Spontaneous abortions are considered a natural screening process to eliminate abnormal conceptuses (zygotes or early embryos) that may be incompatible with life (Moore & Persaud, 1998).

An abortion can occur in a number of ways. It is important for NICU therapists to be familiar with these, as many parents of NICU infants have experienced a previous pregnancy loss:

- A *spontaneous abortion* (or miscarriage) occurs naturally, most often 3–12 weeks after fertilization.

- A *missed abortion* is an intrauterine fetal death that is not immediately expelled from the uterus.

- An *induced abortion* is caused by the use of drugs or the removal of the fetus by vacuum curettage before it is viable (prior to 20 weeks). Therapeutic abortions

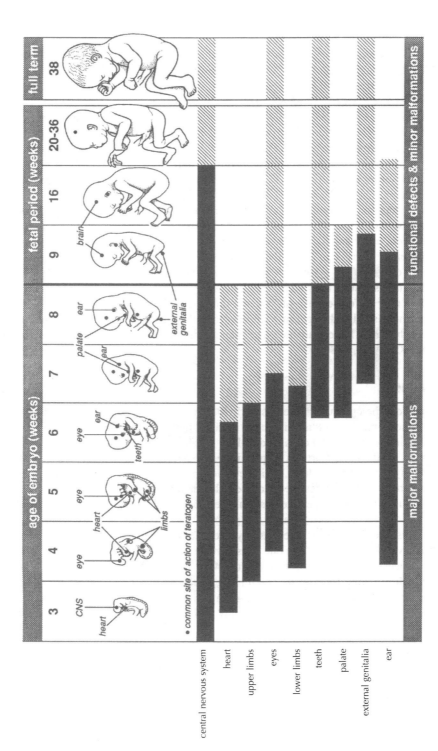

Figure 17. Critical periods of development. (From Moore, K.L., & Persaud, T.V.N. [1993]. *Before we are born: Essentials of embryology and birth defects* [4th ed., inside back cover]. Philadelphia: W.B. Saunders; adapted by permission.)

fall under this category and are usually done to restore/maintain the mother's health or to prevent the birth of an infant with a known fatal condition or severe anomalies (e.g., anencephaly).

- In a multiple pregnancy, a *reduction* is the removal of a fetus before viability to enhance the potential for survival of the remaining fetuses.

NEWBORN CLASSIFICATIONS AND RISK ESTIMATES

Hospital nurseries classify infants according to various parameters to facilitate description of the infants during case discussions and report writing. The most common parameters used for classifying newborns include GA, birth weight, and weight-by-age relationship. Another classification often used in NICUs relates to whether the infant is the product of a single or multiple pregnancy. The latter has become a necessary classification in the United States as a result of the dramatic increase (up 344% since 1980) in the incidence of twins and higher order—triplets and above—births (National Center for Health Statistics [NCHS], 1998b). Using descriptive classifications provides more precise communication among health care providers. A summary of the classifications most used in NICUs is presented next.

Gestational Age Assessment

Newborns are most commonly classified on the basis of their fetal age. A variety of methods for estimating the age of a fetus are available and used. The previously mentioned Carnegie Stages system is one such method (O'Rahilly & Muller, 1987). The Carnegie Stages system is a very reliable method for estimating the age of a developing embryo from the moment of conception based on certain physical characteristics. This is the system most commonly used by embryologists. Although this system is more precise than other GA estimates, it is less used clinically. Age estimated on the basis of this method is often called postconceptional age (PCA).

The method used for estimating GA in most clinical settings begins counting the age of the fetus from the mother's last menstrual period (LMP). During the first prenatal visit, the obstetrician calculates the GA of the embryo or fetus and the estimated date of delivery on the basis of the mother's LMP (Gomella, 1999). This form of assessment gives a practical estimate of GA, although it is somewhat crude and imperfect, particularly if the exact date of the LMP is not known. Because conception typically occurs approximately 2 weeks after the LMP, this form of estimation adds 2 weeks to the real age of the fetus from conception. The entire duration of a pregnancy would be approximately 40 weeks based on GA or the LMP, whereas it would be only 38 weeks based on PCA. A 4-week embryo on the Carnegie Stages would thus be considered a 6-week GA embryo based on the LMP.

Another term often used in NICUs to refer to the age of a fetus or premature infant is *age-by-dates*. This term also counts fetal age from the LMP. Although the systems most commonly used in NICUs estimate fetal age based on the LMP, it is important to understand these differences, particularly in interpreting literature that may present information based on PCA instead of GA. The issue becomes more relevant with the increase in infants conceived through in vitro fertilization. In reality, the age of a fetus conceived in vitro should be calculated from the moment of implantation in the utero, which approximates the PCA. To avoid the confusion that would result from using two different measures of age estimation, obstetricians and neonatologists calculate the GA of infants conceived in vitro by artificially adding 2 weeks to the age from the moment of implantation, regardless of the real date of the mother's LMP. The gestational ages reported in this book are based on the LMP unless otherwise indicated.

Other Age Estimates

The term *GA* is generally used in the NICU to estimate the number of weeks that an infant had spent in utero by the time he or she was born. In other words, GA measures the infant's age in weeks at any point throughout the pregnancy, from the LMP up to the moment of birth. The GA classification is used predominantly to determine how close the infant is to completing the pregnancy or how premature the infant is at birth. GA assessment, although important throughout the entire pregnancy, becomes especially meaningful around the time of delivery if a preterm birth is suspected or anticipated (Dodd, 1996).

Gestation can also be estimated from the date of first reported fetal activity and heart sounds. Ultrasound examination performed around the second trimester of the pregnancy may be used when a more precise calculation of GA is needed, such as in making decisions about an infant's maturity and readiness for delivery. Age is calculated on the basis of the biparietal diameter of the skull or the length of the femur on the ultrasound. Accuracy of GA estimates based on skull measurements decreases with GA (mainly after 20 weeks of gestation) because of fetal growth and head shape variability (Gomella, 1999). Femur measurements are more reliable toward the end of the pregnancy or when measuring the skull either is not possible (e.g., the head is engaged) or would give an incorrect maturity estimate (e.g., in cases of hydrocephalus) (Wilkins-Haug & Heffner, 1997). Because GA estimation is not always exact regardless of the calculation method used, it may be reported as a 2-week range (e.g., "a 24–25 weeker").

Fetal lung maturity improves steadily with increasing GA. Readiness for delivery and extrauterine life prior to 37–38 weeks of gestation should be determined through multiple estimates of GA and lung maturity. Under such circumstances, amniotic fluid samples may be drawn to measure the level of pulmonary surfactant in the fluid, the best indicator of the infant's lung maturity. A variety of surfactant tests are available to determine lung maturity with greater precision in anticipation of a preterm delivery (Richardson, 1997).

GA may also be determined postnatally through physical examination of a number of characteristics indicative of the infant's neuromotor and physical maturity. The New Ballard Score (Ballard et al., 1991) is a standardized GA assessment instrument that expands the original Dubowitz Gestational Age Assessment (Dubowitz, Dubowitz, & Goldberg, 1970) by including more specific definitions as well as criteria for assessing extremely premature infants (see Figure 18). Criteria for neuromotor maturity include measures of posture and joint flexibility (passive tone). Physical maturity examines the appearance of the skin and organs (e.g., breasts, genitalia, eyes, ears) (Ballard et al., 1991). Ultrasonographic and physical examination methods provide the most reliable GA estimates.

Infant Classification by Gestational Age

Institutions vary slightly in their definitions of infant classification by GA. The following are the most commonly used GA categories (Pursley & Cloherty, 1997):

NEUROMUSCULAR MATURITY

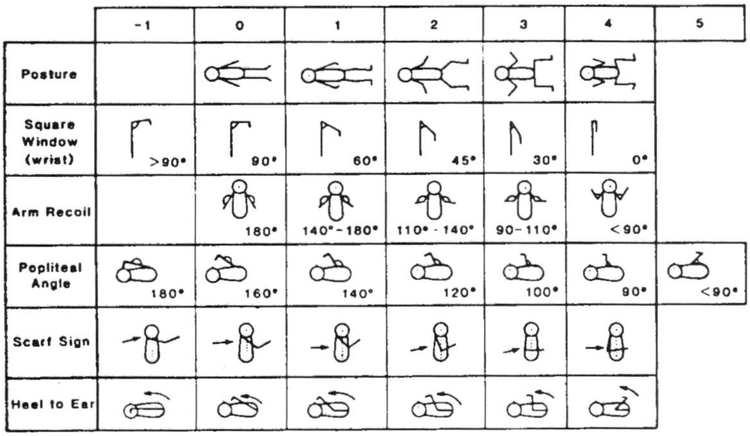

	-1	0	1	2	3	4	5
Posture							
Square Window (wrist)	>90°	90°	60°	45°	30°	0°	
Arm Recoil		180°	140°-180°	110°-140°	90°-110°	<90°	
Popliteal Angle	180°	160°	140°	120°	100°	90°	<90°
Scarf Sign							
Heel to Ear							

PHYSICAL MATURITY

Skin	sticky friable transparent	gelatinous red, translucent	smooth pink, visible veins	superficial peeling &/or rash, few veins	cracking pale areas rare veins	parchment deep cracking no vessels	leathery cracked wrinkled
Lanugo	none	sparse	abundant	thinning	bald areas	mostly bald	
Plantar Surface	heel-toe 40-50mm: -1 <40mm: -2	>50mm no crease	faint red marks	anterior transverse crease only	creases ant. 2/3	creases over entire sole	
Breast	imperceptible	barely perceptible	flat areola no bud	stippled areola 1-2mm bud	raised areola 3-4mm bud	full areola 5-10mm bud	
Eye/Ear	lids fused loosely:-1 tightly:-2	lids open pinna flat stays folded	sl. curved pinna; soft; slow recoil	well-curved pinna; soft but ready recoil	formed &firm instant recoil	thick cartilage ear stiff	
Genitals male	scrotum flat, smooth	scrotum empty faint rugae	testes in upper canal rare rugae	testes descending few rugae	testes down good rugae	testes pendulous deep rugae	
Genitals female	clitoris prominent labia flat	prominent clitoris small labia minora	prominent clitoris enlarging minora	majora & minora equally prominent	majora large minora small	majora cover clitoris & minora	

MATURITY RATING

score	weeks
-10	20
-5	22
0	24
5	26
10	28
15	30
20	32
25	34
30	36
35	38
40	40
45	42
50	44

Figure 18. New Ballard Score system to assess newborn infants. (From Ballard, J.L., Khoury, J.C., Wedig, K., Wang, L., Eilers-Walsman, B.L., & Lipp, R. [1991]. New Ballard score, expanded to include extremely premature infants. *Journal of Pediatrics, 119,* 418; reprinted by permission.)

- Preterm: Less than 37 weeks
- Full term: 37 weeks to less than 42 weeks
- Postterm (or postmature): 42 weeks or above

In 1997, 11.4% of all live births in the United States were preterm births (all subtypes) (NCHS, 1999), an increase of more than 4% from 1989 (U.S. Department of Health and Human Services [USDHHS], 1999). Black (African American and other) women had approximately twice the risk of having a preterm infant as Caucasian women (USDHHS, 1999). Some institutions use *extremely preterm* as an additional category to identify infants born before 28 weeks of gestation (USDHHS, 1999).

This type of classification is used as a rough estimate of an infant's developmental maturity and potential medical and nursing needs associated with gestational development.

Although the need for intensive medical and nursing care for preterm infants is well known to the general public, postterm infants, especially those born at or beyond 43 weeks' GA, also may have serious medical issues requiring special care at birth. For example, the intrauterine crowding that occurs toward the end of pregnancy may cause compression of the umbilical cord. The infant may begin to receive insufficient nutrients as a result of the pressure on the cord. As the pressure continues or increases the infant loses soft tissue, especially subcutaneous fat, and overall weight. Although individuals not in the medical field may think that postterm infants will be "big" or macrosomic, the reality is that they lose weight toward the end of the pregnancy. It is not unusual to find a postterm infant who is SGA.

Persistent cord compression depletes glycogen storage and, if severe, may cause the infant to experience neonatal hypoglycemia (Beers & Berkow, 1999). Amniotic fluid also decreases in volume and becomes more concentrated (Fox, 1997). The infant may also experience hypoxia and pass meconium, which becomes very toxic as it dilutes in the concentrated amniotic fluid (Fox, 1997). Meconium aspiration may lead to severe perinatal asphyxia or death of the postmature infant, either in utero or during the birthing process (Campbell, Ostbye, & Irgens, 1997). The changes observed in postmature infants have also been attributed to placental insufficiency or aging of the placenta (Beers & Berkow, 1999), but a number of studies in the 1990s failed to demonstrate evidence of placental degeneration (Fox, 1997). Therefore, placental degeneration or the role that such degeneration may play on the changes that occur in postmature infants, although widely accepted, remains inconclusive.

This GA classification system is useful for informing parents of an infant's potential risk regarding his or her overall maturity, specifically if birth was premature or postmature. Postnatal age (corrected age) is also commonly reported in describing preterm infants. It is measured by adding an infant's chronological age in weeks (age from birth) to the GA at birth. The use of GA is often continued until the child reaches at least term age (40 weeks GA) or the expected due date.

Birth Weight

Birth weight classification is predominantly used for describing LBW infants, although it applies to all infant weight groups. As with GA, there is no universal agreement on the definition or interpretation of the birth weight classification across institutions. The most common birth weight classification includes four categories (Pursley & Cloherty, 1997):

1. Macrosomia: 4,000 g or more
2. Normal birth weight (NBW): 2,500 g–3,999 g
3. Low birth weight (LBW): 1,500 g–less than 2,500 g
4. Very low birth weight (VLBW): less than 1,500 g

A fifth birth weight category, extremely low birth weight (ELBW), is used in many institutions to classify infants weighing less than 1,000 g. Likewise, infants born weighing less than 750 g are classified in some institutions as "micropreemies." These categories have become essential for describing these increasingly growing and unique subtypes of VLBW infants, who require the most specialized level of neonatal care.

Birth weight is considered one of the most important predictors of an infant's health and survival (NCHS, 1998a). In 1997, the median birth weight in the United States was 3,000 g–3,499 g; 7.5% of the infants born were LBW and 4.2% were VLBW (NCHS, 1999). There has been a marked improvement in the mortality rate of LBW infants, especially among infants weighing between 750 g and 1,499 g (a decrease greater than 50% from 1985 to 1995) (NCHS, 1998b).

It should be noted that birth weight and GA, although interrelated in most cases, are separate entities and should be assessed and interpreted independently. Although most LBW infants are also preterm, LBW is not equivalent to premature gestation. For example, an infant born at 38 weeks of gestation with a birth weight below 2,500 g would be considered LBW but would not be considered preterm. This infant would be at greater risk than an infant born NBW. Likewise, an infant born before 36 weeks of gestation and weighing more than 2,500 g would be classified as preterm but not as LBW. The greater birth weight gives this infant an advantage over a preterm who is also LBW. Both classifications are typically used in combination when describing infants and analyzing potential risk.

Both classifications—GA and birth weight—serve as rough indicators of the infant's anticipated perinatal and postnatal needs. Infants who are ELBW are generally the most fragile preterm infants because of the immaturity and profound instability of their body systems. These infants usually require prolonged tertiary-level neonatal intensive care. The other two LBW groups—LBW and VLBW—may be cared for in either a Level II or Level III NICU depending on their medical status, stability, and life-support needs. In some community hospitals, after a brief postnatal observation period, stable LBW infants who do not require specialized care at birth may remain in the Level I (normal newborn) nursery or in their mother's room until discharge. Infants with mild macrosomia may also be cared for in the Level I nursery, whereas those with more severe cases of macrosomia may require intensive care management, depending on the etiology of the above-average intrauterine weight gain and the infant's perinatal or postnatal course. These infants may be admitted to either a Level II or Level III nursery based on the degree of specialized care that they require. Infants with severe asphyxia who require ECMO therapy receive care in a specialized setting.

Weight-by-Age Relationship

Weight-by-age relationship is a classification that establishes whether an infant's weight at birth falls within the average range, below average, or above average for his or her GA. The newborn's weight is plotted by GA on a standardized graph that displays the normal weight distributions by percentiles, or by standard deviations (or both) (see Figure 19). Weight appropriateness for GA is determined on the basis of the point on the graph where a score falls, which is described as follows:

- *Appropriate for gestational age (AGA):* between the 10th and the 90th percentile or between plus or minus two standard deviations from the mean
- *Small for gestational age (SGA):* below the 10th percentile or more than two standard deviations below the mean
- *Large for gestational age (LGA):* above the 90th percentile or more than two standard deviations above the mean

LGA does not necessarily imply that an infant is very heavy, and *SGA* does not necessarily imply that an infant is very small. Regardless of absolute weight, a small

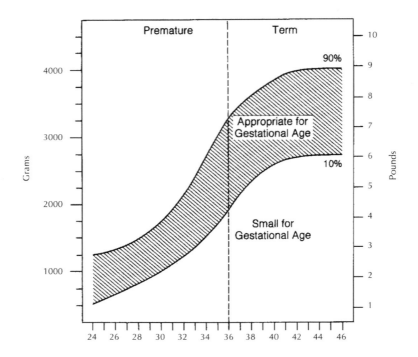

Figure 19. Newborn weight by gestational age. The shaded area between the 10th and 90th percentiles represents infants who are appropriate for gestational age. Weight below the 10th percentile makes an infant small for gestational age (SGA). Prematurity is defined as being born before 36 weeks' gestation. (From Lubchenco, L.O. [1976]. *The high risk infant.* Philadelphia: W.B. Saunders; reprinted by permission.)

premature infant who weighs more than what is appropriate for gestational age would be classified as LGA, whereas a heavier infant whose weight is lower than what is appropriate for his or her gestation would be classified as SGA. The term SGA applies only to weight/age discrepancy at birth and should not be used when describing infants with postnatal weight gain disorders. Thus, if the weight of an infant born AGA drops below the 10th percentile after birth, he or she is not considered SGA despite meeting all other criteria.

Weight-by-gestation classifications do not take into consideration the etiology of the weight gain deviation from the normal range. Although weight gain is most often influenced by genetic or demographic/socioenvironmental factors, a number of maternal and infant disorders also affect weight gain. Infants born SGA or LGA, either because of constitutional or demographic factors, usually do not present significant problems at birth unless the weight-by-gestation discrepancy is major. Conversely, infants whose weight-by-gestation discrepancy results from medical or physiologic factors (e.g., factors interfering with placental blood flow and oxygenation, metabolic disorders) may experience more serious issues at birth, requiring specialized medical or nursing care. For example, maternal preeclampsia and exposure to teratogens tend to cause intrauterine growth restriction (IUGR) that may lead to an SGA birth (Feinberg & Repke, 1997; Wilkins-Haug & Heffner, 1997). Such SGA infants typically require closer attention and more intensive care than infants with familiar- or demographic-type SGA. Likewise, diabetic mothers have a higher incidence of LGA births than mothers without diabetes (Cloherty, 1997). Their infants may present serious neonatal metabolic and feeding problems that require specialized care, perhaps including developmental or therapeutic intervention. Very SGA infants are at high risk for perinatal problems and even neonatal death, regardless of the cause of their growth restriction. Very LGA infants also tend to have a higher morbidity and mortality risk than AGA infants.

In general, infants born SGA or with IUGR have higher morbidity rates in the first few months of life and experience a higher incidence of neurologic, neurophysiologic, and heart rate alterations in the neonatal period in comparison with AGA infants (Curzi-Dascalova, Peirano, & Christova, 1996). Studies suggest that healthy SGA infants also experience immaturity or dysregulation of respiratory function control (Curzi-Dascalova et al., 1996). Respiratory rhythm alterations include delayed establishment of neonatal breathing patterns, higher incidence of respiratory pauses, and more time spent in periodic breathing (Curzi-Dascalova et al., 1996). Curzi-Dascalova and colleagues speculated that such respiratory variations may result from decreased brain stem blood supply and chronic hypoxia. Respiratory difficulties associated with SGA may alter the infants' overall physiologic functioning.

Infants who begin to gain weight appropriately shortly after birth have a better prognosis than those who continue to have postnatal weight-gain problems (Pursley & Cloherty, 1998). Those with persistent weight-gain problems may benefit from early intervention services that are geared to enhance their procuring abilities and feeding success.

Multiple Births

Infants may be classified as *singleton*, *twins*, or *higher order* (triplets, quadruplets, or above) according to the number of embryos that results from a pregnancy. Twins are the most frequent product of multifetal pregnancies in the United States, with an incidence of 11 per 1,000 pregnancies (Powers, 1997) and a 4% rate increase from the year spanning 1995–1996 (NCHS, 1998b). Higher order births have increased even more steeply since the 1970s than twins. Between 1995 and 1996, the number of live multiple gestation births of three or more infants increased by 19% (NCHS, 1998b). The increased incidence of multifetal pregnancies has been associated with infertility treatment and delayed childbearing (NCHS, 1998b; Powers, 1997; USDHHS, 1999). Other factors associated with multiple gestation include race (i.e., a higher incidence among African Americans) and parity (Powers, 1997). Although the mortality rate of multiple gestation infants remains high, survival has improved considerably as a result of enhanced fetal monitoring and other technological advances.

Multiple gestation infants can be classified by zygocity as *monozygous* (the product of one fertilized egg) or as *dizygous* or *multizygous* (the product of more than one fertilized egg). A natural higher order pregnancy can include both monozygous and multizygous fetuses. Monozygous infants who share placental vascularization (i.e., the division occurred 3 days or more after fertilization) have a higher mortality rate than dizygous infants (Powers, 1997). Likewise, monozygous infants who share the amniotic sac—the least common type—have a 50%–60% perinatal mortality rate, usually because of cord entanglement or knotting (Powers, 1997). Dizygous fetuses have one amniotic sac and one placenta per fetus, although sacs may fuse when fetuses are implanted too closely. These infants almost always have individual placental vascularization and a lower mortality and morbidity risk (Powers, 1997).

Multifetal gestation is associated with numerous maternal and infant risks. Most multifetal pregnancies result in premature labor probably as a result of intrauterine crowding and other factors (Gomella, 1999; Twinstuff, 2002). Mortality risk increases proportionately to the number of fetuses and with each week of shortened gestation of the pregnancy (Powers, 1997). With few exceptions, the majority of infants of multifetal pregnancies are born LBW as a result of prematurity complicated by fetal weight-gain disorders, particularly in the third trimester, and many are likely to require NICU care at birth. Perinatal death of higher order infants increases with the number of fetuses. In twins it is 4–11 times higher than in singletons (Powers, 1997); in triplets it is as high as 25.5%, and it is even higher for pregnancies above three fetuses (Gomella, 1999). Discordant weight gain among twin fetuses is common; when the weight discrepancy between fetuses is greater than 25%, the mortality rate can be as high as 80% (Powers, 1997). Furthermore, the mortality rate of surviving twins continues to be approximately three times higher than that of singletons throughout the first year of life (Powers, 1997). Multiple birth infants also have a higher risk of deformational plagiocephaly or the development of an abnormally shaped head because of in utero constraint and prematurity (Littlefield, Kelly, Pomatto, & Beals, 1999, 2002). Brain trauma may result if deformational forces are severe.

Combined Use of Classifications

Classifications are generally used in combination when describing NICU infants. A typical NICU medical record describes infants by their gender, GA, maturity (preterm, full term, or postterm), and weight-by-age relationship; multiple birth is included when appropriate. The most frequently combined factors include maturity and weight-by-age relationship, resulting in nine possible combinations: term, preterm, or post-term infants who can be AGA, LGA, or SGA. The following examples show how classifications are used in combination:

- A 28-week GA infant weighing 1,300 g would be described as VLBW, AGA, preterm
- A 43-week GA infant weighing 4,400 g would be described as macrosomic, LGA, postterm (some hospitals do not routinely use the term *macrosomia*)
- A 40-week GA infant weighing 2,200 g would be described as full-term, SGA (could also be classified as LBW)
- A 34-week GA infant weighing 1,200 g would be described as LBW, SGA, preterm
- A 26-week GA infant weighing 900 g would be described as ELBW, AGA, preterm

GA is often used in combination with the other factors during an infant's perinatal phase. Later, GA may be used to reflect the infant's developmental level as well as his or her chronological or extrauterine age, and it is often expressed as the infant's "corrected age." For example, a preterm infant born 5 weeks ago may be described as an ex-24 week AGA preterm, day of life 35, with a corrected age of 29 weeks.

CONCLUSION

A general understanding of embryologic development is essential to promote best practice in the developmental management and care of NICU infants, particularly as it relates to critical or sensitive developmental periods and to potential developmental consequences of embryologic alterations. An extensive exposition of these topics is beyond the scope of this book. Readers should refer to Bailey et al. (2001) and Moore and Persaud (1998) for a comprehensive discussion of the literature.

Thorough familiarity with the typical newborn classification systems and the parameters associated with each classification system are of utmost importance for comprehending infant behavior and estimating an infant's potential developmental risk. Also important for best practice in the NICU is a broad understanding of the specific capabilities of full-term and preterm infants. The latter content is expanded in Chapters 8 and 9.

8

Developmental Capabilities of Full-Term NICU Infants

OVERVIEW

This chapter presents a review of the performance abilities of full-term newborns. Special emphasis is given to their physiologic capabilities (i.e., respiratory, cardiovascular, temperature regulation, spontaneous crying, and perinatal arousal), as well as to the effects of the environment on newborn physiologic functioning. Other neonatal capabilities reviewed include neuromotor functioning, regulation of states of arousal, interactive skills, self-regulation, and sensory functioning. This section of the chapter concludes with the proposal of a model of occupational performance development in newborns based on the progressive emergence of fetal capabilities.

The remainder of the chapter discusses the potential impact of illness and medical instability on the capabilities of newborns. The effects of transient and serious or prolonged medical issues are compared. Particular emphasis is given to how neonatal illness may affect infants' neurobehavioral functioning and, ultimately, their capacity to self-regulate. The chapter describes behaviors that may signal that an infant's neurobehavioral status is at risk. Also described is the impact of neonatal illness on the development of sensorimotor and sensory processing abilities. The chapter concludes with examples of subtle signals that could indicate deterioration of the infant's condition or the presence of less obvious problems.

OBJECTIVES

- Describe the typical physical characteristics of healthy full-term newborns
- Identify the physiologic abilities that enable healthy infants to survive independently from the intrauterine environment at birth (respiration, spontaneous crying, cardiovascular functions, temperature regulation, and perinatal arousal) and recognize how environmental influences may support or interfere with a newborn's physiologic functioning
- Describe the typical postural patterns, motor behaviors, and reflexes of healthy newborns, recognizing the lack of correlation between the reflexes and motor development
- Describe the typical states of arousal, and explain the importance of protective arousal responses of newborns and their relation to sleep behavior in the prevention of sudden infant death syndrome (SIDS)

- Describe the developmental and social relevance of neonatal interactive skills and infant, caregiver, and physical environment factors that may interfere with an infant's engagement in interactive behaviors
- Identify behaviors that are believed to indicate an infant's self-regulation abilities, and compare both types of behaviors (approach and coping signals)
- Describe the sensory abilities of healthy neonates within the various modalities (i.e., tactile, olfactory, vestibular, visual, and auditory) as well as the interrelation of infants' sensory and performance abilities
- Compare the developmental consequences of transient and severe or prolonged illnesses in infants
- Identify behavioral signals that suggest that an infant's neurobehavioral system has experienced stress, and explain the potential life-threatening and developmental consequences of prolonged or severe exposure to physiologic stress
- Identify general strategies for decreasing stress in the NICU

HEALTHY NEWBORNS

Green noted that the healthy newborn "is born full term, with an appropriate weight and free of infection, severe trauma, or congenital disabilities" (1994, p. 3). Shortly after birth, a healthy newborn begins to display the richness of behaviors that he or she had been mastering for months in utero. After 40 weeks of intrauterine development, the healthy full-term infant has achieved the most remarkable milestone in the life of a human being: the capacity to live as an independent being. Transition to life outside the womb involves the greatest change in life support that a human being ever experiences. Within a few seconds, the infant must assume a large number of body functions previously accomplished through the mother's body. The ease with which an infant masters the transition to and begins interacting with the extrauterine environment is indicative of his or her capacity to self-regulate internal functions. A well-regulated healthy full-term infant possesses the necessary physiologic stability at birth to control multiple body processes independently from his or her mother, without undue stress to his or her neurobehavioral system (Als, 1986).

Physiologic Processes

Respiration

One of the first functions that newborns must take over is breathing. The mechanical squeeze and sensory input that the fetus receives during labor is believed to arouse the infant and facilitate breathing (Ronca, Abel, & Alberts, 1996). A well-regulated infant begins to breathe spontaneously when exposed to the extrauterine environment at birth, at a rate of approximately 40–60 breaths per minute (Cochran, 1997). The lungs undergo much preparation in utero for postnatal functioning. Amniotic fluid and infant urine in utero fill the lungs, producing internal transpulmonary pressure that promotes lung growth and elasticity (Hutchinson, 1989). Infants with fetal kidney disorders and urinary dysfunction often experience problems with postnatal lung expansion. Lung growth is also enhanced through the negative intrathoracic pressure caused by fetal breathing movements of the diaphragm, particularly toward the end of the pregnancy. The absence of fetal breathing can alter the physiology of lung development and affect the initiation of respiration at birth. Neurological mechanisms, a variety of neurochemicals, and other mechanical factors are also necessary for the lungs to expand adequately at birth (Hutchinson, 1989).

Surface tension within the lungs must be sufficiently low to allow the lungs to inflate and deflate without much effort. A specific type of alveolar cell produces and secretes a protein and lipid compound that reduces lung surface tension and promotes alveolar stability, thereby facilitating lung inflation. This surface-active, tension-lowering compound is called *pulmonary surfactant*. The presence and adequate distribution of surfactant are essential for the initiation of spontaneous, unassisted ventilation as well as for adequate oxygenation. Although surfactant production begins early in development, it is spread throughout the lungs by motion and certain agents toward the end of pregnancy. Elevated adrenergic and steroid hormones during labor increase surfactant production and release it (Liley & Stark, 1997). Once released and spread, surfactant helps distribute air uniformly inside the lungs, improving oxygenation. It also reduces the likelihood of air-sac collapse during expiration by lowering the surface tension of the sacs, and it promotes absorption of lung liquid, helping to keep the lungs dry after birth. Infants born before term or through cesarean section often experience respiratory difficulties, partly because of insufficient or inadequately distributed pulmonary surfactant (Liley & Stark, 1997).

Despite the complicated lung development that occurs inside the womb, the lungs must undergo additional developmental changes postnatally. One of the most important postnatal changes involves a 20-fold increase in the number of alveoli and in the total lung surface area (Hutchinson, 1989). Periodic breathing observed in many healthy newborns may in part be explained by lung immaturity (Cochran, 1997). Infants with periodic breathing breathe in cycles consisting of about 1 minute of fairly regular respirations interrupted by pauses of 5–10 seconds. After each brief pause, infants reinitiate breathing on their own by taking a few more breaths followed by another pause, and the process is repeated until it is replaced by regular respiration. This type of breathing pattern is seen in some full-term newborns, but it is more prevalent in premature infants. Periodic breathing must be distinguished from apnea, which involves abnormally prolonged (longer than 20 seconds) respiratory pauses during periodic breathing episodes (Cochran, 1997).

Along with taking their first breaths, most healthy full-term infants begin to cry shortly after birth as an automatic reaction, perhaps to the extreme change in environmental temperature and other birth-related stress (Ronca et al., 1996). Crying in healthy infants should be robust. It is widely believed that crying helps expand and clear the lungs of amniotic fluid and secretions and that infants who fail to cry at birth may experience delayed lung expansion and transient respiratory distress. Gentle shaking or slapping, although not a current practice, was used in the past to get newborns to expand their lungs at birth by crying. However, Ludington-Hoe, Cong, and Hashemi (2002) pointed out that several studies have demonstrated that infants who do not cry at birth and those who do cry at birth have similar pulmonary function. Crying full-term newborns may exhibit minor chest retraction, but no expiratory grunting and only minimal nostril flaring should be observed during their crying spells (Cochran, 1997).

Cardiovascular Functioning

Circulation and other cardiovascular functions are also intimately related to respiration. Normal cardiovascular and respiratory functioning requires integrity of the nervous system at many levels, from the neocortex to the spinal cord (Harper, 1996). Cardiorespiration is an extremely sophisticated and complex process that requires integration of the breathing and cardiovascular reflexes and involuntary control of numerous muscles within seconds from birth. Healthy full-term newborns typically master this neonatal milestone without problems.

The infant's first sighs trigger a series of events that initiate the shift from fetal circulation to, within minutes to hours after birth, an approximation of adult circulation (Gomella, 1999). At the onset of respiration, the lungs expand, oxygenation begins, pulmonary vascular resistance decreases as the lungs inflate, concentration of peripheral arterial oxygen (PaO_2) increases (constricting the ductus arteriosus), systemic vascular resistance increases, and the foramen ovale closes functionally (Harper, 1996). Closure of the ductus arteriosus and the foramen ovale marks the transition to mature circulation and postnatal oxygenation. A transient heart murmur may be heard as the ductus is closing and is normal in the absence of other signs (Cochran, 1997).

An evenly distributed pinkish pigmentation of the skin within a few minutes or hours after birth is indicative of adequate blood circulation, oxygenation, and temperature regulation. (Mild temporary cyanosis of the hands, feet, and the perioral area or jaundice are considered normal in the newborn period; Cochran, 1997). Adequate circulatory perfusion and oxygenation require the infant to maintain a fairly regular heart rate between 120 and 160 BPM (Wilkins-Haug & Heffner, 1997).

Temperature Regulation

Healthy full-term infants provided with reasonable warmth are able to maintain adequate body temperature without significant loss of the calories necessary for weight gain and growth (Chatson, Fant, & Cloherty, 1997). Heat generation in newborn full-term infants results primarily from lipolysis, reesterification, and oxidation of sympathetic-innervated brown-fat tissues (Chatson et al., 1997). If exposed to excessive cold, any infant—especially one who is premature or sick—will experience protective peripheral vasoconstriction that may lead to hypoxia, anaerobic metabolism, acidosis, and even death. Most premature infants have difficulty with temperature regulation because of the immaturity of their systems and a lack of body fat.

Crying

The quality of the infant's cry is another indicator of autonomic regulation and central nervous system integrity. High cry threshold, longer latency to cry, shorter first cry sound, and shorter overall crying bouts have been associated with disrupted autonomic regulation in infants (Zeskind, Marchall, & Goff, 1996). In addition, healthy newborns whose crying acoustics present a certain characteristic (i.e., "high first formant") are more likely to die of SIDS than infants without this characteristic pattern (Corwin et al., 1995). Healthy newborn cries are typically strong and may vary in their characteristics, based on the context (i.e., cries that occur "spontaneously" versus those that occur in response to a painful stimulus) (Clarici, Travan, Accardo, DeVonderweid, & Bava, 2002).

Perinatal Arousal

After the early crying phase, most healthy full-term newborns exhibit a period of heightened alertness for a few minutes or even hours, enabling them to engage in the first interactive exchanges with their parents (Ronca et al., 1996). Nature-enhanced arousal primes infants to take advantage of their parents' emotional sensitivity during the perinatal period. Positive initial interactive exchanges have been associated with early maternal bonding (Harrison & Kositsky, 1987) but are not essential for bonding to occur. Cold, illness, physiologic instability, or sedation may curtail perinatal arousal, hindering the infant's participation in such a monumental event for the family. Initial alertness is often followed by a period of deep sleep that may last for several hours.

Other Physiologic Processes

Metabolic, digestive, and other physiologic processes also become operational at birth but are less evident. Functional operation of the autonomic neonatal processes requires highly refined stability and control of the infant's autonomic/physiologic subsystem (Als, 1986). In addition, the environment may support or interfere with the infant's physiologic functioning. Central nervous system maturity and exposure to a supportive environmental context enable most healthy full-term infants to assume the necessary physiologic functions at birth. This process may be less smooth when environmental conditions are unfavorable, such as when sick or premature infants have to be exposed to extensive and disruptive life support equipment and procedures. Infants who do not have physiologic stability will require environmental modulation to reduce stress and enhance physiologic functioning.

Neuromotor Control

By term age, the healthy infant has achieved sufficient postural and motor control to maintain the extremities in a symmetrical pattern of total flexion when at rest and to move in and out of the flexed position (with fairly smooth movements) when awake and active. Similar organized movements are also seen when the infant is in a state of light or active sleep. Smooth motor activity is a major indicator of infant well-being at birth (Brazelton & Nugent, 1995). Motor activity may be more disorganized when the infant is drowsy, agitated, fussy, or crying. Brief startles and jitteriness after stretching movements are normal in newborns (Brazelton & Nugent, 1995).

The typical postural pattern of full-term newborns is called *physiologic flexion*; it is characterized by strong flexor muscle tone of the extremities and increased stretch reflexes. Intrauterine posturing and crowding are partially responsible for the increased flexor tone and postural patterns seen in full-term newborns (Maekawa & Ochiai, 1975). Physiologic flexion with head turning is a comforting position for most infants; it approximates bringing the hands to the face, thereby facilitating hand-to-mouth self-calming behaviors. Smooth motor activity, the ability to resume a physiologic flexion posture after being disturbed or handled, and the ability to produce self-regulation behaviors such as hand to mouth are indicative of good motor and physiologic stability and control.

Reflex Development

A variety of automatic reflex behaviors develop in utero and are present at birth. It is believed that reflexes enable the infant to actively participate in the labor and delivery process (Brazelton, 1998). Reflex development helps determine a newborn's motor competence and serves as a measure of perinatal central nervous system integrity (Brazelton & Nugent, 1995). Although there is some controversy in the literature regarding specifically when many primitive reflexes emerge, there is consensus on which reflexes should be present in full-term newborns. Examples of commonly assessed newborn reflexes include the palmar grasp, the plantar grasp, the asymmetric tonic neck reflex, automatic stepping, rooting, sucking, swallowing, the gag reflex, proprioceptive placing, and the Moro reflex. Some of the neonatal reflexes (i.e., rooting, sucking, gag, and swallow) have survival implications for the infants. Absence of neonatal reflexes is a sign of dysfunction or depression of the central nervous system. However, studies in the 1990s suggest that the presence of primitive reflexes does not necessarily predict attainment of early motor milestones in healthy infants (Bartlett, 1997) or in infants with mild brain damage (Cioni et al., 1997).

Motor Development

Primitive spontaneous movements may be more indicative of neurological maturation than the presence of reflexes. Two organized motor behaviors in newborns—hand to mouth and defensive reactions—are important indicators of central nervous system integrity. Both behaviors reflect infants' ability to protect themselves. Hand to mouth enables an infant to self-organize, self-console, and even facilitate sucking, whereas defensive reaction protects the infant from airway occlusion. In the latter movement, the infant responds with swiping motions of the arms to push away any stimuli covering his or her face (Brazelton & Nugent, 1995). The potential significance of protective mechanisms such as defensive reactions for preventing SIDS is discussed below under the States of Arousal subsection.

Infants who lack neuromotor stability at birth may require external motor support to engage in more mature forms of behaviors, such as shifting between states of arousal, falling into deep sleep, or becoming alert. This assistance can be in many forms, including positioning with boundaries, tactile containment (e.g., holding, swaddling), provision of a pacifier, or facilitation of nutritive sucking on the breast or nipple.

States of Arousal

Development of states of arousal follows a somewhat predetermined ontogenetic sequence, with continuity from fetal through neonatal periods and major subsequent changes throughout infancy (Scher, 1998). Neonatal sleep patterns are established by 36–38 weeks GA (Groome, Swiber, Atterbury, Bentz, & Holland, 1997). Healthy full-term infants sleep an average of 16–20 hours per day (Brazelton, 1998). Within a few hours from birth, infants fall into a deep sleep phase that lasts for a few days. During this deep sleep phase, they typically only wake up for feeding and usually fall asleep while feeding. This phase is believed to work as a protective mechanism to shut out environmental stimuli as the infant gradually adjusts to extrauterine life (Brazelton, 1998). *Habituation*, the ability to inhibit a response to irrelevant stimuli, is another important indicator of an infant's well-being and nervous system integrity. The stress of a difficult or prolonged labor may cause temporary disruption in a newborn's habituation (Brazelton, 1998). Newborns with habituation difficulties are more sensitive to environmental stimuli and may experience difficulty maintaining a sleep state.

After the neonatal deep sleep phase, periods of alertness increase as a 2- to 3-hour sleep–wake cycle is established. Healthy newborns are quite able to regulate their state of arousal to wake up when approaching a feeding, fall asleep at the end of a feeding, or cry to signal the need for attention or care. They are capable of demonstrating the full spectrum of states of arousal from deep sleep to active awake and crying (see Table 8).

Healthy newborns often have discernible diurnal/nocturnal sleep patterns, with significantly more sleep occurring during nighttime than during daytime (Sadeh, Dark, & Vohr, 1996). The ability to reach and maintain lower states of arousal, especially deep sleep, helps infants conserve energy for weight gain and growth and is believed to promote neurobehavioral recovery after stress. Infants who cannot habituate or adequately modulate their state of arousal tend to be more vulnerable to stress and may experience difficulty with weight gain (Brazelton, 1998; Sadeh et al., 1996). Failure to demonstrate the typical sleep patterns of newborns may be indicative of brain dysfunction (Scher, 1998).

Arousal is considered an important survival response in infants (McNamara, Wulbrand, & Thach, 1998). Stimulus-induced arousal in healthy sleeping infants follows a sequence of behavioral manifestations that begins 2–4 seconds prior to a full arousal response: An augmented breath (a sigh), accompanied by a startle, is followed by stereotypic thrashing movements of the arms (Thach & Lijowska, 1996). A more thorough study by McNamara and associates (1998) found that these behavioral observations corresponded with progressively ascending central nervous system activation beginning with a withdrawal reflex at the spinal level, followed by brain stem respiratory and startle responses, and ending with cortical arousal. Startles and

Table 8. Neonatal states of arousal

State of arousal	Description
Deep sleep	Eyes closed, no eye movements under closed eyelids; regular breathing; relaxed facial expression; no spontaneous motor activity other than startles
	Deep, motionless sleep predominates in the full-term newborn
	Also called State 1, quiet sleep, non-REM (non–rapid eye movement) sleep, or regular sleep
Light sleep	Eyes closed, rapid eye movements under closed eyelids, irregular respirations, low-amplitude motor activity, occasional mouthing and sucking movements
	Also called State 2, active sleep, REM sleep, or irregular sleep
Drowsy	Semidozing, eyes closed or open, fluttering eyelids, variable activity level, fussing, whimpering, and facial grimacing
	Also called State 3 or transitional sleep
Quiet alert	Awake, "bright-eyed" appearance; apparent visual focusing and processing of information; minimal motor activity
	Also called State 4 or awake
Active awake	Clearly awake and aroused, but eyes may be opened or closed; high level of motor activity; may fuss without crying
	Also called State 5
Crying	Audible, robust, rhythmic crying
	Also called State 6

Source: Brazelton & Nugent (1995).

thrashing arm movements were found to be significantly associated with partial occlusion of the airway and, thus, are believed to have a protective function during mild asphyxia (Thach & Lijowska, 1996). Arousal threshold is significantly higher from a state of deep sleep than from light sleep (Read et al., 1998). Adequate arousal threshold and responses may be crucial in the prevention of SIDS. Based on these findings, an infant who has difficulty becoming aroused or waking up (e.g., infants in deep sleep, sedated infants, small preterm infants not connected to a monitor) may be more likely to experience asphyxia or SIDS than an infant who is easily aroused.

Well-regulated infants are generally able to make smooth transitions between states, may self-calm and self-console when under minor distress, and may arouse themselves when necessary. Their ability to become alert, although still limited, enables them to visually scan the immediate surroundings and to engage in brief interactive exchanges with humans and nonhuman objects. For example, an infant may be able to fixate on a black and white design, without external assistance, by maintaining a quiet alert state and a flexed posture. Less regulated healthy infants may need assistance from their caregivers to move between states of arousal. For example, an infant may need to be rocked, contained, or swaddled to fall asleep or calm down after a crying spell or to engage in feeding. An infant who has difficulty waking up may need to be uncovered, talked to, or given tactile and vestibular stimulation to become alert.

Interactive Abilities

The ability to register stimuli and attend enables healthy newborns to react to human and nonhuman sensory stimuli. Alertness is the precursor of attentional and interactive abilities. Infants who can maintain at least brief periods of alertness demonstrate that they have achieved sufficient control and stability in the physiologic, motor, and state subsystems to engage in social interaction with their caregivers. Most healthy full-term neonates can engage in interactive processes with their caregivers and with their environment shortly after birth to the extent of their self-regulation abilities and the support provided by contextual elements.

Healthy newborns are strongly attracted to the human face; the preference for a facial image over a non–face-like stimulus has been repeatedly demonstrated in the literature (Slater & Kirby, 1998; Valenza et al., 1996). This strong attraction entices the infant to participate in social interaction beyond the initial interaction that occurs during the perinatal arousal period. Social interaction, as a dyadic process, is heavily influenced by neonatal capabilities as well as by the environmental context. Although neurobehavioral stability gives infants the capacity to alert and attend to the caregiver, the caregiver's response, as the most important component of the infant's environmental context, either supports or dissuades the infant's interaction efforts. For example, Figure 1 in Chapter 1 illustrates that the interactive process between a newborn and her toddler sibling is supported by the sibling's social encouragement.

The mother's psychological state is perhaps the most pervasive environmental influence on an infant's ability to socially interact. Depressed mothers, for example, tend to be poorly attuned to, less affirming of, and more neglectful of their infants (Murray, Fiori-Cowley, Hooper, & Cooper, 1996). Adversity and postpartum depression have been associated with dysfunctional infant attachment (Murray et al., 1996). Maternal psychiatric illness affects the infant's social and emotional functioning (Weinberg & Tronick, 1998). In such cases, the mother's inconsistent availability or responsiveness may curtail the infant's interaction attempts. In these situations, the father's or a sibling's participation in the interactive process is essential to support the infant's attachment efforts. Full expression of a healthy infant's interactive capacities is therefore determined by the dyadic interrelation between intrinsic (infant) and extrinsic (environmental) factors, particularly the infant's mother or father.

As language skills develop, infant interactions become more complex, integrated, and rich. Infants who are less healthy and less stable or who are developing slowly may experience greater difficulty engaging in social interaction and other mature behaviors. These infants may benefit from external motor supports to promote arousal and alertness and from environmental modulation to decrease unnecessary, overloading, or distracting stimuli—thereby enabling the infants to optimize their functional capabilities.

Self-Regulation

Self-regulation is the culmination of the neurobehavioral developmental process. Neurobehavioral stability and control of the underlying subsystems—physiologic (autonomic), motor (neuromotor), state of arousal, and attentional/interactional—undergo progressive intrauterine refinement, with self-regulation, the fifth subsystem, as the end product (Als, 1986). It gives an infant the capacity to modulate his or her own systems as necessary to engage in infant occupations; to interact more effectively with human and nonhuman stimuli; to inhibit or withdraw from stressful stimuli; to maintain a state of homeostasis when confronted with stress; and to self-calm, self-console, or reorganize when stress exceeds his or her capacity to self-regulate. Self-regulation in early infancy involves the infant's ability to influence his or her pattern of arousal throughout the day (Rothbart, Derryberry, & Posner, 1994). Self-regulation implies that the infant is able to achieve a healthy balance in states of arousal (e.g., alertness versus sleep) and in activity and exploration (e.g., approaching and withdrawing appropriately from stimulation). Sometimes self-regulation is accomplished independently, and sometimes the infant requires assistance. Caregivers learn from experience to use only as many comforting strategies as necessary for their infants to regain a calm, alert, or sleeping state and/or to modify sensory aspects of the environment to make it easier for infants to modulate their own responses (i.e., regulate themselves).

Self-regulation is related to the construct of temperament. The developmental literature defines these two constructs in a number of ways, depending on the age range of the infants or children to whom the term *temperament* is being applied. Temperament refers to constitutionally based individual differences in emotion, motivation, and attention (Bates, 1987) that sometimes translate into individual variation in reactions or reactivity to sensory experiences. Reactivity is the somatic, endocrine, and/or autonomic nervous system response to sensory events (Rothbart et al., 1994). It depends on the individual sensory threshold (e.g., how much is too much for the particular infant), the type of event (e.g., touch, movement, sights, sounds, or combinations), and the timing of the event.

A well-regulated infant may interrupt an interaction containing a stimulus that he or she perceives as too stressful or exceeding his or her self-regulation capacities in various ways. For example, an infant with good coping skills who is in a brightly lit room may cover his or her face to withdraw from the stress of the lights. Similarly, an infant who is not ready for visual interaction may shift to a lower state of arousal or may avert eye contact to avoid interaction. Such behaviors are called *self-regulation coping signals*. Self-regulation also enables an infant to interact with stimuli that he or she interprets as pleasant or non-stressful. An example is the infant who immediately gazes at his or her caregiver's face and makes sucking movements when enticed by the caregiver to engage in social interaction. The latter behaviors are called *self-regulation approach signals*.

Approach and coping signals give caregivers an indication of the infant's self-regulation status at any point in time. Approach signals imply that the stimulus is not stressful and, therefore, that the infant is ready for the interaction. In contrast, coping signals imply that the stimulus is perceived as stressful but that the infant has the capacity to tolerate or decrease the impact of the resulting stress. Although both approach and coping behaviors suggest that an infant is coping well with the situation, the caregiver must immediately recognize coping signals because they indicate an increasingly stressful interaction. Coping signals alert caregivers that the stress of the stimulus could reach or exceed the infant's self-regulation limits. Table 9 presents examples of self-regulation behaviors.

Self-regulation decreases the infant's degree of dependence on external environmental support. Although individual variability exists, by term age, most healthy infants have achieved sufficient self-regulation to perform a wide range of tasks and activities characteristic of newborns (see Chapter 1).

Specific Sensory Abilities

A variety of rudimentary sensory processing abilities have been identified in newborns. Sensory skill assessment examines another functional aspect of the nervous system and is a major component of most neonatal assessments. The following subsections describe the sensory abilities of healthy newborns and the influence of sensory abilities on infants' interactive skills and participation in age-appropriate occupations.

Tactile Responsiveness and Discrimination

The skin is perhaps the most important avenue for interaction between caregivers and newborns. The tactile system is one of the first sensory systems to develop and

Table 9. Approach and coping self-regulation signals

Approach signals	Coping signals
Smiling	Averting gaze
Mouthing	Leg bracing
Cooing	Hand-on-face movement
Relaxed limbs	Sucking
Minimal motor activity	Hand or foot clasp
Smooth body movements	Grasping
Alertness	Fisting
Soft, relaxed facial expression	Assuming a flexor posture
	Bracing body against crib (searching for boundaries)
	Shifting to lower states of arousal (drowsy or light sleep)

Sources: Als (1986); Als et al. (1982a, 1982b).

is the most mature sensory system at birth (Gottfried, 1990). Intrapair tactile responses have been documented in twin fetuses as early as 8–10 weeks after conception (Piontelli et al., 1997). By term age, most reflexes are elicited by tactile input, with tactile awareness and discrimination emerging first in the body regions involved in exploratory functions (e.g., the mouth, the hands). Rooting, a fully functional tactile reflex in most full-term newborns, reflects tactile system maturity and responsiveness around the mouth: Tactile stimulation of the corner of the mouth triggers a reflex, whereby the infant turns his or her head and opens the mouth in search of the source of the feeding. The palmar grasp reflex is evidence of tactile sensitivity in the hand. Palmar grasping may serve as a way for infants to "connect" with young siblings and other caregivers. It is interesting to note that in newborns, the top of the head and the shoulders are much less sensitive, perhaps as a natural mechanism to protect infants from the strong tactile input of the birthing process (Birren, Kinney, Schaie, & Woodruff, 1981).

Avoidant tactile responses (turning away from the stimulus) prevail in utero, whereas approach reactions (turning toward the stimulus) to tactile stimuli predominate by term age, provided that the stimulus is not stressful (Prechtl et al., 1979). Avoidant and approach responses serve as procuring signals by which infants communicate to caregivers the way that tactile stimuli are being tolerated. Avoidant reactions in newborns may discourage social interaction if caregivers interpret the reactions as disinterest or rejection (Biringen & Robinson, 1991). Avoidant reactions to painful or stressful stimuli, however, are appropriate and tend not to be regarded as rejection. Approach reactions, in contrast, may facilitate ongoing contact with a comforting tactile stimulus and potentially foster caregiver–infant interaction. For example, physical contact (human touch) and swaddling (nonhuman input) are known to promote soothing, consoling, and cuddling in newborns (Candilis-Huisman & Bydlowski, 1997; Hubin-Gayte, 1997). Contact with the caregiver increases when the infant cuddles, perpetuating the calming response for as long as the infant tolerates the tactile input. Cuddling gives a feeling of comfort to caregivers and reassures them of their infant's well-being. Thus, cuddling may encourage caregiver–infant interaction through the tactile system.

Animal and human studies suggest that normal functioning of the tactile system and appropriate tactile stimulation are extremely important for the infant's emotional development and for development of healthy caregiver–infant interaction (Gottfried, 1990). Human touch is also believed to organize the infant's development and learning (Gottfried, 1990). The effects of nonhuman touch are less clear.

Olfactory Responses

Olfactory abilities have been studied minimally in infants. The few studies available suggest that newborns are capable of perceiving and processing olfactory stimuli, may discriminate between certain olfactory stimuli, and show preference for certain smells. In a classic olfaction study, MacFarlane (1975) found that breast-feeding infants turned their head more frequently toward a nursing pad impregnated with their mother's milk than toward a similar pad impregnated with breast milk from another woman. Schaal et al. (1998) found that 3-day-old breast- or bottle-fed infants showed preference for the smell of familiar amniotic fluid than nonfamiliar amniotic fluid or a control stimulus. Marlier et al. (1997) found that in the first 3 days of life, breast-fed infants had no olfactory preference for either amniotic fluid or maternal milk. A significant preference for maternal milk appeared on days 4 and 5, suggesting that development of olfactory preference requires experience with the stimulus. An alternative explanation proposed for the infant's milk preference on the later days was a change in the quality and taste of the breast milk over the studied period—that is, it becomes a body fluid considerably different from amniotic fluid. Olfactory preference for breast milk may be a natural survival mechanism to enhance feeding success. This type of discrimination suggests sophisticated olfactory sensory processing.

Anecdotal reports suggest that many infants, especially those with nervous system immaturity, tend to exhibit avoidance reactions to strong scents. Although these observations have not been scientifically documented, as a preventive measure, NICU personnel should avoid the use of strong perfumes when working with sensitive infants.

Vestibular Responses

The vestibular system is a phylogenetically older system located in the lower, central regions of the brain. It is considerably mature, both structurally and functionally, in a full-term neonate. The fetus is exposed to almost constant vestibular input in utero from either fetal or maternal movements. Oculomotor responses to vestibular input (e.g., nystagmus, doll's eye reflex) are present and often tested at birth to determine vestibular system maturity (Brazelton & Nugent, 1995). The vestibular influence on a newborn's arousal is well known: Gentle, rhythmic rocking is soothing, whereas fast, arrhythmic movements increase overall activity and agitation. For ages, mothers have used slow rocking to calm and comfort their infants and help them fall asleep. Passively rocked preterm and near-term infants have been found to synchronize their breathing with the rocking rhythm (Sammon & Darnall, 1994). The regularity of respiration induced by rocking may be part of a more generalized calming effect of vestibular stimulation.

Immaturity of other systems may preclude full expression of an infant's vestibular capabilities. An example of this is a newborn's inability to sustain antigravity head righting. Although righting efforts are present, the weight of the head and lack of extensor tone prevent head raising.

Taste Discrimination and Preferences

Most development of the gustatory system occurs postnatally. Fetuses are known to swallow amniotic fluid throughout the pregnancy, but taste discrimination in utero is not clear. Anecdotal evidence suggests that some pregnant women report experiencing fetal movement alterations depending on the type of food ingested, suggesting some degree of taste discrimination. (An alternative interpretation is that the fetus physically responds to certain substances ingested by the mother, such as sugar or caffeine.) For years, it has been known that full-term newborns have certain taste preferences. Sweet-tasting liquids appear to be the most preferred and most organizing for newborns. Studies have shown that newborns prefer sweet water to plain or sour water and milk to plain water (Desor, 1973). Sucrose has been found to reduce crying and facilitate hand-to-mouth activity (Blass, 1997; Graillon, Barr, Young, Wright, & Hendricks, 1997); it also increases the strength and frequency of sucking (Maone, Mattes, Bernbaum, & Beauchamp, 1990). Sucrose, in association with sucking, has also been found to inhibit crying and distress in newborns, during and after painful procedures (Barr et al., 1994). Studies with methadone- and cocaine-exposed infants suggest that sucrose responses are mediated centrally by endogenous opioids (Blass & Ciaramitaro, 1994; Maone, Mattes, & Beauchamp, 1992). The taste of milk has also been found to reduce crying (Blass, 1997). Discrimination of bitter and salty tastes is less clear, but by term age, discrimination for these tastes appears to be less developed than for other taste stimuli (Beauchamp, Cowart, Mennella, & Marsh, 1994; Desor, 1975; Kajiura, Cowart, & Beauchamp, 1992). The gustatory system, nevertheless, is far from being fully developed in neonates.

Visual Sensory Processing

The visual system develops later in the fetus, partly because of the limited intrauterine visual experiences. Contrary to previous beliefs, evidence suggests that newborns possess somewhat refined and organized visual sensory processing abilities (Slater & Kirby, 1998). They are able to orient to, fixate on, and scan a stimulus as well as to visually track a moving object (Muir, Humphrey, & Humphrey, 1994). In addition, they can discriminate between different visual images, demonstrating visual preference for certain images, especially the human face (Slater & Kirby, 1998). Visual pattern recognition is more limited in the newborn but increases rapidly after the first month of life (Muir et al., 1994). Full-term neonates can fixate for as long as 10 seconds and may reestablish eye contact with a stimulus within 1–1$^{1}/_{2}$ seconds after losing eye contact (Dayton & Jones, 1964). Other visual preferences of neonates include the following:

- High-contrast (black-and-white) images over monochromatic images (Fantz & Miranda, 1975)
- Detailed, complex patterns over simple patterns or plain stimuli (Morante, Dubowitz, Leverne, & Dubowitz, 1982)
- Large designs over small designs (Hainline & Lemerise, 1982)
- Normal facial figures over scrambled facial figures (Fantz, 1973)

Skoczenski and Norcia (1998) found that visual contrast sensitivity in newborns is affected by "neural noise" that is nine times higher than in adults. Contrast sensitivity and visual discrimination abilities improve proportionately to the decrease in neural noise in early infancy. Improved visual discrimination increases the complexity of visual interactions.

Auditory Responsiveness and Discrimination

Healthy newborns are able to hear, recognize, and respond to an auditory stimulus by opening their eyes for alerting, startling, or turning their eyes or head to localize the stimulus. The auditory discrimination abilities of full-term neonates have been demonstrated through numerous studies. Readiness for auditory discrimination begins in utero as the fetus is exposed to sounds amplified within the fluid-filled amniotic chamber. The earliest documented auditory discrimination abilities show an alteration in the responses of 30- to 35-week PCA fetuses when presented with a change in an auditory signal composed of repetitive vowel sounds (Cheour-Luhtanen et al., 1996). Toward the end of the pregnancy, many women often report that listening to fast, heavy-percussion music tends to agitate their fetus, whereas listening to classical or soft music tends to have the opposite effect. Fetuses must perceive the different qualities of the stimuli to respond differently. By term age, infants have had considerable familiarity and discriminatory opportunities with a wide range and variety of auditory input, especially heartbeat, other intrauterine sounds, and their mother's voice. Full-term infants can distinguish between certain auditory stimuli and respond differently according to the properties of the stimulus and familiarity with the sound. One of the most striking auditory discrimination abilities of newborns is their preference for female voices (Ecklund-Flores & Turkewitz, 1996). The exact time at which these sophisticated forms of discrimination emerge is not known.

Auditory stimulation is strongly associated with arousal. Exposure to continuous noise (e.g., white noise, the humming noise of mechanical equipment) has been found to decrease arousal. Neonates manifest auditory-induced decrease in arousal by decreased heart rate and motor activity (Brackbill, 1970; Schmidt, Rose, & Bridger, 1980), deeper and more regular sleep, and decreased crying (Murray & Campbell, 1971). The effects of intermittent noise are less clear. Depending on the properties of the stimulus, intermittent noise may arouse (Brackbill, 1970), calm (Field, Dempsey, Hatch, Ting, & Clifton, 1979), or not alter the state of arousal of a newborn. The sound of a heartbeat is a specialized type of intermittent auditory stimulus that has powerful calming and soothing effects on most newborns (Murray & Campbell, 1971). Familiarity with the heartbeat stimulus and the comfort associated with prior exposure to its sound are believed to induce calming, although the common reaction to most other intermittent auditory input is increased arousal. Another impressive auditory capacity of healthy newborns is their ability to rotate their head to localize an auditory stimulus presented to one side (Ecklund-Flores & Turkewitz, 1996). Auditory localization is a complex behavioral response that requires integration of auditory, motor, and visual abilities. Most neonatal assessments contain elements of sound localization as a measure of the infant's nervous system integrity and maturity. Auditory processing and discrimination abilities improve in infancy and childhood as primary auditory pathways and central processes mature (Werner, 1996).

Neonatal Occupations

Well-regulated infants are able to participate in many expected newborn activities, or occupations, such as procuring, feeding, socially interacting, and exploring (refer to Chapters 1 and 3). However, individual variability exists in neurobehavioral control at birth and in the extent to which healthy full-term infants can participate in neonatal occupations or activities. As discussed in Chapter 1 and previously in this chapter, contextual elements may support or interfere with an infant's occupational performance, regardless of his or her underlying capacities. An infant may have underlying strengths in some areas that enable him or her to engage in some forms of occupations but not in others, and the environment may support engagement in some occupations and not in others. Thus, the inability to participate in certain newborn occupations is not necessarily an indication of neurobehavioral immaturity or that the infant is not healthy.

Clinical observation suggests that participation in neonatal occupations within a supportive environmental context is a progressive process consistent with self-regulation (i.e., achieving control and stability of the various subsystems). Figure 20 shows the developmental progression of procuring, exploring, feeding, and interactive abilities in relation to the development of self-regulation in the various subsystems. The following discussion explores the interrelation of these factors.

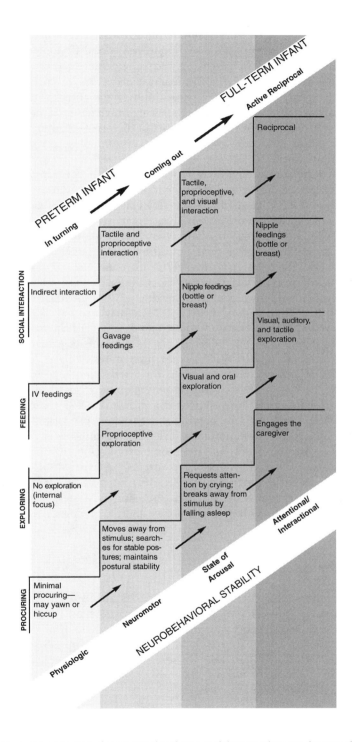

Figure 20. Developmental progression of occupational performance abilities in infants as a function of self-regulation.

Infants who possess only physiologic stability—with no neuromotor, state, or interactional stability—have very limited ability to engage in neonatal occupations. They will be in an in-turning phase of neurobehavioral development (see Chapter 3), with all energy directed inward as they strive to achieve increased physiologic and motor control (Gorski et al., 1979). Minimal procuring is possible; however, caregivers may discern the need for comforting, repositioning, and increased physiologic support through the infants' motor behavior (e.g., flailing movements of the extremities, facial grimacing) or through physiologic indicators of distress (e.g., apnea and bradycardia, oxygen desaturation, frequent yawning or hiccuping). These infants cannot explore, interact, or nipple feed.

As physiologic control and neuromotor stability improve, infants begin to enter the coming-out phase, during which brief periods of interaction with the environment become possible (Gorski et al., 1979; see also Chapter 3). Infants gain the ability to procure by moving away from a stimulus, engaging in tactile and proprioceptive exploration by rubbing against bedding, "searching" for physical boundaries (stable postures), grasping and sucking, and exhibiting a wider range of facial expressions. During this phase, infants are more likely to maintain a stable posture at rest when provided with appropriate boundaries. When infants in this phase must be fed by gavage because of inability to coordinate sucking and swallowing, they seek and benefit from opportunities to suck nonnutritively. They may also have very brief periods of visual alertness and may respond to voices and sounds with increased alertness.

Increasing stability of state of arousal enables infants to procure through crying, breaking away from a stimulus by shifting to lower states, initiating active oral feeding, and adding visual and oral exploration to their emerging repertoire of exploration skills. This stage initiates the transition from the coming out to the active reciprocity phases of neurobehavioral development (Gorski et al., 1979; see also Chapter 3). Interactional/attentional stability heightens the infants' procuring abilities, engaging the caregiver more directly in interactive exchanges. Simple visual, auditory, proprioceptive, tactile, vestibular, and minimal motor exploration are now possible.

Most healthy full-term infants have reached at least the coming out stage at birth, provided that the environmental context supports their efforts. Some have even reached active reciprocity at birth. Prematurity, illness, sedation, or lack of environmental support may limit a newborn's abilities to engage in neonatal occupations.

SICK FULL-TERM INFANTS

Medical instability can affect the neonatal abilities of full-term infants who are sick. Although most of these infants may have adequate organ maturity and structural development, the disease process or the medical management of their condition may render them functionally unable to make full use of their capabilities. Regardless of the structural maturity of their body systems, medically unstable infants may revert to an immature, internally focused, in-turning mode as they struggle to maintain physiologic stability during their illness.

Transient Medical Issues

At birth, full-term infants may have medical issues that require brief NICU admission until their condition is stabilized. Common neonatal transient conditions include exposure to minor maternal infection, minor respiratory distress or tachypnea, moderately low Apgar scores at 1 and 5 minutes, temporary temperature regulation problems, transient metabolic disorders, neonatal hyperbilirubinemia, or sedation. Such conditions usually resolve within 1–2 days and typically have no long-term consequences. In these cases, problems with neonatal abilities are almost always temporary and unlikely to require developmental intervention. During the initial distress phase, these infants should be allowed to recover, postponing engagement in neonatal occupations until their condition has stabilized. They might benefit from external support such as motor containment (e.g., swaddling, using rolled blankets or Bendy Bumpers from Children's Medical Ventures, http://www.childmed.com/products) and modulation of environmental stimuli to decrease physiologic stress. Transient feeding problems may occur but usually resolve by the time that IV feedings are discontinued. Infants with transient conditions may be referred for therapy, depending on the type and duration of their presenting problems, to promote achievement of stability. An infant will probably be referred for therapy if a need for developmental follow-up is identified. The therapist may also be asked to provide consultation regarding feeding, positioning, or environmental modulation while the infant is in the NICU, and to collaborate with the developmental team on discharge planning and family recommendations.

Serious or Prolonged Medical Issues

The functional capabilities of seriously ill full-term newborns are usually compromised by the medical or physiologic instability that results from neonatal disorders. These infants generally require longer NICU admission, closer medical and nursing management, and possible developmental monitoring. Infants with certain conditions may be too sick to engage in traditional neonatal activities: perinatal asphyxia; meconium aspiration; cardiorespiratory disorders; congenital anomalies involving major organs (e.g., heart, liver, intestines); brain or chromosomal abnormalities; moderate to severe metabolic disorders; or conditions resulting from maternal factors such as preeclampsia, severe diabetes, or placental insufficiency. By term age, these infants should be ready to engage in externally focused occupations such as procuring, exploring, socially interacting, and feeding; however, their need to maintain or regain physiologic and motor stability instead focuses them internally, thus limiting their neonatal abilities (Gorski et al., 1979). The interaction among medication, medical instability, life-support measures, the disease process, and management of the disease may result in regression to more primitive levels of neurobehavioral functioning (see Figure 20). As factors related to illness begin to affect an infant's neurobehavioral homeostasis, he or she becomes less able to self-regulate and more likely to become dangerously stressed when exposed to sensory stimuli.

Sick or healthy infants who experience stress when exposed to a sensory stimulus begin to display characteristic behaviors that signal the extent to which the interaction causes neurobehavioral stability. These behaviors are called *stress reactions*. Stress reactions vary in severity according to the degree of stress, the status of the infant's neurobehavioral system, and the subsystems being affected. The most subtle stress reactions are those affecting the state or the attentional subsystems. These reactions are usually observed in infants who have adequate physiologic and motoric stability but insufficient energy and alertness to tolerate caregiving and social interaction. Although state-related or attentional stress reactions interfere with an infant's participation in neonatal activities, they are not likely to compromise the infant's well-being.

Motor stress reactions are more disruptive than state-related stress reactions. They increase the infant's energy consumption, potentially affecting weight gain and growth, and may alter the infant's physiologic homeostasis. Prolonged stress reactions eventually compromise the infant's physiologic integrity and stability. Lack of physiologic stability is potentially life threatening and should be avoided by all possible means. Physiologic stress reactions are the most severe and the most likely to affect the infant's well-being. Table 10 lists common stress reactions, beginning with the more subtle attentional reactions and ending with the more life-threatening physiologic reactions.

Infants who are physiologically unstable are usually incapable of engaging in social interactions without a further loss of physiologic stability. Such interactions must be modulated to the individual tolerance of each infant to avoid potentially life-threatening consequences. For example, an infant who is sick and physiologically unstable may experience a decrease in oxygen saturation as a result of sustained interaction efforts. If the interaction demands continue, the infant's loss of stability may progress to a more serious stress reaction, such as an apneic episode or bradycardia. This stress reaction may be avoided if the interaction is minimized, paused, or stopped altogether, based on the infant's tolerance.

Although stress reactions are discussed in this section about sick full-term infants, it should be noted that stress reactions can appear in any preterm or full-term infant who is unable to self-regulate when exposed to an environmental stimulus. Stress reactions occur more frequently in preterms and in sick infants.

Table 10.   Types of neurobehavorial instability and potential stress reactions

Types of instability	Possible stress reactions
Attentional/interactional	Inability to integrate social interaction with other sensory input
	Avoidance of social interaction
State	Gaze aversion or gaze locking
	Glassy eyes
	Irritability
	Lack of alertness
	Diffuse sleep states
Motor	"Sitting on air"
	Saluting
	Finger splaying
	Squirming
	Frantic, disorganized movements
	Trunk arching
	Gaping facial expression (low tone, open mouth)
	Generalized hypotonia
Physiologic (autonomic)	Yawning
	Burping
	Hiccuping
	Gagging
	Spitting up
	Sneezing
	Color changes (paleness, mottling, flushing, cyanosis)
	Changes in vital signs (heart rate, respiration rate, oxygen saturation)

Sick infants, especially those experiencing stress reactions, may benefit from direct developmental intervention throughout their NICU stay. A medically fragile infant's ability to conserve energy and preserve physiologic homeostasis may be enhanced thorough stress-reduction environmental modulation techniques (e.g., dimming the lights, lowering ambient noise, decreasing activity level, planning the timing of care), proper positioning, and limited situations that demand interaction. The infant's performance abilities will improve as physiologic stability and medical status improve. Proprioceptive exploration and motor procuring efforts will emerge first, followed by more concerted procuring, visual and oral exploration, and oral feeding. (Although oral feeding is demanding for many infants, its importance supersedes other infant occupations.) Social interaction is a more demanding task that requires a greater degree of attentional stability. Self-regulation and nonstressful participation in social interaction will become possible only when the infant's condition has almost fully stabilized.

Neonatal illness may also affect the development of motor and sensory processing abilities. A prolonged illness or compromised central nervous system may disrupt or delay spontaneous development of sensory processing and sensorimotor skills. For example, a sick infant's struggle to achieve or maintain physiologic or medical well being may thwart his or her efforts to engage in the exploratory play likely to promote sensory processing skill development. A longer illness may have a more permanent effect on sensory processing development unless appropriate intervention is provided. The application of developmentally supportive care and neurodevelopmental and sensory integration principles in the recovery phase, when physiologic stability has improved, may enhance the infant's sensorimotor and sensory processing abilities. Proper positioning is vital to optimize the infant's short- and long-term participation in age-appropriate, family-expected occupations.

Careful observation of an infant's abilities during the first few days of life is essential for the detection of less obvious conditions. For example, a progressive deterioration in physiologic status, crying pitch, or sucking and swallowing patterns can be early signs of certain congenital cardiovascular conditions (Kessel & Ward, 1998). Infants with brain alterations or malformations may present with less variable postures, a characteristic extended posture, poor behavioral state organization, excessive wakefulness, and abnormal quality and poor repertoire of movement (Ferrari et al., 1997). These infants will also exhibit limited ability to engage in neonatal occupations. Therapists who are sensitive to behavioral observations can play an important role in the early identification of conditions that are difficult to identify.

Some conditions, particularly those involving the central nervous system, tend to cause developmental sequelae that may interfere with functional performance. In these cases, infants may present with irritability, sensory defensiveness (especially oral), abnormal posturing, decreased or increased muscle tone, jerky movements, the inability to fixate on or follow visual stimuli, dysfunctional interactions with caregivers, dysfunctional feeding, or delayed developmental milestones. Once the infants' physiologic status is stabilized, traditional developmental early intervention is indicated to optimize development of performance abilities.

CONCLUSION

The developmental capabilities of full-term infants are remarkable. By the time that most full-term infants are born, they are capable of engaging in a wide array of occupations to satisfy their caregivers' expectations. Sick newborns, in contrast, may be less able to engage in their families' expected occupations because illness may limit optimal use of their capabilities. A thorough understanding of the capabilities of healthy newborns, along with a general knowledge of the impact of illness on a newborn's capabilities, is essential for helping sick infants to engage in occupations throughout their recovery process.

9

Developmental Capabilities of Preterm and Low Birth Weight Infants

<hr>

OVERVIEW

This chapter presents a synopsis of the functional abilities of infants born prematurely. It begins by noting that the infants' performance abilities are strongly dependent on their GA and age from birth, as well as their birth weight and neurobehavioral stability (see Chapters 7 and 8). Premature infants have extrauterine experiences that influence their development in ways that differ from those of healthy full-term infants. As a result, by the time many premature infants reach term age, their functional performance varies considerably from that of healthy newborns who are born after a complete pregnancy. The functional performance of healthier, more mature, and stable preterm infants ultimately closely resembles that of healthy full-term infants.

Whenever possible, this chapter compares development of the functional capabilities of premature infants across the various neurobehavioral subsystems with the development of healthy full-term infants (as described in Chapter 8). Physiologic processes reviewed include cardiorespiratory functions, crying, temperature regulation, and the effect of the environment on physiologic functioning. Areas of neuromotor control include reflex development, muscle tone, and motor activity. Other areas include states of arousal, interactional/attentional development, self-regulation, and specific sensory abilities. Particular emphasis is given to development of pain sensitivity and multimodal sensory integration.

OBJECTIVES

- Identify the factors that may influence the development of functional capabilities of premature infants
- Understand how an unsupportive environment, an illness, and/or medical or nursing interventions may compromise the well-being of small or premature infants
- Recognize the impact that the premature infants' early exposure to extrauterine experiences may have on the infants' neonatal development and functional performance by the time they reach term age
- Describe intrauterine development of cardiorespiratory functioning, crying, and temperature regulation and functional differences observed in premature infants reaching term age

- Describe the developmental progression of neuromotor control and states of arousal in utero and in infants born prematurely
- Identify the developmental stages of interactive capabilities and the underlying capabilities infants need to have to engage in attentional and interactive activities
- Describe the development of self-regulation and sensory functions in premature infants

CAPABILITIES OF PRETERM OR LOW BIRTH WEIGHT INFANTS

The neonatal capabilities of infants born prematurely depend on multiple factors. The factors that most influence performance of preterm infants who are otherwise healthy and exposed to a supportive environment are GA, age from birth, and birth weight. These three factors affect an infant's performance abilities because of their direct association with neurobehavioral stability. Healthy preterm infants of higher weight and GA tend to be more mature and stable and, as a result, have more advanced neonatal abilities than the more premature, lower birth weight, smaller infants. Factors such as medical and nursing procedures, environmental stress, illness, sedation, side effects of medication, and an unsupportive environment further compromise premature infants' limited self-regulation and performance abilities regardless of GA or weight, but these factors affect smaller infants more seriously.

The effect of extrauterine experiences on the development of preterm infants complicates the discussion of their functional capabilities. A prematurely born infant whose fetal development is completed outside the womb exhibits different functional capabilities than a normally developing fetus of comparable GA. The NICU environment exposes the infant to overwhelming stimulation of the less mature distance sensory receptors (i.e., hearing and vision) while limiting exposure to and affecting the quality of stimulation of the more mature contact sensory receptors (tactile and vestibular) (White-Traut, Nelson, Burns, & Cunningham, 1994). The capabilities of preterm infants at term age differ considerably from those of the healthy full-term newborns in several areas. For example, a preterm infant who was born at 28 weeks GA and is reaching term age will likely be able to visually track a caregiver's movements more closely than a newborn full-term infant. This preterm infant may respond negatively to being touched if he or she has experienced frequent disruptive or painful tactile experiences, whereas the newborn full-term infant without disruptive tactile experiences may respond positively to being touched. The discussion that follows focuses primarily on intrauterine development, with reference to postnatal fetal development whenever available and appropriate.

Physiologic Processes

Cardiorespiratory Functioning

Perinatal cardiorespiratory responses of healthy preterm infants born close to term age (after 36 weeks GA) are comparable to those of full-term infants, although responses may be slightly attenuated. Healthy preterm infants with minor immaturity of respiratory control at birth may present with transient respiratory distress requiring short-term assistance with their initial respirations (e.g., bagging, oxygen blown on face). Within a few minutes, healthy infants should begin to breathe unassisted. Preterm infants with marked lung immaturity and/or serious illness usually require intubation and mechanical ventilation within a few minutes from birth.

The respiratory activity of preterm infants differs considerably from that of full-term infants. Preterm infants who are able to breathe on their own often exhibit irregular breathing patterns, with frequent respiratory pauses and higher respiratory rates than those of full-term infants (Avery, 1987). Periodic breathing (i.e., respiratory bouts interrupted by somewhat regular pauses) is common, presenting in 30% of infants born prematurely (Cochran, 1997). If respiratory pauses are brief and sporadic, infants may receive adequate oxygen from room air without ventilator support. More serious periodic breathing may require medical intervention and ventilatory support (see Chapter 6).

Apnea, or respiratory pauses lasting more than 20 seconds, may interfere with occupational performance in preterms. Apnea of prematurity occurs most often in infants younger than 34 weeks GA and weighing less than 1,800 g, presenting in 50%–65% of preterm infants (Gomella, 1999). Apnea may present with bradycardia. Apnea spells are longer and occur more frequently in preterms during quiet sleep and at higher environmental temperatures (Bader, Tirosh, Hodgins, Abend, & Cohen, 1998). Healthy preterm infants often recover spontaneously from apneic spells, but stimulation may be necessary to reinitiate breathing during more serious episodes. Mild, short-duration, sporadic apnea is considered normal in preterm infants and usually does not interfere with their functioning. Prolonged or frequent apnea and apnea accompanied by bradycardia or requiring stimulation are considered serious respiratory problems that interfere with engagement in neonatal occupations and require medical attention (see Chapter 6). Infants with these conditions are not considered healthy preterms and should not be encouraged to engage in interactive exchanges during their periods of instability.

Respiration rate remains virtually unchanged in utero between 31 and 38 weeks. Healthy preterm newborns who need to take over breathing functions while their lungs have not fully matured compensate by accelerating the rate of their breathing pattern. Consequently, preterm and VLBW infants approaching term age usually have higher respiratory rates than their full-term counterparts (Prechtl et al., 1979). Respirations become slower and more regular, and respiratory pauses decrease in number and duration as the lungs mature. Regular respirations are a prerequisite for the achievement of quiet alertness (Als et al., 1982b), for coordination of breathing with sucking and swallowing (Daniels, Devlieger, Minami, Eggermont, & Casaer, 1990), and, ultimately, for engaging in neonatal occupations.

Preterm infants in general have higher and more irregular heart rates than full-term infants. Their heart rate fluctuates between 120 and 160 BPM. Fluctuations are usually associated with sleep and activity. That is, they are lower and more regular during deep sleep, higher and more irregular during light sleep, and higher and somewhat regular during quiet alertness. Their overall higher heart rate is in part attributed to increased time in light sleep. Cardiac neuroregulatory control is stable in healthy preterms, and a certain amount of heart rate variability is a normal feature of the neuroregulatory process. Important to this process is the function of the vagus nerve, which reduces the heart rate and restores it to baseline after an increase (e.g., after a stressful procedure). When the vagal response is working appropriately, there is reciprocity of action between parasympathetic and sympathetic nervous systems, and homeostasis is maintained. However, the immature nervous systems of many preterm infants do not provide for efficient maintenance of homeostasis, and there is excessive heart rate variability, which is associated with increased perinatal risk (DiPietro, Caughy, Cusson, & Fox, 1994). The shift from fetal to adult circulation may be slower than in full-term infants and may be accompanied by a minor asymptomatic delay in the closure of the ductus arteriosus. Vasomotor responses resemble those of full-term infants but are more attenuated and immature (Jahnukainen, van Ravenswaaij-Arts, Jalonen, & Valimaki, 1993). Prolonged delay or failure of closure of the ductus arteriosus is a serious condition that usually requires surgical intervention.

Crying

Crying is one of the most effective procuring strategies available to newborns. As previously discussed, perinatal crying may help in lung expansion at the onset of respiration. Many preterm infants either do not cry at birth or have weak crying and sighing. Lack of crying is associated with the degree of prematurity. Crying efforts without an audible sound can result from nervous system immaturity, low muscle tone and strength, sedation, intubation, or damage to the vocal cords as a result of intubation. Preterm infants also may exhibit less frequent and less intense crying than full-term infants, which is usually associated with preterm infants' overall strength, lung maturity, and limited ability to achieve higher states of arousal. However, the duration of preterm infant crying does correlate with pain profile scores (Johnston, Sherrard, et al., 1999), suggesting that crying should be factored into such scores in the NICU. By term age, the crying patterns of healthy preterm infants usually resemble those of full-term newborns, regardless of the preterm infants' GA at birth (Barr, Chen, Hopkins, & Westra, 1996). Even infants with diagnosed respiratory and neurological problems have cry characteristics that resemble those of healthy newborns (Robb & Goberman, 1997), suggesting that the acoustical and temporal features of the newborn cry are shared by both healthy and at-risk newborns.

Temperature Regulation

As discussed in Chapter 5, poor temperature regulation is an important indicator of lack of physiologic stability in preterm infants and is one of the most serious problems they face at birth (Gomella, 1999). Most preterm infants must be exposed to a neutral thermal environment immediately after birth. Gomella defined a neutral thermal environment as the "external temperature range within which metabolic rate and hence oxygen consumption are at a minimum while the infant maintains a normal body temperature" (1999, p. 38). The neutral environmental temperature must be determined individually for each infant according to his or her GA and body weight. Younger, smaller infants have more immature thermoregulatory abilities and, thus, require higher environmental temperatures than older, heavier infants. Air drafts cause skin cooling and evaporative heat loss and must be avoided when working with infants who have poor thermoregulation. Readers are referred to Chapter 5 for a detailed explanation of the different types of heat loss experienced by preterm infants. Thermoregulatory capabilities improve as the infants grow and become more physiologically stable.

Effect of the Environment on Physiologic Functioning

Preterm newborns are more susceptible to environmental influences, have more immature physiologic subsystems, have poorer self-regulation abilities, and, thus, need more environmental support than healthy full-term newborns. Contextual supports that enhance their physiologic stability can optimize their overall functioning. For example, providing motor containment through boundaries reduces the infants' motor activity and conserves energy for physiologic stability and growth. Extreme caution must be taken, however, to avoid misinterpreting the infants' improved self-regulation under external assistance as real readiness for interaction. Although it is possible to prolong interactions in infants who are still somewhat physiologically unstable by providing external support, this may come at a high physiologic cost (Lester, Boukydis, & LaGasse, 1996). Conversely, an environment that does not offer the contextual support that these preterm infants need would perpetuate their loss of stability and also threaten their well-being.

Approach signals observed in a preterm infant who is exposed to a sensory stimulus indicate that the infant is physiologically stable, that the infant is tolerating the stimulus well, and that the interaction may continue. Approach signals include smiling, cooing, quiet alertness, or active alertness with smooth body movements (see Figure 21; also refer to Chapter 8). These signals are seen in the healthier, larger, or older preterm infants. Self-regulatory coping signals imply that an infant has perceived stress and is becoming somewhat unstable but is still capable of responding adaptively to the stimulus to reestablish or prevent further loss of stability. Coping signals include taking the hand to the mouth, touching the face with the hand, searching for boundaries, and tucking into a flexion position (see Chapter 8). Coping signals are seen in slightly less stable infants or in infants experiencing an increasingly intense or prolonged stimulus (see Figure 22). They serve as a warning that additional exposure to the stimulus could exceed stress tolerance, jeopardizing homeostasis. When the

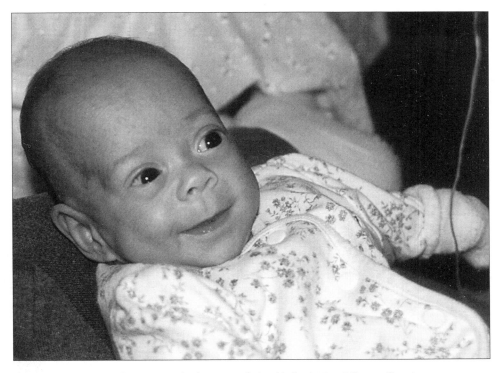

Figure 21.   This infant's smile is an example of an approach signal indicating her ability to self-regulate.

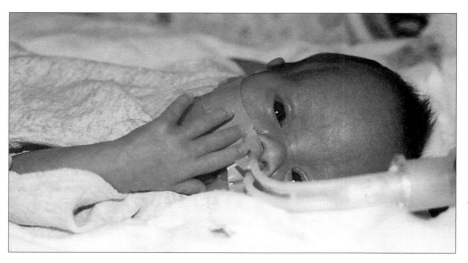

Figure 22. Bringing the hand to the mouth suggests that this infant is coping with environmental stimuli. He may need a break to regain neurobehavioral stability if the stressful stimuli persist.

stimulus is reaching an infant's self-regulation and stress tolerance limits, the attentional/interactional subsystem becomes unstable and stress reactions begin to appear. Attentional or interactional stress reactions such as gaze aversion may appear first, followed by state changes (e.g., shifting to lower states, displaying restlessness or agitation) (Figure 23), motor stress (leg extension, finger splaying, trunk arching) (see Figure 24), and, eventually, physiologic stress reactions (e.g., spitting up, voiding) as stress intensifies (Als, 1986) (see Chapter 8).

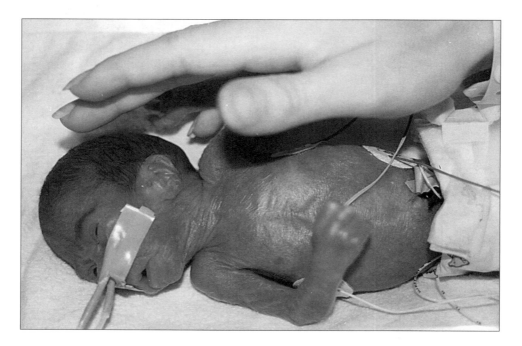

Figure 23. Facial grimacing and gape face behaviors suggest that this infant was stressed beyond her ability to cope.

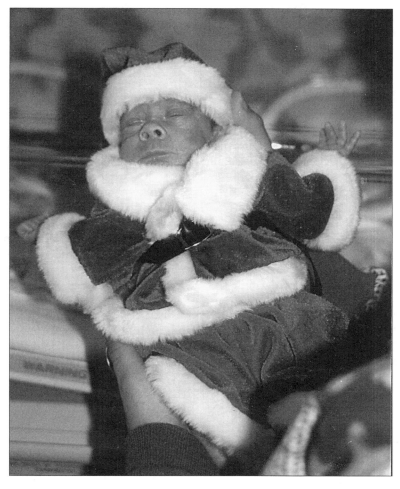

Figure 24. An infant displaying motor stress after being dressed for the holidays by her parents.

Subtle stress reactions such as gaze aversion serve as "time-out" signals that communicate to the caregiver the infant's need to break away from the stimulus, at least momentarily, to reorganize. For example, an infant who is becoming stressed during social interaction with a caregiver may respond with gaze aversion. If the caregiver looks away momentarily, then the infant may be able to regain sufficient stability to continue interacting. If the momentary interruption is not sufficient to reorganize the infant, the caregiver may try providing additional support during the time out, such as containing the infant in flexion. If a time-out break or external support to prevent further stress is not provided or is not sufficient to reorganize the infant, stress reactions may escalate until a dangerous state of autonomic instability is reached. Environmental support should be offered as soon as subtle stress reactions appear or even before, when coping signals become more frequent and intense. Stress reactions are listed by subsystem in Chapter 8, under the Sick Full-Term Infants heading.

An unsupportive or detrimental environment affects infants with immature nervous systems more severely than it affects more mature infants. Stress prevention should be a priority when working with preterm infants.

Neuromotor Control

Reflex Development

A number of primitive reflexes may be absent in preterm infants depending on their central nervous system maturity. There is some discrepancy in the literature concerning the time at which various reflexes appear. Studies of prenatal reflex development are few and inconclusive. Current understanding of late-term fetal reflex development is based primarily on premature infants' responses to stimuli under extrauterine conditions, instead of under real fetal conditions in utero. D'Argassies (1977) conducted the most comprehensive study on reflex and postural development of preterm infants. D'Argassies studied healthy and sick preterm infants as young as 23 weeks post conception. The findings, however, have been criticized because some of the infants studied were critically ill and a few died soon after testing. It has been argued that the behaviors of these infants were not necessarily representative of those of healthy preterms or fetuses. Despite the controversy, D'Argassies's study is still the best available exposition of premature reflex development. Table 11 is a summary (based on D'Argassies's study) of the time of emergence and developmental progression of the primitive reflexes. As indicated on the table, prior to 37 weeks, preterm infants' reflex behavior differs from that of full-term infants. Most of the primitive reflexes begin to appear at approximately 28 weeks and continue to evolve until approximately the 37th week. By 40 weeks corrected age, preterm infants should display most primitive reflexes. Clinical observations and a study by Allen and Capute (1990) support some of these findings.

Muscle Tone

D'Argassies (1977) and Dubowitz and Dubowitz (1981) described the development of muscle tone and primitive reflexes as progressing in a caudo-cephalic direction. Amiel-Tison and Grenier (1986) reinforced those early observations when they found that in preterm infants, tone and tonic/proprioceptive reflexes appear first in the legs, with extensor and flexor control progressing to the trunk and ultimately extending to the head and neck. Thus, the ability to bear weight on the legs appears at an earlier age than trunk control or the ability to right the head. (Dubowitz & Dubowitz, 1981, had found a similar developmental progression.) Allen and Capute (1990) provided further confirmation of previous findings, as seen by the following summary of their study's major findings:

- Flexor tone begins to emerge first in the lower extremities, at approximately 29 weeks.
- Upper extremity recoil appears at approximately 35–37 weeks, 2–3 weeks later than in the lower extremities.
- Knee tone precedes hip tone; in turn, hip tone precedes shoulder tone.
- Trunk tone appears near term, between 36 and 40 weeks.
- Neck tone remains underdeveloped by term age.

In preterm infants, the developmental progression of tone beyond 40 weeks appears to follow the same course as that of full-term infants. Passive flexor tone decreases as extensor tone improves in a cephalo-caudal (instead of caudo-cephalic)

Table 11. Reflex development in premature infants (based on D'Argassies, 1977)

Reflex	Gestational age (in weeks)						
	23–24	25–26	27–28	30	32	35	37
Palmar grasp	Slight, latent	Improving	Localized	Less latency, vigorous in fingers and wrists	Stronger traction begins	Firm, effective, head does not follow traction	Vigorous except for neck
Galant	Strong	Strong	Strong	Strong	Strong	Strong	Strong
Rooting	Incomplete	Slight, yawn, upper lip and sides	Yawn, 3 phases, no lower lip	Incomplete 4th phase, poor head extension	Complete, intense, long lasting	Perfect, head extension still weak	Perfect, weak head extension
Sucking	Arrhythmic, brief	Improving	"Chewing" motions	Better synchrony	Active, good	Better, expresses hunger	Like full-term
Gag/swallow	Absent	Absent	Tongue protrusion	Suck/swallow not coordinated with breathing	Active, fair	Better	Like full-term
Moro	Minimal (hand only)	Better, slight upper extremity extension	Present, upper extremity extension, no abduction	Vigorous, easily elicited	Complete abduction/extension upper extremities	Complete, brisk	Perfect
Plantar grasp	Absent	Constant	Constant	Constant	Constant	Constant	Constant
Automatic walking	Absent	Trace	Improving	Improving	Present, tip-toes	Present, not sustained	Automatic, full plantar support
Crossed extension	Absent	Questionable	Contralateral defense reaction	Improving	Flexion/extension good, abduction beginning	More like full-term	Complete, begins toe fanning
Doll's eye	Absent	Absent	Absent	Absent	Beginning	Present	Present
Placing	Absent	Absent	Absent	Absent	Absent	Weak	Appears

direction (Amiel-Tison & Grenier, 1986). Development of active tone also progresses cephalo-caudally beyond 40 weeks, with head extensor control emerging first, followed by trunk control, and, ultimately, by hip and lower extremity control (Amiel-Tison & Grenier, 1986).

Despite some controversy, most clinicians agree on the following points:

- Premature infants tend to exhibit low muscle tone.
- Muscle tone increases as preterm infants approach term age.
- After term age, muscle tone appears to develop in preterm and full-term infants in a cephalo-caudal pattern.
- Preterm infants often exhibit postural patterns by term ages that differ from those of full-term newborns, possibly because of the difference in their postural experiences.

- Preterm infants who are assisted to maintain postures comparable to in utero postures tend to develop muscle tone and postural patterns more similar to those of full-term infants.

Motor Activity

The motor activity of preterm infants also differs from the usual motor activity displayed by full-term infants or from movement patterns of fetuses in utero. Intrauterine body movements decrease as fetuses approach term age. This decrease in motor activity has been attributed to intrauterine constriction resulting from fetal growth or longer periods of quiet sleep. A longitudinal study conducted by Ten Hof and associates (2002) confirmed that between 24 weeks and 36 weeks, overall motor activity of fetuses decreases in utero because movement bursts become more spaced out, although the duration of the movement bursts remains unchanged. Ten Hof et al. found high intrafetal consistency in the movement patterns displayed by the fetuses studied. That is, fetuses that moved minimally at 24 weeks also did so at 36 weeks and vice versa. There was great variability across the fetuses because some simply moved more than others, but they did so consistently at least throughout the last trimester in utero. However, the authors found that the decrease in movement was not associated with prolonged periods of quiescence. Rather, the movement decrement observed appeared to parallel the decrease in motor activity found in premature infants approaching term age. The authors concluded that the decrease in motor activity that occurs as fetuses approach term age is the result of developmental maturation and changes in movement parameters rather than intrauterine crowding or increased duration of quiet states.

A comprehensive review of the literature shows some consistent differences between the motor activity of preterm and full-term infants:

- Preterm infants move more and have brief periods of inactivity. They exhibit motor activity during more than 80% of their sleep time.
- Motor activity is state related. Movements in light sleep tend to be more localized and uncoordinated, whereas generalized phasic movements and startles predominate during deep sleep.
- Preterm infants' movements tend to be less modulated and less coordinated because of the immaturity of their central nervous system, their limited proximal stability, and the predominance of light sleep. As preterm infants approach term age and proximal stability improves, movements become more coordinated.
- With increasing age, there is a decrease in startles and extraneous movements of the extremities and an increase in organized movements, such as bringing the hand to the face or mouth.
- Healthy preterm and full-term infants have a more extensive repertoire of movements and better quality of motor activity than preterm infants who are smaller and sicker.

Preterm infants are capable of producing quite sophisticated actions in response to certain stimuli (Als et al., 1982b). Younger preterm infants first exhibit protective and avoidant responses to tactile, vestibular, and auditory input. For instance, a 28-week GA preterm infant may startle or display flailing extensor arm movements when moved or gently touched, whereas a 34-week GA infant may orient toward the stimuli, possibly displaying smooth flexor movements. Avoidance responses are primitive, spontaneous procuring efforts that although interfering somewhat with functional performance, communicate to the caregiver that the infant is stressed and needs assistance. Avoidance responses are gradually replaced by approach responses as the nervous system matures with age and the infant gains increased physiologic control (Als et al., 1982b). The enhanced motor development of older, healthier preterm infants and their ability to self-regulate and respond with approach behaviors give them an advantage over the sicker or younger infants in their interactions with the environment and, ultimately, their functional performance.

State of Arousal

It is commonly agreed that most preterm infants do not possess a full capacity for control over states of arousal until after 36 weeks and that consistent periods of focused alertness emerge after 37 weeks. The following list describes the developmental progression of state behavior in preterm infants (summarized from Als et al., 1982b; Barr et al., 1996; Doussard-Roosevelt, Porges, & McClenny, 1996; and Prechtl et al., 1979):

• Preterm infants sleep longer than full-term infants.

• The sleep of preterm infants is characterized by much motor activity.

• On average, preterm infants spend approximately 80% of their sleeping time in the more disorganized state of light sleep compared with full-term infants, who spend 50% of their overall sleeping time in either light or deep sleep.

• The proportion of time spent in deep and light sleep changes as the infants mature.

• Time spent in light sleep decreases as neurobehavioral organization improves and is replaced by increasingly long periods of alertness.

• Vagal maturation, an indicator of physiologic stability in infants, has been associated with less light sleep in preterm infants approaching term age.

• Periods of alertness are brief and sporadic in preterm infants.

• Before term age, healthy preterm infants tend to cry less than full-term infants.

• After 40 weeks corrected age, preterm infants cry more than before term age, resembling the crying patterns of full-term infants.

Als and associates (1982b) adapted the Brazelton's (1973) state classification system to more clearly describe the poorly differentiated states of arousal of preterm infants. This scale includes Brazelton's six original, easily differentiated states ("B" states) as well as seven more diffuse states that are characteristic of preterm infants ("A" states). This scale forms part of the Assessment of Preterm Infants' Behavior (APIB) (Als et al., 1982b). See Table 12 for a summary of the APIB state definitions.

Illness and physiologic instability affect state behavior in preterm infants. Thus, healthy preterm infants exhibit more "B" states, whereas smaller, sicker preterm infants demonstrate more "A" states. Higher-risk preterm infants spend more sleep time in light sleep than healthier preterm infants do (Doussard-Roosevelt et al., 1996).

The ability to maintain periods of quiet alertness is a high-level task for premature infants. Good quality alertness appears closer to term and is only seen in the healthiest preterm infants who have achieved physiologic and motor stability. Physiologic stress signals may be observed as infants try to achieve a quiet alert state, reflecting the physiologic cost that they have to pay for their alertness efforts. Such signals must

Table 12. State definitions from the Assessment of Preterm Infants' Behavior (APIB)

	"A" states	"B" states
Sleep states		
Deep sleep (State 1)	Sleeping with momentary regular breathing, eyes closed, and no eye movements under closed lids; relaxed facial expression; no spontaneous activity; movements oscillating fairly rapidly with isolated startles; jerky movements or tremors and other behavioral characteristics of State 2 (light sleep)	Sleeping with predominantly regular breathing, eyes closed, and no eye movements under closed lids; relaxed facial expression; no spontaneous activity except isolated startles
Light sleep (State 2)	Sleeping with eyes closed (or partially open) and rapid eye movements observed under closed lids; low activity level with diffuse or disorganized movements; irregular respirations and many sucking movements, many whimpers, much facial twitching, and much grimacing; the impression of a "noisy" state is given	Sleeping with eyes closed and rapid eye movements observed under closed lids; low activity level with movements and dampened startles; movements are likely of lower amplitude and more monitored than in State 1; infant displays dampened startles in response to various internal stimuli, respirations are more irregular; mild sucking and mouthing movements off and on; one or two whimpers may be observed, as well as an isolated sigh or smile
Transitional states		
Drowsy (State 3)	Semi-dozing; eyes may be open (with an open, glassy look) or closed (with eyelids fluttering or exaggerated blinking); activity level is variable, with or without interspersed, mild startles from time to time; diffuse movements; fussing and/or much discharge of vocalization, whimpers, facial grimacing, and so forth	Same characteristics as the drowsy "A" state but with less discharge of vocalization, whimpers, facial grimacing, and so forth
Awake states		
Quiet alert (State 4)	Low alert (4AL): Awake with minimal motor activity (eyes half open or open but with glazed look, giving impression of little involvement and distance, or focused, yet seeming to look through, rather than at, an object or the examiner) or clearly awake and reactive but eyes open intermittently. Hyperalert (4AH): Awake with minimal motor activity (eyes wide open); "hyperalert" or giving the impression of panic or fear; may appear to be "hooked" by the stimulus and unable to modulate or break the intensity of the fixation	Awake with bright, shiny look; seems to focus attention on source of stimulation and appears to process information actively and with modulation; motor activity is at a minimum
Active awake (State 5)	Eyes may be open but infant is clearly awake and aroused, as indicated by motor arousal, tonus and mildly distressed facial expression, grimacing, or other signs of discomfort; diffuse fussing	Eyes may be open but infant is clearly awake and aroused, with considerable, well-defined motor activity; clear fussing, but no crying
Crying (State 6)	Intense crying, as indicated by grimacing and "cry face," yet crying sounds very strained or weak or is even absent	Rhythmic intense crying that is robust, vigorous, and strong in sound

Source: Als, Lester, Tronick, & Brazelton (1982a).

be monitored, recognized, and respected even in the most stable preterm infants to preserve the infants' well-being and optimal functioning.

Interactional/Attentional and Self-Regulation Capabilities

Preterm infants develop the ability to self-regulate and socially interact as their nervous systems mature and as they achieve neurobehavioral stability. Readers are referred to this chapter's previous discussions on the topic, as well as to Chapter 7 for an extensive discussion of the neurobehavioral development of preterm infants. The following points serve as a reminder of the major principles related to the interactive capabilities of preterm infants (see also Figure 20 in Chapter 8):

- Only infants with state of arousal stability who are able to sustain alertness have the underlying capacities for engaging in prolonged interactional or attentional activities.
- Infants in the in-turning phase are physiologically unstable; interaction activities during this stage should be avoided to the extent possible.
- Infants in the coming-out phase have achieved a degree of physiologic and motor stability that enables them to engage in limited social interaction activities, provided that there is close monitoring to prevent stress reactions and that concurrent stimulation is avoided.
- Infants who have reached the final stage of reciprocity are stable and can safely tolerate moderate amounts of social interaction.
- Regardless of the level of stability, infants' responses to stimulation, particularly self-regulation coping signals and stress reactions, should always be monitored.
- Premature or prolonged engagement in interactional activities can have detrimental consequences for unstable infants.

Specific Sensory Abilities

A review of the literature suggests that fetuses have primitive ability to perceive touch, sound, movement, and light as early as 23 weeks (McVey, 1998). Processing of sensory information, however, is an interactive skill that requires an underlying foundation of capacities similar to those required to engage in social interaction. Although some preterm infants are capable of discriminating and responding to some forms of sensory stimulation, interpreting and appropriately responding to sensory input occurs at a high physiologic cost for them. Therefore, to preserve a preterm infant's physiologic well-being, intentionally imposed sensory stimulation should be avoided prior to achievement of self-regulation. Sensory experiences beyond the essential stimuli provided within the NICU environment should be individualized to the infant's tolerance and should be limited to experiences that may enhance the infant's physiologic stability. For example, cuddling, tactile containment, deep touch, massage, and gentle rocking may be used to promote alertness for essential activities such as breast or bottle feeding. There is no consistent scientific evidence to support sensory activities that mimic the intrauterine environment, such as heartbeat sounds, vibratory or oscillating beds, or water beds. Moreover, it should be stated that unstable infants should not be exposed to any unnecessary stimulation. Sensory interventions for these infants should take the form of environmental modification to reduce unnecessary stimulation and promote energy conservation.

Pain Sensitivity

Preterm infants' abilities to perceive and respond to pain have been studied extensively. For years, health care personnel interpreted preterm infants' dampened crying efforts as inability to perceive pain. There is little doubt, however, that preterm infants respond to noxious stimuli with clear flexor withdrawal as early as 26 weeks postconception, suggesting that they are able to perceive and move away from a nociceptive stimulus (Andrews & Fitzgerald, 1994).

Determining whether a preterm infant perceives pain depends in part on how pain is defined. If pain is defined as a motor reaction associated with exposure to a noxious stimulus, then most people would agree on the basis of infants' withdrawal responses and facial expressions that preterm infants *do* experience pain. Conversely, if feeling pain is defined as the conscious awareness and interpretation of a sensory stimulus as an uncomfortable and emotional experience, then it could be argued that preterm infants *do not* feel pain (Lloyd-Thomas & Fitzgerald, 1996). Studies in the 1990s demonstrated that these infants do feel pain (Committee on Fetus and Newborn, 2000). McVey (1998) found that although the preterm infants' motor abilities for pain expression may be immature, the mechanisms that mediate pain perception appear to be functional at very early GAs. Menon, Anand, and McIntosh (1998) found that the behavioral, metabolic, and endocrine responses to painful stimuli are similar in preterms and older infants but that preterms tend to be more sensitive to pain and to have heightened responses to successive painful stimuli, perhaps because of poorer habituation abilities. Anand (1998) also described increased sensitivity to pain in preterm neonates. Lloyd-Thomas and Fitzgerald clarified that although "noxious stimuli frequently produce a biochemical stress response, such a response does not necessarily indicate pain" (1996, p. 798). Neonatal therapists need to recognize and respect these infants' increased sensitivity to noxious stimuli and the subtle reactions that might indicate that they are experiencing discomfort and stress, although maybe not at a conscious level.

The following list presents important research findings in relation to pain in preterm infants:

- Facial expressions and body movements are strongly associated with exposure to a painful stimulus (i.e., a heel stick) as early as 23 weeks postgestation (Hadjistavropoulos, Craig, Grunau, & Whitfield, 1997; Lindh, Wiklund, Sandman, & Hakansson, 1997; Rushforth & Levene, 1994).
- Facial grimacing responses to noxious stimuli are more frequent than actual crying (Rushforth & Levene, 1994). Also, facial reactions to noxious stimuli are milder in younger GAs, suggesting decreased ability to display complex responses (Stevens, Johnston, & Horton, 1994).
- Facial expression of pain is influenced by behavioral state (Stevens et al., 1994), with infants having milder reactions to pain when they are in sleep states, especially deep sleep. This finding explains in part the lower incidence of pain responses in younger infants who spend most of their time in sleep states. Facial activity and state are moderately correlated with heart rate changes at 32 weeks (Morison, Grunau, Oberlander, & Whitfield, 2001).
- Invasiveness of a particular procedure and GA are less predictive of an infant's responses to pain than facial and body activity (Hadjistavropoulos et al, 1997).
- Exposure to a painful stimulus increases heart rate (Lindh et al., 1997; Van Reempts, Wouters, De Cock, & Van Acker, 1996) and reduces heart rate variability (Lindh et al., 1997), especially in stressed preterm infants.

- Although biobehavioral and physiologic reactivity to pain is highly correlated in most preterm infants, individualized responses are not uncommon, especially at very young GAs—that is, high biobehavioral with low physiologic reactivity or low biobehavioral with high physiologic reactivity (Morison et al., 2001).

- The duration of crying among preterm infants has been positively correlated with pain scores (Johnston, Sherrard, et al., 1999).

- Exposure to pain (i.e., a heel stick) and the severity of illness alter cry acoustics (i.e., increase the fundamental frequency, harmonic structure, and peak spectral energy) (Stevens et al, 1994).

- Crying associated with a routine heel stick procedure decreases when infants are given a 24% sucrose solution; plain water or an 18% solution are not effective (Abad, Díaz, Domenech, Robayna, & Rico, 1996; Stevens, Taddio, Ohlsson, & Einarson, 1997).

- Repeated doses of sucrose are more effective in decreasing crying than a single dose (Johnston, Stremler, Horton, & Friedman, 1999).

- Sucrose offered through a flavored pacifier (Maone et al., 1990) also decreases facial expressions of pain in preterm infants.

- Sucrose administration has no effect on the infant's heart rate (Johnston, Stremler, Stevens, & Horton, 1997).

- Infants exposed to chronic pain have higher morbidity and mortality rates (Menon et al., 1998).

Although the nature of the NICU environment demands frequent exposure to stressful and painful stimuli, neonatal therapists should identify and recommend ways to minimize exposure to nonessential aversive or novice stimuli and strategies to modulate infants' responses to unavoidable painful stimuli.

Tactile Sensitivity

Most tactile responses of preterm infants are reflexive. Reflex testing is conducted on a routine basis to determine the maturity and central nervous system integrity of preterm infants. Prior to an infant's achievement of stability, reflex testing should be performed only when absolutely necessary for diagnostic or treatment planning purposes. Deep touch sensitivity is also present in preterm infants. Deep touch (i.e., swaddling or contained holding) is calming and organizing for most preterm infants (Browne, 2000). Palmar tactile input through grasping (e.g., holding on to the caregiver's finger) is also organizing for many infants and may enhance flexor tone through its influence on the traction reflex. Responses to light touches tend to be more individualized: Some infants appear to enjoy light touch whereas other infants may respond with stress, especially if the stimulus is applied repeatedly on a small area of the skin.

Taste Sensitivity

Preference for sweet taste has been well documented, even in very small preterm infants. Sucrose administration decreases crying and facilitates calming behaviors such as mouthing and hand-to-mouth maneuvers in preterm infants (Barr et al., 1994).

Auditory and Visual Sensitivity

Chapter 8 discusses auditory and visual sensitivity. Although preterm infants possess rather sophisticated sensory processing abilities, activities requiring complex sensory processing of auditory or visual stimuli should be postponed until infants have achieved adequate physiologic, motor, state, and attentional/interactional stability.

Multimodal Sensory Integration

Preterm infants have limited abilities for multisensory processing. Complex multimodal sensory integration is believed to develop later in infants (Ayres, 1972). Exposure to multimodal stimulation—for example, speaking to the infant (auditory input) while holding the infant (tactile input) and establishing eye contact and smiling (visual input)—may be too difficult and stressful for preterms who are not ready for such a complex integration process. Individual tolerances for combined stimuli should always be assessed prior to making recommendations for feeding, handling, and social interaction. The presentation of stimuli through one modality at a time is more effective and less disorganizing for most preterm infants.

CONCLUSION

This chapter has described the development of premature infants' capabilities. Emphasis has been given to the behavioral responses of premature infants at term age, which differ qualitatively from those of full-term infants. Early interventionists working with infants born prematurely must become well familiarized with these infants' behavioral patterns and differences, as well as their strengths and limitations, to address the infants' needs more effectively.

10

Evaluation of Infant Behavior and Development in the NICU

OVERVIEW

This chapter covers the basic elements of behavioral and developmental evaluation of NICU infants, giving particular emphasis to the assessment of the premature infant. The complexity of the evaluation process and the importance of team collaboration in the evaluation of these infants are underscored. The interrelation of the various team members throughout the evaluation process is described.

A variety of commonly used assessment instruments are referenced, with training requirements indicated when appropriate. Guidelines for the selection of assessment instruments are also provided, as well as a thorough description of the essential components of a neonatal evaluation—namely physiologic stability and homeostasis, organization of states of arousal and neurobehavioral organization, and the effects of the physical and social environments.

OBJECTIVES

- Recognize the complexity and continuity of the evaluation process of NICU infants
- Describe the ways by which the various team members, including family members, can share and consult with each other throughout the assessment process to obtain the most comprehensive picture of an infant
- Identify the data that can be collected through reviewing an infant's medical and social history, and recognize the importance of conducting a thorough review of the history in preparation for the assessment of a NICU infant
- Identify the major precautions that should be taken by the evaluator to ensure that an infant's presenting problems are well understood and that the infant can be safely evaluated
- Identify the most common neonatal assessment instruments, indicating which instruments require formal training or certification
- List the considerations for selecting an assessment instrument for a NICU infant
- Describe the essential components of a neonatal evaluation in terms of physiologic homeostasis, neurobehavioral organization (states of arousal and self-regulation), motor organization and postural reflexes, participation in infant occupations, and active engagement with the physical and social environments

GENERAL CONCEPTS OF NEONATAL ASSESSMENT

Evaluation of infant behavior and development in the NICU is a complex process involving integration of information from a variety of sources and interaction with a number of team members, including primary nurses and the infant's family. To achieve an accurate picture of the infant's functioning, it is necessary to do much more than administer an assessment tool or battery. Learning what information has already been gathered about the presenting problem and planning the evaluation accordingly are of primary importance to the NICU therapist. This approach makes appropriate use of assessments completed by other team members and prevents the additional stress imposed by unnecessary handling.

The NICU therapist must be adept at modifying any assessment tool to meet the individual demands imposed by an infant's medical condition and by the infant's thresholds for particular types of handling and stimulation. Although one could argue this is necessary for all pediatric evaluations, it is most critical in the NICU, where a momentary loss of physiologic stability can be life threatening.

The evaluation process in the NICU must be continuous to accommodate the constantly changing medical conditions of the neonates. It is not unusual for infants in the NICU to change from stable to critical condition in a matter of hours or minutes. Thus, the NICU therapist must always be prepared to adapt, postpone, or abandon planned assessments or care recommendations based on an infant's current status.

As discussed in Chapter 4, gaining the respect and trust of NICU staff involves time and experience. When NICU staff are familiar with the therapist's approach to infants and families and confident in the therapist's ability to conduct an evaluation appropriately and safely, they are more likely to refer infants for assessment, share important information, and collaborate with the therapist in evaluating the infant's needs and capacities. One of the best ways to instill such confidence is through a consistent professional demeanor and through an approach that is respectful of other team members and of the infant's family (see also Chapter 11). The therapist's credibility is also enhanced when he or she uses assessment instruments and methods that are based on existing evidence and are reliable, valid, and safe for use with NICU infants.

PRELIMINARY DATA COLLECTION AND TEAM COLLABORATION

When making an initial response to a referral, the NICU therapist must be certain that the presenting problem is understood by communicating directly with the referring attending neonatologist, neonatology fellow, or his or her appointee (e.g., resident, nurse practitioner). A thorough review of the medical record should follow, including

- The infant's birth date and GA at birth
- Maternal age, education, primary language, marital status, number of pregnancies, live births, and losses
- History of previous siblings in the NICU
- Prenatal course and any complications or issues that may affect current functioning in the infant (e.g., premature rupture of membranes, oligohydramnios, antenatal medications and/or procedures, in utero substance exposure)

- Perinatal history: mode of delivery; Apgar scores at 1, 5, and 10 minutes (if applicable); and complications at the time of delivery (e.g., a prolonged resuscitation, meconium aspiration)

- Birth weight and growth parameters at birth (e.g., restricted growth in addition to prematurity, being large and born to a diabetic mother)

- Medical history: diagnoses, history of medical and surgical interventions. (e.g., cardiac anomalies; neurologic, metabolic, or cardiorespiratory compromise; possible continuing recovery from a recent surgery or invasive procedure)

- Medication history and current medications, particularly those affecting arousal, muscle tone, regulation of cardiorespiratory functions, and antireflux medication

- Pattern of weight gain and growth (e.g., difficulty gaining weight, clues in the infant's history regarding the cause of slow growth)

- Feeding history, including length of time on parenteral and gavage feedings, tolerance of feedings, and current feeding regimen (see Chapter 13 for further recommendations for gathering specific information prior to a feeding evaluation)

- Make up and ages of the immediate family (parents and siblings), grandparents, and others living in the home

- Cultural background of the family

- Family history, including involvement with child protective services

- Psychiatric or psychosocial history of the family, including any history of substance abuse or physical or emotional abuse by the parents or by a partner

When there are complex social issues regarding the family, social work notes are a valuable source of information. Direct contact with the social worker who knows the family best is recommended prior to meeting with the family. The social worker may provide additional insights into the family's current level of coping and need for psychosocial support. Sometimes, a psychologist and/or psychiatrist is already involved with the family. This person's perspectives may also be helpful, if not prior to the evaluation, then at least before the therapist makes repeated contacts with the family. Most families cope appropriately with their infant's NICU stay and look forward to meeting with the therapist as a sign that their infant has the potential to make positive gains.

If the referring physician or practitioner is not available and the need for evaluation is not clearly stated in an infant's medical record, the therapist's next sources of information for the presenting problem are the nurse manager, the bedside nurse, and the parents. If there are contraindications to handling or other safety issues that have not been cleared through the primary medical or nursing personnel, the therapist should consider postponing the evaluation until the safety of the infant is ensured.

As noted previously, being respectful of other team members includes calling ahead or visiting the nurse at the infant's bedside to arrange an evaluation time that fits the infant's care plan and schedule. Doing this achieves two very important goals. First, it increases the odds that family members will be available to participate in the evaluation process Second, it ensures that the evaluation is scheduled for a time that will optimize the infant's state of arousal and performance.

The importance of teaming with parents and other significant family members in observing their infant's behavior and development is described in Chapters 4 and 11 and bears repeating here. Participation during observation and evaluation informs family members of their infant's vulnerabilities and strengths. Repeated observations, particularly during routine nursing or medical procedures, provide opportunities to reinforce parents' role as the experts on their child (Nugent, 1985). Parent participation in evaluation also provides a realistic view of the infant's progress, preparing the family for team decision making regarding early versus late discharge.

ASSESSMENT TOOLS

There are a number of assessment tools for use with preterm infants and full-term neonates. Most cover similar areas of performance: maturity of neurobehavioral, sensory, and motor systems as well as reflex development. All require training for reliable administration and interpretation, and most require certification.

The most useful protocol for an individual therapist is the one that best fits his or her knowledge base and skills. Information obtained from an assessment tool is only helpful when it can be interpreted appropriately. For that reason, no specific recommendations for assessment tools are made in this chapter. Rather, the reader is encouraged to consider the following questions in selecting an assessment tool:

- Is it age appropriate for this particular infant?

- Is it standardized? Is it criterion and/or norm referenced?

- Does the instrument have good reliability and validity? Is there evidence to support its use with this particular type of infant?

- Does it cover the specific domains needed to answer the questions of greatest concern to the family and the medical team?

- How much energy will the assessment require the infant to expend? Does the infant have sufficient medical stability to endure administration of the items, in their usual form or with modifications? Does the assessment have to be administered in one session, or can it be divided based on the infant's tolerance? Does it have to be administered according to a predetermined sequence?

- Has the examiner learned to administer the items reliably (i.e., has the examiner undergone the required training and certification in the use of this instrument)?

- Does the examiner have the knowledge base to interpret the infant's responses appropriately?

- Are the recommendations yielded by the assessment likely to enhance the infant's care and well-being and/or the caregiver's well-being? For example, recommendations should result in one or more of the following: reduced energy expenditure, improved infant–caregiver interaction, improved participation in age-appropriate activities, and/or enhanced family involvement in the infant's care.

Standardized assessment tools can be very useful. In some instances, however, the best assessment protocol is constructed by the therapist to suit a particular infant's individual needs and capacities as well as by the questions that the caregiving team asks at that point in the infant's NICU stay. The following section highlights specific areas that should always be addressed when evaluating infants in the NICU.

ESSENTIAL COMPONENTS OF A NEONATAL EVALUATION

The purpose of a neonatal therapy evaluation is to assess an infant's capacities and his or her participation in the essential developmental tasks and occupations of infancy. The major elements of a neonatal therapy evaluation are

- Medical considerations and stability
- Physiologic homeostasis
- Neurobehavioral organization: organization of states of arousal to support feeding, sleeping, and taking in information from the environment; self-regulation abilities
- Motor organization and postural reflexes
- Active engagement with the environment: seeking stimuli (procuring); being receptive to care, feeding, problem solving, and socially interacting

These elements may be assessed using standardized instruments, observation and handling, or a combination of methods.

Medical Considerations and Stability

An infant's reaction to a particular experience can be interpreted in a variety of ways, depending on what is considered appropriate or acceptable, not only for a particular GA but also for the broader context within which the infant is performing. This broader context can be identified through a careful review of the infant's record *and* by checking with the bedside nurse. Two important aspects of the broader context should be considered in interpreting the results of an infant's neonatal evaluation. First, which medications is the infant currently receiving or being weaned from, and what are their potential influences on the infant's behavioral responsiveness? Second, is the infant likely to be fatigued and/or stressed because of medical conditions, routine care, or recent procedures? Some procedures or situations could account for physiologic instability, fatigue, lethargy, or irritability. Examples include recent surgery; a heel stick; IV or percutaneous line placement; multiple or severe episodes of apnea, bradycardia, or oxygen desaturation; an eye examination; a lengthy family visit; or multiple interruptions of rest by NICU staff for examinations or tests. Lack of medical stability often leads to difficulty maintaining physiologic homeostasis.

Physiologic Homeostasis

Infants in the NICU may initially require mechanical ventilation and other similar external supports to maintain physiologic homeostasis. As their health improves, the infants need fewer such supports and become increasingly able to use their internal resources for regulating physiologic functions in response to occasional perturbations (e.g., stress from receiving care or from painful procedures). The following signs of a temporary imbalance in physiologic or autonomic nervous system (ANS) functions may result as a response to handling:

- Changes in skin color: flushing, pallor, mottling, or cyanosis
- Sweating

- Tachycardia or bradycardia
- Tachypnea or apnea
- Oxygen desaturation
- GER (spitting)
- Gassiness or watery stools
- Drop in body temperature

Such physiologic changes are not always stress related. Signs of ANS distress may also be related to specific medical conditions (e.g., cardiac, lung, or gastro-intestinal disease), medications, or abstinence from addictive substances to which the infant may have been exposed in utero or in the course of his or her medical care (e.g., fentanyl or morphine sedation for surgery or ECMO).

The initial observation should *always* include assessment of the infant's physiologic status as well as a review of the infant's physiologic stability throughout that particular day. (This information is found in the bedside chart.) When any of the previously listed signs of distress appear during the course of an evaluation, the therapist should discontinue handling or stimulation and immediately inform the bedside nurse.

Assessment of an infant's ability to recover from ANS distress is an equally important aspect of the therapist's observation and evaluation. Asking the following questions contributes to this assessment:

- Was the infant able to recover spontaneously, or did the infant require assistance?
- If assistance was required, what was the extent? (e.g., Was stimulation required after a bradycardia, and was the stimulation mild, moderate, or vigorous?)
- Once physiologic homeostasis was restored, was the infant's alertness and activity affected? How was it affected (i.e., What did this event cost the infant in terms of energy)?

The NICU therapist must be well familiarized with the infant's past medical history and current care plan to appropriately interpret signs of ANS distress and recovery. When signs of ANS distress occur during an evaluation, the decision to continue the evaluation after recovery depends on the infant's medical condition at the moment and on the judgment of the medical team. It is always appropriate to discuss the medical and physiologic aspects of the infant's assessment with members of the medical team. It may be appropriate to ask the infant's nurse and/or physician to participate in the assessment. Requesting an opportunity to observe the infant's responses to care may be appropriate to enable the therapist to better understand the infant's ability to tolerate handling.

Neurobehavioral Organization

State of Arousal

One element of an infant's neurobehavioral organization is his or her organization of states of arousal. An assessment of the infant's state of arousal provides a baseline and a context for all other behavioral observations. The degree and quality of arousal should be determined from the moment that the infant is initially approached, prior to handling, and should be continuously noted throughout the evaluation.

There are several classifications of neurobehavioral states of newborns (Brazelton, 1973; Prechtl & Beintema, 1968). As of 2003, however, Brazelton's (1984) classification is the one used most commonly for preterm infants 32 weeks of gestation and older and for full-term infants. This system defines six states of arousal (see Chapter 8 for greater detail):

- State 1—Deep sleep: regular breathing, eyes closed, no eye movements, no spontaneous activity except startles or jerky movements at regular intervals
- State 2—Light sleep: eyes closed, rapid eye movements, low activity with random movements and startles, irregular respirations, sucking movements
- State 3—Drowsy: eyes may be open or closed, eyelids fluttering, variable activity level with occasional mild startle
- State 4—Quiet alert: bright look, focused attention on source of stimulation, minimal motor activity
- State 5—Active alert: considerable motor activity with thrusting movements of the extremities
- State 6—Crying: intense crying; requires help to stop crying

Als, Lester, Tronick, and Brazelton (1982a) developed a scale specifically for preterm infants that includes the Brazelton's (1973) six well-organized states ("B" states) and seven less organized states ("A" states). As noted in Chapter 9, this scale forms part of the APIB (Als et al., 1982a). See Table 12 (in Chapter 9) for more information.

State of arousal has a profound influence on passive and active muscle tone, reflex response, sensory and social responsiveness, and feeding. All of these responses and functions are attenuated if the infant is in a drowsy state or are either exaggerated or impeded if the infant is agitated or crying. An infant who is initially asleep, comes to quiet alertness with handling, or cries and is able to self-soothe or be comforted is more likely to participate fully in an evaluation and to demonstrate his or her full range of tone and responses. In contrast, an infant who remains drowsy throughout handling may appear hypotonic, underresponsive to sensory stimuli and may have difficulty with sucking and swallowing. Moreover, an infant who is irritable, cries vigorously, and cannot be easily soothed may appear hypertonic and may be unable to organize a response to visual, auditory, or feeding stimuli. Thus, the infant's state of arousal is a critical component of all neonatal evaluations. Observation of state of arousal should include the following capacities:

- Range of states that the infant is able to achieve
- Quality of each state, especially quiet alertness (e.g., bright, focused eyes)
- Frequency of state changes
- Smoothness with which the infant moves from one state to another
- Physiologic cost to the infant of moving between states
- Degree of irritability experienced by the infant
- Ability to self-soothe or to be consoled

Infants who have difficulty organizing or regulating their state of arousal may experience difficulty interacting with their environment and participating in age-appropriate activities. Ongoing determination of the infant's state of arousal is important as the infant's care or intervention is administered.

Most neonatal assessment instruments specify the states of arousal that are necessary for proper administration of each item. For example, the following instruments specify the required arousal level for each assessment item:

- The Neonatal Behavioral Assessment Scale (NBAS) (Brazelton, 1984)
- The Assessment of Preterm Infant Behavior (APIB) (Als et al., 1982a)
- The NICU Network Neurobehavioral Scale (NNNS) (Lester & Tronick, 2001, in press)
- The Neurobehavioral Assessment of the Preterm Infant (NAPI) (Korner & Thom, 1990)

The APIB, NNNS, and NAPI are designed for preterm infants or high-risk newborns, such as those with prenatal substance exposure, chronic medical conditions, or known neurologic compromise (e.g., hypoxic-ischemic encephalopathy). See Table 13 for more details on these and other assessment instruments.

Ability to Self-Regulate

Another important neurobehavioral consideration is an infant's ability to self-regulate. A complete evaluation of an infant in the NICU always includes an assessment of his or her self-regulatory capacity. Self-regulation includes the infant's ability to

- Habituate to repeated stimuli and to protect his or her sleep
- Tolerate basic care as well as painful or stressful stimuli
- Respond to caregivers' social interactions at a minimum of physiologic cost
- Make active efforts to self-regulate states of arousal

Well-regulated infants often respond to environmental stimuli by adopting and maintaining a relaxed, flexed posture; maintaining a state of quiet alertness; or regulating their own heart and respiration rates to continue interacting with the stimuli if necessary or desired. Well-regulated infants also may initially respond to a stressful stimulus with stress cues, but they may then employ self-regulation strategies (e.g., tucking, foot bracing, bringing the hand to the face, thumb sucking) to calm or reorganize themselves. These infants tend to return to a more balanced posture and to physiologic baseline more readily than infants who are not able to self-regulate. Conversely, infants who have difficulties with self-regulation may respond to environmental stimuli with more sustained stress reactions, such as brisk trunk and extremity extension, gaze aversion, tongue thrust, yawning, spitting up, and increasing or decreasing heart and respiration rates. These infants have greater difficulty with self-calming and may require caregiver intervention to regain physiologic and motor stability (see Chapter 8).

An infant who becomes agitated and restless or begins to arch the trunk during a neonatal assessment is giving signs of self-regulation difficulties. The assessment may have to be stopped, at least momentarily, until the infant regains stability and self-regulation. If the infant still is unable to self-regulate after being given a break, postponing the assessment may be necessary. In contrast, an infant who initially fusses and then cuddles or relaxes when picked up during the assessment is giving signs of adequate self-regulation. These signs suggest that the stimulation is well tolerated and that the evaluator may proceed with the assessment (see Chapter 8).

Table 13.   Neonatal assessment instruments

Instrument	Contact information	Description
Neonatal Behavioral Assessment Scale (NBAS)[a] (Brazelton, 1984)	The Brazelton Institute 1295 Boylston Street, Suite 320 Boston, MA 02215 http://www.brazelton-institute.com	Designed for full-term newborns Contains 28 behavioral items scored on a 9-point scale, 18 reflex items scored on a 4-point scale, and 7 optional "qualifiers" to assess the quality of responsiveness and facilitation required to elicit the response Infant's best performance is scored Used extensively
Naturalistic Observations of Newborn Behavior (NONB)– Newborn Individualized Developmental Care and Assessment Program (NIDCAP) Level I[a] (Als, 1995)	Neurobehavioral Infant and Child Studies Children's Hospital Boston 320 Longwood Ave Room EN-107 Boston, MA 02115 http://www.nidcap.com/ nidcap/ nidcap_trainingcenters.htm	Systematic method of observation of infants up to 42 weeks of gestation Particularly useful for infants younger than 30 weeks Observations focus on the interplay of an infant's autonomic, motoric, state organizational, and attentional functioning as the infant interacts with the caregiver and the environment—usually before, during, and after caregiving
Assessment of Preterm Infant Behavior (APIB)–NIDCAP Level II[a] (Als, Lester, Tronick, & Brazelton, 1982b)	Neurobehavioral Infant and Child Studies Children's Hospital Boston 320 Longwood Ave Room EN-107 Boston, MA 02115 http://www.nidcap.com/ nidcap/ nidcap_trainingcenters.htm	Assessment based on the NBAS, focusing on preterm infants Contains 285 items, which are scored on a 9-point scale reduced into 32 summary scores that are organized into five behavioral systems: physiologic, motor, state, attentional-interactive, and self-regulation Items administered in a progressively challenging and complex order
NICU Network Neurobehavioral Scale (NNNS)[a] (Lester & Tronick, 2001, in press)	Infant Development Center Women & Infants' Hospital of Rhode Island 101 Dudley Street Providence, RI 02905 http://www.infantdevelopment.org	Based on the NBAS to assess the neurological integrity and behavioral functioning of infants 28–46 weeks of gestation who are at high risk or have been exposed to drugs Includes a unique stress scale to document signs of withdrawal common in addicted infants Items are administered in "packages," beginning with a change in focus or position
Neurobehavioral Assessment of the Preterm Infant (NAPI)[b] (Korner & Thom, 1990)	Child Development Media 5632 Van Nuys Boulevard Suite 286 Van Nuys, CA 91401 http://www.childdevelopmentmedia.com	Relatively brief (27 items) test designed to assess infant maturity between 32 weeks of gestation and term age Most items overlap with other assessments (e.g., reflexes, passive/active tone, rotation, orientation, irritability) Items must be administered in a sequence from rousing to soothing to alerting

[a]Training and certification required
[b]Training recommended; certification not required

Motor Organization and Postural Reflexes

Assessment of postural and motor capacities is another essential component of neonatal evaluation, as self-regulatory behavior and infants' capacity to interact with their environment often rely on motor organization. For example, infants with hypotonia require external support to maintain sufficient flexion to bring a hand to the mouth for self-comforting. Infants with increased tone or hyperreflexia may also require external postural support to assume a comfortable flexed posture with their extremities tucked close to the body. Evaluation of motor organization is incorporated to varying degrees in all of the formal neonatal assessment tools. Although the validity of newborn behavior as a predictor of neurodevelopmental outcome remains a matter of debate, a baseline recording of reflexes and responses is recommended for all stable infants in the NICU (Amiel-Tison, 1996) as well as for those with a known risk (Lindeke, Stanley, Else, & Mills, 2002; Molteno, Thompson, Buccimazza, Maganiser, & Hann, 1999). Key components of a neonatal neuromotor assessment include

- Undisturbed posture at rest, including position and symmetry of the limbs
- Response to handling and repositioning (e.g., Moro reflex, prone head lift and turn, efforts to right the head on pull-to-sit movement, ability to cuddle into examiner's shoulder)
- Power and range of active movement (e.g., efforts to right the head on the pull-to-sit maneuver, strength of arm and leg extension against resistance)
- Passive tone and range of motion (e.g., truncal tone, popliteal angles, scarf sign)
- Proprioceptive responses (e.g., asymmetrical tonic neck reflex [ATNR], placing, clonus)
- Primitive reflexes that may influence the infant's ability to interact with the environment in an adaptive fashion—that is, to procure, feed, socially interact, and learn (e.g., rooting, sucking, swallowing, gag, palmar and plantar grasp, blinking in response to threats)
- Reflexes that provide clues to the integrity and/or symmetry of nervous system functioning: stepping, trunk incurvation, Babinski sign, vestibular response (e.g., lateral eye movement after a vertical turn)
- Visual tracking
- Auditory localization
- Response to light touch
- Response to a painful stimulus

A factor of equal importance to an infant's capacity for engaging in developmental tasks and occupations of infancy is the caregiver's ability to respond appropriately to the infant's signals for external assistance. This process, sometimes called *mutual regulation*, can only be assessed within the context of the physical environment and while considering the numerous additional influences shown in Figure 5 (found in Chapter 1). Examples of such influences include characteristics of the physical NICU environment on the day of observation, the culture of the infant's family, the caregiver's cognitive and social competencies, and the social supports available to the family.

Active Engagement with the Environment

Physical Environment

The physical environment is an important consideration in assessing an infant because it provides the context for the observation and can profoundly affect the infant's state of arousal and behavioral organization. Assessing the physical environment's possible influence on the infant's neurobehavioral organization is a very important aspect of neonatal intervention.

From a sensory perspective, the NICU's physical environment is known to provide powerful, often overwhelming experiences for all involved (i.e., patients, staff, and family members). Evaluation is complicated by the fact that the NICU environment is characterized by a number of converging, rather than discrete, stimuli. For this reason, the therapist should begin with a neurobehavioral observation when the infant is undisturbed. The infant will respond to the environment in general, and to specific events occurring around him or her, without the added stress of handling or imposed stimulation. The therapist can then observe while the infant is receiving care and, finally, while he or she is recovering after care. This observation approach enables the therapist to obtain as complete a picture as possible of the infant's ability to maintain and/or regain physiologic homeostasis, to regulate states of arousal, to signal distress or availability for interaction, and to recover from stressful events. Als and Gibes (1986) developed a detailed process for this type of observation within the Newborn Individualized Developmental Care and Assessment Program (NIDCAP). The Naturalistic Observations of Newborn Behavior (NONB) (Als, 1995) is used as part of the NIDCAP assessment. It can be administered to infants through 42 weeks of gestation and is particularly useful for infants younger than 30 weeks of gestation. The NONB consists of structured observations conducted at 2-minute intervals before, during, and after caregiving. Thus, it is sufficiently detailed to provide a thorough understanding of an infant's behavioral patterns and to serve as a source of behavioral research data. The concentrated blocks of time required to complete the NONB may not be practical for day-to-day clinical application. However, the premise that infants should be evaluated prior to, during, and after care has been a significant contribution to neonatal assessment. Als (1986) also reinforced the message that infants should be approached from the perspective of their physiologic stability and state of arousal—that is, their readiness for interaction with the environment.

The attributes of environmental stimuli to which the infant is exposed should be noted throughout the entire observation period. The following are the most important stimuli attributes to consider (Martin, 1991):

- Modality: type of sensation being experienced or sensory system being stimulated
- Intensity: strength of the stimulus required to reach the response threshold
- Duration: length of exposure to the stimulus required to elicit a response
- Location: site or area where the stimulus is perceived; some parts of the body are more sensitive than others to specific sensations (e.g., touch, pain, temperature, proprioception)

Individuals vary in their sensory thresholds, stimulus reactivity, ability to register and to process sensory experiences, and ability to inhibit irrelevant or distracting stimuli. These sources of individual variation help explain the diversity of responses seen among individual infants who are given the same types of sensory experiences. Individual differences in infants' responsiveness need to be assessed and considered to adequately support their performance.

Social Environment

Assessment of an infant's social environment must include various elements of the infant's social transactions. These elements may be related to the infant, the infant's family, or other caregivers. These elements provide the social context for the evaluation, putting the assessment observations into perspective with typical patterns of behavior and with experiences and events that may influence the assessment results. Understanding these elements provides additional opportunities for successful interaction with the infant and for obtaining the most accurate information about the infant's social responsiveness.

Infant Factors

An infant's capacity for social engagement and for responding to the environment is determined by several factors. The first factor to consider is the infant's previous response to social approaches. For example, has the infant been able to tolerate social approaches without a loss of physiologic stability? The second factor is whether the infant has been alert at any time just prior to the assessment. Third, it is important to consider whether the infant is typically more alert at predictable times and, if so, what events usually presage alert periods. It may be necessary to schedule the assessment at the optimal time for the infant. A fourth factor is whether the infant was alert during the care period preceding the assessment and, if so, for how long. Assessment observations represent only a brief period—a snapshot—of the infant's day. It is possible that the infant expended energy responding to a family visit or to a caregiver's interactions shortly before the assessment, potentially limiting the infant's responses to subsequent stimuli. A fifth factor is the infant's typical response to the presence of individual family members and familiar caregivers at the bedside. Particular family members or caregivers may elicit a more optimal response. In addition, a characteristic interaction pattern may bring out the infant's best performance or engagement—or may cause the infant to withdraw.

Family Factors

Certain family-related factors may influence the infant's social interaction and responsiveness as well. One is related to the timing of family visits. At what time of day and how often does the family typically visit? So that family members' interactions with the infant may be observed, the therapist may need to conduct the assessment outside of his or her normal work hours. Another factor is whether family visitation coincides with the infant's optimal time for responding to social approaches. If not, the therapist may recommend modifying the family's visitation schedule to synchronize with the infant's optimal time for interaction. It also is important to consider how family members interact with and/or gain support from each other, particularly at the infant's bedside. Some parents prefer the support of other NICU parents or of NICU staff to members of their family. Others are most comfortable when alone with their infant. When family members visit the NICU together, they may provide the necessary support for optimal comfort at the bedside and, therefore, an optimal approach to the infant. Nevertheless, interactions among family members are not always positive and may distract or stress individual caregivers. When scheduling an assessment during which family members will be present, the therapist must account for these factors. Nurses and social workers are often the best sources of this kind of information. The therapist should ask about family preferences or cultural/ethnic concerns to consider when making suggestions for infant–caregiver interaction. This is particularly important when there are sensitive issues or prohibitions regarding particular aspects of care. For example, the family may have decided not to have their infant use a pacifier, or their religious beliefs may prohibit the use of certain types of toys or holiday-themed items at the infant's bedside.

Other Caregiver Factors

An infant's responsiveness to the social environment also may be influenced by factors connected to caregivers outside of the family (e.g., staff). The therapist needs to determine which staff are involved in the infant's care and whether the assessment can be scheduled so that primary caregivers will be present, thus providing various firsthand insights into the infant's behavior. In addition, a family member sometimes forms a special connection with a particular team member (e.g., physician, primary nurse, social worker). The therapist should consider what insights that team member can offer regarding the family member's coping abilities and information processing style.

CONCLUSION

When the medical, physiologic, and behavioral status of an infant is known and the physical and social contexts for evaluation have been explored, information from observation of and interaction with the infant becomes more useful and relevant. For example, conducting an examination when an infant has been sedated after a large bolus of antiseizure medication would give the therapist the erroneous impression of hyporeflexia and low tone. Similarly, evaluating sensory and behavioral responsiveness of an infant who is agitated or fatigued after a medical or nursing procedure will provide a false impression. All observations and responses need to be considered within the overarching context of the infant's medical and physiologic stability, as well as the characteristics of the social and physical environments at the time of the observation.

Evaluating infant behavior and development is one of the NICU therapist's most challenging aspects of practice. A contextual approach that incorporates direct observation with information from a variety of sources (e.g., the infant's family, other team members, medical records) allows the therapist to obtain the most comprehensive view of the infant's ability and availability to participate in developmentally appropriate tasks. Such an approach also helps ensure the cooperation of the individuals who will ultimately implement the plan for developmental care. Engaging family and other team members in the evaluative process and incorporating their priorities and suggestions when making recommendations allows the NICU therapist to formulate a plan that best addresses the infant's needs within his or her performance context.

11

Family-Centered and Relationship-Based Care in the NICU

Elaine C. Meyer and Rosemarie Bigsby

OVERVIEW

This chapter uses the contextual model for the occupational performance of infants presented in Chapter 1 to describe a model for family-centered, relationship-based care in the NICU. These models illustrate the participation of immediate and extended family and of NICU personnel in an infant's development of apprenticeship and learning occupations. Family-centered care and relationship-based care can contribute to a family's ability to cope with the stress of having an infant in the NICU. A family-centered approach has been described as the preferred approach for optimizing the family's participation in their infant's care and for expanding opportunities for the fulfillment of parental roles.

This chapter presents a comprehensive summary of the literature on family-centered, relationship-based intervention with NICU families. Principles of family-centered care and parent–professional partnerships are summarized, stressing the role of the NICU therapist in family-centered intervention. Guidelines are provided for enhancing infant–caregiver participation from a family-centered perspective. Emphasis is given to parent-identified needs, parental role fulfillment, and the enhancement of parental coping in the NICU. Suggestions are given to help therapists determine when a referral for mental health services might be indicated for the family.

OBJECTIVES

- Identify the basic principles, benefits, and constraints of family-centered, relationship-based care in the NICU
- Identify activities known to promote implementation of family-centered care in the NICU
- Identify false beliefs that preclude adoption of family-based approaches
- Recognize that the ultimate goal of therapy in the NICU is optimizing the participation of the infant and family members in activities that reflect and are valued by the family
- Describe activities that support parental role participation

- Identify the special considerations that therapists must observe in supporting parental role performance and coping in the NICU
- Identify the key personnel in charge of providing psychological support to families of NICU infants
- Describe the main purpose and basic elements of parent–professional partnerships in the NICU

ELEMENTS OF FAMILY-CENTERED CARE IN THE NICU

In theory, the principles of family-centered care are easy for health care personnel to embrace. It is hard to argue against principles such as the primacy of the family in an infant's life and the basic rights of a family to participate in its infant's care. However, actual implementation of family-centered care in the NICU has proven more complicated (Arango, 1999). This chapter takes a closer look at the family of an infant in the NICU, as well as some real and perceived barriers to family participation.

A family-centered approach to care assumes certain core beliefs (Shelton et al., 1987):

- Recognition that the family is the constant in the child's life, whereas service systems and the personnel within those systems fluctuate
- Facilitation of parent–professional collaboration at all levels of health care
- Sharing of unbiased and complete information with parents about their child's care on an ongoing basis and in an appropriate and supportive manner
- Implementation of appropriate policies and programs that are comprehensive and provide emotional and financial support to meet the needs of families
- Recognition of family strengths and individuality and respect for different coping methods
- Understanding the developmental and emotional needs of infants, children, and adolescents and incorporating their families into health care delivery
- Encouragement and facilitation of parent-to-parent support
- Assurance that the design of health care delivery systems is flexible, accessible, and responsive to family needs

A basic tenet of family-centered care is the primacy of the family in the infant's life. Clinical service providers typically change during the course of the infant's development, but the family remains constant. Acknowledgment of racial, ethnic, cultural, and socioeconomic diversity among families is another assumption of family-centered care. Health care should be provided within a flexible framework to be responsive to various needs and coping abilities of families. Most NICU personnel would agree with those principles. The philosophy of family-centered care further asserts that families and clinicians are "partners" in caring for infants. As such, parents deserve to have complete, objective information about their infant. They should be encouraged to participate in decision making about their infant's care. They should be offered opportunities to obtain support and information from other families with similar concerns.

To embrace these principles, health care professionals may need to reconsider and set aside some widely held, incorrect beliefs. For example, participation by the family in the patient's daily care may be viewed as disruptive to the NICU routines; thus, some care providers may curtail the full participation of parents. Clinicians may share information on a need-to-know basis rather than provide the family with complete information. Staff may discourage referrals for parent-to-parent information sharing if they believe that this form of support leads to misconceptions and misinformation. Proponents of family-centered care assert that such prevalent attitudes of health care professionals and styles of interaction with family members deter professionals from providing optimal services to patients and their families (Arango, 1999; Rushton, 1990).

The successful transition of particular NICUs from caregiver-centered to family-centered care has not been well described. Case reports, opinion papers, and how-to articles are more common (Griffin, Wishba, & Kavanaugh, 1998; Heller & McKlindon, 1996; Jarrett, 1996a; McGrath & Conliffe-Torres, 1996; Rushton, 1990; Sweeney, 1997; Thurman, 1991; Ward, 1999). An emphasis on the following elements recurs in the literature:

- Systematic, carefully thought-out training for staff at *all* levels, from attending physicians to housekeeping personnel
- Incorporation of "veteran" parents as educators and supporters for other parents
- Provision of anticipatory guidance to parents as early as possible, including during the mother's prenatal hospitalization
- Ongoing, evaluative feedback (surveys or telephone interviews) from families following their infant's discharge from the NICU

Evaluative feedback from parents and family members has yielded a wealth of information about families' perceptions of the NICU experience. The stress imposed by the physical environment, barriers to parental participation, and sources of support have been richly described (Bass, 1991; Coffman, Levitt, & Deets, 1991; Dobbins et al., 1994; Miles, Fun, & Carlson, 1993; Miles, Funk, & Kasper, 1992; Prudhoe & Peters, 1995; Raeside, 1997; Redshaw & Harris, 1995; Seideman et al., 1997).

The literature highlights the difficulty of educating NICU staff about making the transition to a more family-centered philosophy. Only a few studies, however, have focused on important implementation aspects such as improving the attitudes of nurses toward increased parental participation and the ability of NICU staff to cope with the stresses of the NICU environment (Frank, Paredes, & Curtin, 1997; Rosenthal, Schmid, & Black, 1989). Meyer and colleagues (1996), for example, examined the attitudinal changes and resistance of staff members to the implementation of sibling visitation in the NICU. Prior to visitation, staff members were concerned about the risks of infection, disruption of NICU routines, and supervision issues. Following a well-organized sibling visitation program, the staff acknowledged that these concerns were largely unfounded.

Previous chapters introduced transactional theory and the concepts of risk, resilience, and goodness of fit that could set the foundation for family-centered neonatal care. These concepts provide a psychosocially oriented, developmental framework for neonatal intervention. As increasing numbers of NICUs make the transition to family-centered care, neonatal therapists working in the NICU need to understand the core principles of this approach. Therapists must then incorporate these principles into their interactions and interventions with families and other members of the health care team to promote family participation.

Enhancing Family Participation

Optimal participation of the infant and family members in activities that are valued within the family's culture is the ultimate goal of developmental intervention (Coster, 1996). To achieve that goal, family resources, priorities, and values must be explored (Raines, 1996); existing barriers to family participation must be identified; and the capacity of the infant and family to cope with and/or adapt to the challenges of the NICU must be supported (see Chapter 1). These objectives can best be met through a psychosocially oriented model for service delivery. This is sometimes referred to as the infant mental health model, in which the developmental and behavioral performance of the infant is viewed within the context of family needs, values, expectations and abilities (Olson & Baltman, 1994). In this chapter, the term *relationship-based care* (Holloway, 1998) is used to describe a practical, psychosocially oriented approach for working with family members and other caregivers. The relationship-based approach focuses the therapist on enhancing NICU infants' performance within the most enduring context for development—their relationship with their parents (Holloway, 1998). Rather than taking a prescriptive approach with a preset agenda, Holloway recommended guiding one's actions by parent–infant cues and by the existing circumstances. Holloway (1994) made the following practical suggestions for collaborating with parents to support their successful participation in caregiving activities:

- Create opportunities for a two-way dialogue between the parent(s) and the therapist.
- Address the parents' concerns as well as those identified by the therapist.
- Select methods of interacting with parents that respect their individual role definitions and their values and interests.
- Observe and interpret the infant's behavior jointly with parents, and remain alert and sensitive to the responses of the infant and the parents.
- Acknowledge the parents' skills and successes, and use the parents' expertise.
- Support the importance of parent–infant nurturing in all caregiving activities.

Family involvement is an integral part of neonatal therapy services delivered within a relationship-based model. The initial referral for a particular infant may be generated by members of the medical team, but from that point on, interaction with the family becomes as important as contact with the infant or collaboration with the other team members. Ideally, prior to initiating contact with an infant, the therapist will meet with the infant's parents to discuss visiting schedules. Developmental assessments can often be postponed until the parents can be present. If that is not possible, then the therapist should contact the family and arrange a time to review the assessment findings, jointly observe the infant, and generate suggestions for enhancing and promoting infant–caregiver participation. The following subsections discuss important considerations when first approaching parents and/or family members.

Initial Contact and Assessment

Family members usually focus first on their infant's appearance and the extent of his or her illness (Griffin et al., 1998). Following introductions, including an explanation of the therapist's professional role and of presenting problems that generated the referral, the therapist should turn his or her attention to the infant. Most parents expect the therapist to focus his or her work on the infant. Nonetheless, the therapist must inform the family that although intervention begins with the infant, it must be gradually expanded to include parent–infant interaction and caregiving. When the parents and infant are ready, the skillful therapist makes this transition as seamless as possible.

It is important to refer to the infant positively. Good places to start include pointing out a particularly attractive or endearing trait, such as the infant's eyes or hair, or complimenting the parents on a family photo or toy that they brought in to brighten and personalize the infant's space (see Figure 25). These are more than social gestures. They communicate to the family the therapist's view of their infant as an individual who belongs to a family rather than merely as a patient. This communication sets a tone of respectfulness and honors the parents as being central in the baby's life.

If the infant has been a long-term resident of the NICU, the therapist should look for opportunities to point out the family's beneficial actions on the infant's behalf. Further options for therapy involvement also should be discussed, beginning by asking parents how they are currently involved in their baby's care, how comfortable they are with the level of care that they are offering, and whether there are other areas of care in which they would like to participate (Lawhon, 2002). This information increases the therapist's understanding of the parents' perspectives and priorities for care (i.e., parent identified needs) rather than those hypothesized by professionals or the team (Meyer et al., 1994).

Overall, parents must be made aware that part of the therapist's role is to help facilitate their parental role or involvement in ways that they think are important (see Figure 26). Suggestions gleaned from previous experiences with other NICU infants and their parents form an important component of what therapists have to offer families. It is vital for a therapist to convey availability as a resource person who is attuned to the parents' priorities for care.

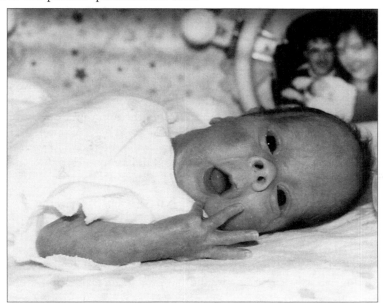

Figure 25. Family photo used to personalize an infant's bed space. Complimenting family members on personal touches such as photos communicates the therapist's acknowledgment that the family is central in the baby's life.

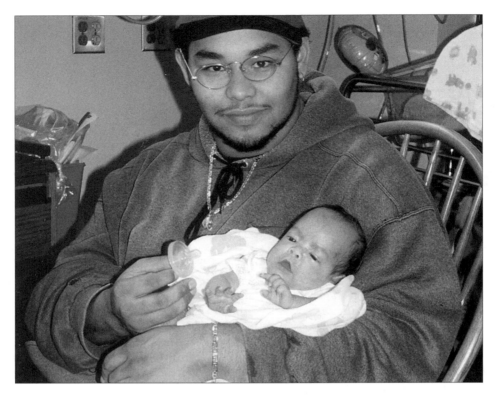

Figure 26.   This proud father is closely involved in his infant's care in the NICU.

Family Visitation and Intervention

The therapist must discuss the family's typical schedule for and engagement during visitation: who visits, when the visit occurs, how long the visit lasts, and which aspects of care include family involvement. Are family members participating in skin-to-skin care? Is their infant being fed at specific times or at a time that is convenient for the family? What are the parents' preferences for privacy and for joint observation with the therapist? This information helps determine the appropriate areas and schedule for assessment and intervention.

Initial interactions with family members provide the therapist with the opportunity to build a therapist–family relationship and to communicate the importance that the therapist places on

- Functioning as a member of the larger NICU team
- Including the family in that team
- Acknowledging the family's primary role in the infant's life
- Recognizing the family's right to privacy and confidentiality
- Identifying what is important to the family and incorporating family priorities into objectives for intervention
- Learning how the family members perceive their infant's needs and which strategies they choose to use to accommodate those needs

- Assessing the family members' desired level of participation in their infant's care and providing the supports that are necessary to enhance their involvement

Accomplishing these objectives is a tall order for the neonatal therapist, requiring a strong psychosocial approach to service provision. Some parents may be hesitant or fearful of becoming more involved in their infant's care. They may have tried and failed, or they may not realize the extent to which they can participate. Several issues must be understood to provide psychosocially sensitive care to parents and family members in the NICU. These issues are explored in the following subsections.

Violation of Expectations

Most parents expect that their baby will be born full term, will be healthy, and will be able to go home within a few days following the birth. Hospitalization in the NICU can violate these parental expectations. Preterm infants are often born before their parents are practically or emotionally prepared for their arrival. What is expected to be a joyous and celebratory time in the family's life can quickly turn into a stressful experience in the NICU. Parents may be fraught with fear and worry about the infant's survival, health, and well-being. An infant's admission to the NICU can immediately derail parental expectations and plans for quiet time with the baby, rooming-in (sleeping in the same room as the infant), breast feeding, nurturing, and introducing the baby to family and friends.

Mothers can be particularly affected by unfulfilled expectations. They may not receive the expected level of care from family or staff because of their infant's critical needs. Mothers, as well as fathers, can experience strong emotions during this time, including sadness, disbelief, failure, shame, disappointment, betrayal, and anger (Bass, 1991; Hughes, McCollum, Scheffel, & Sanchez, 1994; Miles et al., 1992). There may be little time for parents to sort through their feelings because the infant's needs are more immediate and serious and, in most cases, take precedence over the parents' needs. Although staff may try to address the parents' psychological needs by offering reassurance or information, efforts may resemble crisis intervention rather than ongoing psychosocial support to explore, acknowledge, and better understand preterm birth and NICU hospitalization.

Loss of Control and Emotional Responses

Loss of control, and the emotional disequilibrium that it engenders, has been identified as a central issue for families facing medical crises (Pollin, 1995). In the NICU, parents may feel a loss of control over the most basic issues, including their infant's survival, protection, and well-being. Parents generally take for granted that they will make decisions about who cares for their child, but this is not so in the NICU. Parents find themselves dependent on individuals previously unknown to them—NICU staff members, with their expertise, availability, and familiarity with the hospital culture. The parents' loss of control in the NICU often stands in stark contrast to the careful planning and preparation exercised throughout the pregnancy, such as eating well to ensure good nutrition, keeping prenatal appointments, assembling the baby's nursery, making a birth plan, and choosing a community pediatrician.

As noted in the previous section, parents also can experience many strong emotions. Some parents describe a profound sense of vulnerability and sadness and an abrupt loss of innocence surrounding their childbirth experience (Affleck & Tennen,

1991; Harrison, 1983; Madden, 2000). For other parents, anger and betrayal are the predominant emotions surrounding the NICU experience. Anxiety and worry can be significant when there is uncertainty surrounding the infant's survival and outcome. How a parent responds emotionally to the NICU is multifactorial, reflecting not only the circumstances of the birth and the infant's condition but also the parent's character style, previous experiences with illness and loss, and attributions regarding the situation. Previous pregnancy loss, in particular, can influence and intensify parental emotional responses to the birth and hospitalization. In these cases, unresolved feelings and grief over the previous loss(es), in addition to the fear of a potential new loss, can be rekindled and affect the parent's attachment to, relationship with, and interactions with the baby.

The infant's needs remain foremost in the parents' thoughts and concerns, so the parents' emotional experience and expression often are yoked to the infant. In general, most parents become less emotionally reactive as their infant's medical course stabilizes and improves. Simply stated, when the baby does better physically, then the parents do better emotionally. In most cases, parents put their own needs behind those of the child and rate their own personal needs as less important than any child or parent–child needs (Kirschbaum, 1990). Although most parents acknowledge their physiologic and psychological needs, some are seemingly unaware of their own needs (Kasper & Nyamathi, 1988). Parents may be helped by simple suggestions to take care of themselves or to pace themselves so that they do not become overly fatigued or ill. They can benefit from hearing that one of the best ways for them to help their infant is to take good care of themselves. Maternal postpartum status and needs should also be recognized and accommodated.

Threatened Parental Roles

Traditional parental roles include protecting, caring, educating, and providing for their children. Most parents—and most societies—expect that parents will act as the primary care providers, advocates, and decision makers for their children. Admission to the NICU can seriously threaten parents' ability to fulfill these important and familiar roles (Miles et al., 1992; Seideman et al., 1997). The NICU can undermine the sense of competence, confidence, and control of even the most experienced, dedicated parents. First-time parents struggle with trying to learn and to fulfill these new and daunting roles. Parents may find themselves vulnerable and, in many cases, unable to protect or even comfort their infant, who must endure necessary but painful procedures (Seideman et al., 1997).

The lack of clear parental roles, the lack of privacy, and the intensity of the NICU environment are not conducive to parental feelings of self-efficacy and self-esteem, or to early parent–infant interactions. Often, parental opportunities to learn about the baby are limited, which can further compromise parental confidence, participation, and pride in caregiving.

Parents need to know that they have special attributes to offer their infant that cannot be provided by staff, such as their touch, their voices, and the mother's breast milk. Staff recognition of the parents' contributions signals validation and respect and conveys to the parents that they are vitally important to their infant. As the infant stabilizes and caregiving opportunities increase, parents generally are ready to participate in the infant's care. Some parents, however, may be reluctant to participate in caregiving because of vivid recollections of their infant's earlier fragile health status and/or their perception of the neonatal staff's superior skills and efficiency (McGrath & Meyer, 1992). Whenever possible, NICU personnel should refrain from "doing for" parents, which may diminish the parents' sense of competence. Professionals need to be aware that they may unwittingly intimidate or inhibit parents. An environment that is conducive to learning—one that is nonevaluative, supportive, and not rushed— must be created.

In a study by Seideman and colleagues (1997), parents of infants in neonatal and pediatric intensive care units placed high value on problem-focused coping strategies, such as being near their child as much as possible, making sure their child receives proper care, and learning as much as possible about their child's situation. Increased participation in caregiving places parents in an ideal position to share observations with other staff and to recognize both positive and negative changes as they occur (Lawhon, 2002). Feeding, in particular, can be a very satisfying aspect of care for parent participation. Yet, feeding can also be anxiety producing for parents, given the considerable emphasis on oral intake and weight gain; the use of these indicators in determining progress and readiness for discharge; and the feeding difficulties of some infants. Beyond learning opportunities, parents may benefit from "agenda-free" down time with their infant. This can be a time when they are free to hold, snuggle with, and get to know their baby without the demands of being taught about caregiving, feeling in the "spotlight," or having to interact with the staff.

Parent-Identified Needs

Although parental needs can vary during the course of hospitalization, parents have identified some important common needs. They consistently highlight the need for obtaining accurate information, ready access to their infant, and meaningful participation in the infant's care. When asked to identify more specific needs, parents cited a belief that there is hope in the knowledge that the child is receiving expert care, and the belief that they have been provided with all available information (Frank et al., 1997; Kirschbaum, 1990). Parents require information to understand and form opinions about the situation, to ascribe meaning to their infant's illness, and to participate in decision making (Bass, 1991; Curley & Meyer, 1996). Similarly, Kasper and Nyamathi (1988) identified common parental needs as proximity to the child; frequent, accurate, and truthful information about the child's condition; participation in the child's care; sleeping accommodations near the child; and reassurance that the child is receiving expert care and treatment.

Parental Coping in the NICU

When faced with the acute stress inherent in intensive care admission, most parents try to cope by relying on previously used strategies for handling stress in their lives (Meyer, Snelling, & Myren-Manbeck, 1998). If parents find that their usual coping strategies are not sufficient, then they may be open to trying new suggestions. It is important to remember that there is not one way to survive a NICU hospitalization, nor is there a ready blueprint for parents to follow. As clinicians, it is advisable to be respectful and supportive of the parents' efforts to cope and to remember that they are doing the best that they can. There may be times when parents struggle to cope by clinging to familiar but ineffective coping strategies. In these situations, coping advice or direct help can be offered if requested by the parents. It is advisable to first join with the parents by identifying the common goals of fostering the well-being of the infant and their success as parents. Ideas can then be generated together, or suggestions can be offered—particularly those that previous NICU parents have found helpful (Lawhon, 2002). Parent support groups and parent-to-parent support from veteran parents can be offered if parents are interested and such programs are available. Many parents whose infants have required NICU hospitalization wish to speak to other parents who have been there and survived (Jarrett, 1996b; Roman et al., 1995). Certainly, veteran parents have important perspectives to share and, by virtue of their status as parents, they possess an unmatchable authenticity. It must be ensured that veteran parents have had the time and opportunity to resolve their own emotional issues and that they have been trained and supervised in providing parent-to-parent support (Jarrett, 1996a).

Although there is wide variability among parents in their responses to the NICU, there are some shared characteristics. When their infant is hospitalized, parents may exhibit shock and disbelief, feelings of helplessness, and loss of power (Graves & Ware, 1990). Almost immediately, they begin to search for explanations to understand the baby's prematurity or illness and to implement coping strategies that have previously served them well. A study by Hughes and colleagues (1994) highlighted the many and varied coping strategies employed by parents in the NICU. Mothers reported using 135 different coping strategies, and fathers reported 70 strategies. Although the frequency with which coping methods were used varied between men and women, the most commonly reported strategies were positive communication/ social support, escape/avoidance, relying on religious faith, crying, taking care of oneself, focusing on the infant, generic emotion-focused strategies (e.g., looking on the bright side), and problem solving. Seeking social support was the most important coping strategy cited by both men and women. Mothers relied most heavily on their spouses, whereas fathers relied most heavily on staff. Discussions about the range of coping styles and preferred methods of coping can be useful to parents, especially when parents cope differently from each other, when there are undercurrents of disapproval about how some family members cope, or when one spouse holds unrealistically high expectations for the other's coping ability.

Meeting the Family's Psychosocial Needs and Initiating Mental Health Referrals

Several staff members within the NICU environment may play a role in psychosocial service delivery to families. Traditionally, social workers are viewed as the primary care providers and advocates for family members. To sustain a viable psychosocially sensitive milieu, however, all staff members need to value and embrace psychological principles. In most units, social workers are assigned to each family and fulfill varied roles, including psychosocial assessment, family support and advocacy, instrumental support, and legal and protective services, if required. Although there is considerable variability among units, other hospital-based professionals who may be available to meet the needs of families include psychologists, psychiatrists, child life specialists, chaplains, discharge planners, ethicists, child abuse specialists, and parent volunteers.

In most cases, the nurses and social workers can adequately address the family's psychosocial needs. When the family's psychological needs demand more intense or more complex services, however, mental health staff should be readily consulted and included in the caregiving team. The expertise of mental health professionals can be particularly useful when working with families that have multiple problems; families with members facing anxiety, depression, suicidal tendencies, or bereavement; and families with members who have preexisting psychiatric conditions. Referrals should be generated if there are concerns that a parent's emotional issues and behavior are interfering with early attachment, visitation, parent–infant interactions, and/or participation in infant caregiving and discharge preparation. For example, a mother who has a history of depression and is withdrawn, tearful, and anxious at the infant's bedside should receive early and coordinated mental health care. Mothers who experience life-threatening childbirth complications and family members who suffer neonatal deaths should be referred. Mothers who require psychotropic medication such as antidepressants, antianxiety medication, or neuroleptic medication may benefit from review of their psychopharmacological management, especially if there are any plans to breast feed. Parents with histories of substance abuse, domestic violence, or protective service involvement should also come to the attention of the unit's mental health consultant.

Parents and Professionals as Partners

Family-centered care models emphasize forging partnerships between parents and professionals in health care planning and delivery. It is advisable to ask parents what their preferences are for the delivery of information and how they would like to be involved in the baby's care and in decision making (Meyer et al., 1998). Rather than having a one-way conveyance of information from staff to parents, a regular forum must be provided for parents and staff to exchange information. Professionals must ask parents about their perceptions of the infant's progress; use understandable language; and offer to write down new terminology, developmental milestones, or findings for parents (McGrath & Meyer, 1992). If the parents seem unable to ask questions or to raise concerns, then it may be possible to facilitate dialogue by sharing common concerns and modeling the questions and comments of other parents. For example, the developmental therapist might say, "Sometimes parents wonder how their baby's prematurity might affect his or her development." Such comments can normalize or decrease parental concerns, facilitate discussion, and demonstrate understanding of parental perspectives.

There is considerable variability among parents regarding their expectations and wishes for parent–professional relationships and collaborative decision making. Affleck and Tennen (1991) found that mothers rarely desire exclusive personal control over their child's hospital care. They reported that 25% of mothers in the NICU sought an active role in decision making when care providers gave adequate information and actively solicited parental participation. A second group, comprising approximately half of the mothers, was reported to be uninterested in participatory control in the infant's medical treatment. These parents willingly relinquished control to the medical staff, whose competence they trusted. A final group of mothers were reluctant to cede control of medical decisions to staff but also were unable to achieve a satisfactory level of participatory care.

CONCLUSION

Within the NICU, therapists must remain receptive to different parental perceptions and choices in degree of participation. The NICU therapist must recognize the need to adapt his or her parent–professional communication style to meet the needs of families, not vice versa. Families of infants in the NICU generally are in crisis. Each family's coping strategies are influenced by the family members' educational and cultural backgrounds, personalities, and past events. The challenge of optimizing infant outcomes after NICU discharge goes beyond the care of the infant. It involves building trusting relationships with families and entering a partnership with them that optimizes their ability to cope with this stressful experience (Van Riper, 2001).

12

Elements of Neonatal Positioning

OVERVIEW

This chapter presents an overview of neonatal positioning and its influence on an infant's well-being and developmental outcomes. The typical postural patterns of healthy full-term infants are described, and the importance of flexion is emphasized. Benefits and disadvantages of prone, supine, and sidelying positioning are discussed. Readers are strongly cautioned about the life-threatening risks of prone positioning, especially during sleep or unsupervised periods. The supine position is recommended by the American Academy of Pediatricians to prevent SIDS, although this position may be disorganizing for some infants. Strategies for decreasing the potential negative effects of supine positioning and for enhancing the infant's tolerance of the position are recommended.

The most prevalent positioning issues in the NICU are discussed in this chapter, and possible causal explanations are given for the most common positioning problems. The chapter reviews potential effects of poor positioning on an infant's developmental outcome. General principles of adaptive positioning are highlighted and followed by detailed discussions of the advantages, disadvantages, and risks of positioning NICU infants in the different positions (prone, supine, sidelying, and head elevated). Emphasis is given to the value of postural supports for promoting the adequate positioning of infants in the NICU.

OBJECTIVES

- Describe the common postural patterns of healthy full-term infants
- Describe the benefits and risks or disadvantages of the various positioning arrangements of healthy full-term infants and NICU infants, recognizing the importance of offering a variety of positioning alternatives
- Identify factors and medical conditions that challenge ideal positioning of infants in the NICU
- Recognize the potential short- and long-term risks associated with inadequate positioning of NICU infants and the most common postural deformities that may result from poor positioning
- Identify the basic principles of adaptive positioning, the positioning equipment and arrangements used in the NICU, and the methods of providing postural support in the different positioning arrangements used in the NICU

- Recognize that the best posture for newborns is symmetric physiologic flexion, with the neck in slight flexion, shoulders protracted, pelvis elevated, and hands in midline, close to the face
- Recognize the importance of offering infants opportunities to explore a variety of positions
- Recognize the importance of maintaining proper positioning when handling an infant
- Identify other issues and considerations related to NICU positioning, including the appearance, cleanliness, and safety of the positioning equipment and the texture and density of materials used

POSITIONING HEALTHY FULL-TERM INFANTS

Positioning and handling are two essential components of the care of newborns in the NICU. With the exception of the transitional full-term infants and the larger, healthier preterm infants, most infants in the NICU typically require specialized and developmentally appropriate positioning and handling. In most hospitals, these two aspects of neonatal care are primary responsibilities of NICU developmental personnel. Positioning concerns are not limited exclusively to the NICU, however. Research findings during the 1990s linked sleeping position with SIDS, raising awareness about the importance and safety of proper positioning for all infants.

The posture of healthy full-term newborns is symmetrical and predominantly flexed, with shoulder protraction and a posterior pelvic tilt (Vergara, 1993). The strong flexor pattern is sometimes referred to as *physiologic flexion* because it has been attributed to the typically flexed position held by most fetuses during their third trimester in utero. This flexed position enables newborns to remain motorically and physiologically organized when they are not being held, regardless of how they are positioned (Chapter 8).

Healthy full-term newborns adopt various typical postures in the prone, supine, and sidelying positions. In the prone position, they adopt a flexed posture, bearing weight unilaterally on the face, upper chest, forearms (generally close to or under the trunk), anterior aspect of the knees, and the feet. The pelvis is usually elevated, and the hips and knees are flexed to about 90° (see Figure 27). In the supine positions, these infants bear weight on the posterolateral aspect of the head (usually the right side), the entire back, and the sacrum. The strong influence of physiologic flexion enables them to maintain the extremities flexed against gravity for the first few days of life, with the scapulae and shoulders protracted, and the hips elevated (see Figure 28). Physiologic flexion prevents adoption of neck hyperextension patterns. Healthy full-term infants also may lie fairly stable in a sidelying position, maintaining the trunk laterally perpendicular to the supporting surface; keeping the neck, trunk, and extremities flexed; and bearing weight on the entire supporting side (see Figure 29).

Unless agitated, healthy newborns who are physiologically and motorically stable can tolerate any position—prone, supine, or sidelying—without undue stress. Prone was once considered the best position for promoting sleep and neuromotor development in infants. Positioning healthy infants in prone for sleeping, however, is now discouraged because of the mounting evidence suggesting increased risk of SIDS in prone (American Academy of Pediatrics [AAP], 1996; Galland, Bolton, Taylor, Sayers, & Williams, 2000; Stark, 1997). The main factor associated with a greater risk

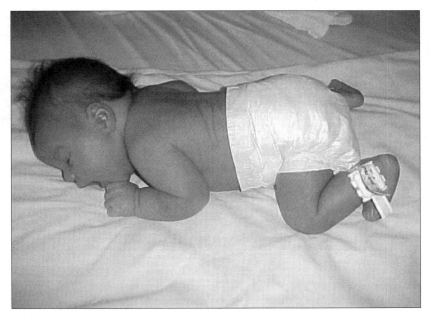

Figure 27. This full-term newborn is only 3 days old. Strong physiologic flexion in his upper and lower extremities is observed in the prone position.

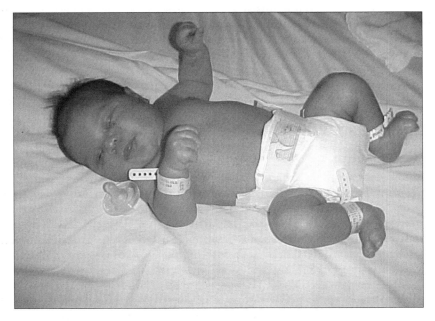

Figure 28. This full-term infant is still showing strong physiologic flexion in the supine position by his third day of life.

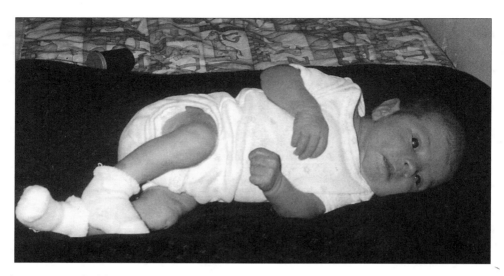

Figure 29. Typical sidelying posture of a 4-day-old full-term infant.

of SIDS in prone is that compared with supine, prone positioning raises thresholds for arousal and wakening; thus, prone sleeping infants have a greater difficulty waking up if they experience respiratory distress (Galland, Taylor, & Bolton, 2002). Effect on the diaphragm is another factor that potentially associates prone positioning with a greater risk of SIDS in full-term infants. The strength of the diaphragm may be affected because the diaphragm is significantly shorter and thicker when an infant is placed in the prone position (Rehan, Nakashima, Gutman, Rubin, & McCool, 2000).

SIDS occurs more commonly after the newborn period. Nevertheless, as a preventive measure, the AAP strongly recommends supine or sidelying positioning of infants birth through 8 months for sleeping or unsupervised periods (Spieker & Brannen, 1996; Willinger et al., 1998). A 38% decrease in the incidence of SIDS over a 4-year period after the original AAP recommendations (Willinger et al., 1998) and accumulating research evidence (AAP, 1996; Spieker & Brannen, 1996) strongly support supine sleeping as the position with the lowest risk for SIDS. Even after accounting for maternal prenatal smoking, SIDS decreased by more than 33% between 1989 and 1996 (Pollack & Frohna, 2001). Sidelying sleeping is considered safer than prone, but not as safe as supine (Spieker & Brannen, 1996). The "Back-to-Sleep" (supine sleeping) campaign of 1994 initially received much resistance from developmental personnel because of fear that supine positioning would be detrimental to the infants' neuromotor development. As of 2003, however, studies have failed to identify serious neuromotor consequences of supine positioning (Ratliff-Schaub et al., 2001). The most notable neuromotor disadvantage is a slight delay (still within the normal range) in the acquisition of several gross motor milestones: head control (Ratliff-Schaub et al., 2001); rolling over (Davis, Moon, Sachs, & Ottolini, 1998; Jantz, Blosser, & Fruechting, 1997); and tripod sitting, creeping, crawling, and pulling to stand (Davis et al., 1998). Such minor and transient neuromotor issues are not of long-term concern, particularly when an infant's survival would otherwise be at risk (Davis et al., 1998; Jantz et al., 1997).

Even the healthiest newborns may experience periods of agitation that may require the use of adaptive positioning strategies. For many infants, the supine position tends to be more stressful and physiologically disorganizing than the prone or sidelying positions. When compared with prone positioning, the following factors associated with supine positioning may be disorganizing for newborns:

- The weight-bearing area is smaller in supine, so limited contact with the supporting surface could cause postural instability and increased startles (Vergara, 1993).
- Infants tend to move more, change postures more frequently, and exhibit less organized movements (i.e., jerky, twitching) in supine than in prone (Hashimoto et al., 1983); movements in supine have a "writhing" quality and "tight" appearance (Hadders-Algra & Prechtl, 1992).
- The supine position facilitates extensor patterns (Fiorentino, 1965).
- Maintaining a flexed posture in supine against the constant pull of gravity on the extremities requires ongoing neuromuscular effort and considerable use of energy, particularly after the first 2 days of life (Maekawa & Ochiai, 1975; Vergara, 1993).
- Respiratory activity is more labored and less coordinated in supine (Adams, Zabaleta, & Sackner, 1994; Hashimoto et al., 1983), whereas the thoracoabdominal musculature is in a position of mechanical advantage in prone (Adams et al., 1994). However, the improved stability of respiratory physiology in prone has "no proven clinical benefit" in healthy infants (AAP, 1996, p. 1216).
- Sleep epochs are shorter and more interrupted in supine (Hashimoto et al., 1983).
- Auditory arousal threshold during sleep is lower in supine (Franco et al., 1998).
- Periods of alertness and arousal (wakefulness) tend to be longer in supine (Amemiya, Vos, & Prechtl, 1991; Hashimoto et al., 1983).

Perhaps the most serious negative effects of supine positioning are decreased sleep and increased energy consumption. In contrast, the supine position is more beneficial than prone in several aspects. For instance, supine sleeping is associated with a lower heart rate and better alertness and arousal (Amemiya et al., 1991). In addition when crying, supine infants have improved pulmonary function (i.e., better lung capacity) (Shen, Zhoa, Huang, Lin, & Wu, 1996). Many of the seemingly negative factors associated with supine sleeping, therefore, may have a protective function against suffocation and SIDS (AAP, 1996). Although the specific mechanisms that explain the lower incidence of SIDS in supine are not known, the lower arousal threshold and heightened arousal observed when infants sleep in supine are believed to be crucial protective elements.

The potential life-saving value of the supine position outweighs by far any minor disadvantages or inconveniences. Well-regulated, physiologically stable infants tolerate and quickly adapt to the potentially disorganizing effects of the supine position. Conversely, infants who are less regulated or who become agitated in supine may require external support to adapt to the stress and challenges of this position.

Sidelying positioning also can be disorganizing for infants who cannot maintain a stable posture. Unstable sidelying infants who are not offered external support may develop increased neck and trunk hyperextension patterns (Vergara, 1993). For many infants, however, sidelying tends to be less disruptive than supine (Grenier, Bigsby, Vergara, & Lester, 2003). Stressful positioning becomes a more serious issue for infants whose health and growth could be compromised by physiologic instability or excessive energy expenditure. For these infants, an individualized evaluation of their responses to caregiving is the only way to determine which positioning and handling strategies reduce stress and promote physiologic and behavioral organization.

A number of simple strategies are effective for enhancing neurobehavioral organization in healthy infants who experience positioning stress. Swaddling has been used for centuries to promote calming and physiologic and motoric stability in newborns in supine, prone, or sidelying positions. Swaddling is generally well accepted by infants (Gerard, Harris, & Thach, 2002). The deep tactile and proprioceptive support offered through swaddling resembles the intrauterine containment lost at birth, possibly helping infants feel secure (Short, Brooks-Brunn, Reeves, Yeager, & Thorpe, 1996) and experience greater comfort sleeping in supine (Gerard et al., 2002). It also helps promote self-calming behaviors (e.g., hand-to-mouth movements, hand-on-face movements, hand clasping, sucking) (Short et al., 1996). Nonnutritive sucking may also comfort and facilitate flexion and neurobehavioral organization in newborns (Pickler, Higgins, & Crummette, 1993). Forming boundaries or "nests" with rolled blankets or stuffed toys is another external-support technique for promoting flexion in infants stressed by positioning (Vohr et al., 1999). Infant hammocks and polystyrene-filled cushions can be calming and organizing but are *extremely dangerous* and should *never* be used without close supervision (Kemp & Thach, 1991). The use of positioning pillows or hammocks with unsupervised infants is *strongly discouraged.*

Healthy full-term infants with serious postural disorganization issues may be referred for positioning consultation, especially if positioning interferes with self-regulation and participation in neonatal tasks and activities. The most common indications for postural intervention are lack of physiologic flexion, strong extensor patterns, and postural asymmetries with lack of midline control.

An additional, longer-lasting concern is the increased incidence of posterolateral deformational plagiocephaly (flattening of the skull), which sometimes occurs in infants with a strong preference for keeping or maintaining the head turned to one side while sleeping in supine. This condition is thought to be more prevalent among infants with localized cranial flattening at birth, which then progresses to posterolateral deformational plagiocephaly (Peitsch, Keefer, LaBrie, & Mulliken, 2002). This type of flattening is particularly common among infants of multiple gestation pregnancies (Littlefield, Kelly, Pomatto, & Beals, 2002). Infants may also develop a flattened skull in the NICU secondary to limited options in positioning after surgical procedures for hydrocephalus or during prolonged periods of intubation. In addition to the misshapen appearance of the skull, the plagiocephaly, if allowed to progress, may result in alteration of the skeletal-facial structures, including displacement of the temporomandibular joint (St. John, Mulliken, Kaban, & Padwa, 2002) and asymmetry of the orbits, with potential disruption of the visual field. Infants with plagiocephaly should be evaluated by a pediatric neurosurgeon or plastic surgeon who may prescribe progressive skull shaping with a helmet or surgical intervention.

POSITIONING IN THE NICU

Positioning influences numerous areas of functioning in developing infants, so proper positioning is critical for the short- and long-term well-being of the infants in the NICU. Positioning can affect an infant's body systems (e.g., autonomic/physiologic, neuromotor, state, interactive, self-regulation) positively or negatively. Proper positioning promotes self-regulation and facilitates the infant's participation in normal sensorimotor experiences, such as bringing the hand to the mouth and face, whereas inappropriate positioning may contribute to physiologic distress and behavioral disorganization (Bellefeuille-Reid & Jakubek, 1989; Fay, 1988; Hallsworth, 1995; Updike,

Schmidt, Macke, Cahoon, & Miller, 1986; Vohr et al., 1999). Soft tissue integrity, postural alignment, and shoulder and pelvic girdle activity can also be affected (Vohr et al., 1999). The long-lasting postural and motor consequences of inappropriate positioning are potentially the most severe in infants with central nervous system disorders (Bellefeuille-Reid & Jakubek, 1989). VLBW and sick infants may be affected by poor positioning in more complex ways. Poorly regulated states of arousal, physiologic instability, and inadequate postural control may occur (Brandon, Holditch-Davis, & Beylea, 1999; Harrison, 1997). This affects the infant's ability to respond adaptively to positive and negative experiences, thereby interfering with the infant's active participation in developmentally appropriate activities.

Infants in the NICU face many issues that hinder their ability to adopt typical newborn flexor postures at a time when flexor patterns should prevail (Hallsworth, 1995). Ideal positioning is challenged by the type and severity of conditions presented by infants within the NICU context. The goal of positioning management in the NICU is to provide postural and self-regulatory supports that normalize infants' sensorimotor experiences as much as possible while accommodating the many constraints imposed by their medical conditions and environment.

Etiology and Outcomes of Poor Positioning

Factors such as neuromotor and physiologic immaturity, illness, genetic or congenital conditions, medication, sedation, life-support equipment, and medical and surgical procedures predispose infants to assume postures likely to interfere with function and development. Neonatal hypotonia is the most common factor that prevents infants from achieving the typical newborn postures of weight bearing and physiologic flexion. Neonatal hypotonia occurs most frequently in preterm infants as a result of neuromotor immaturity and decreased (or lack of) exposure to the flexion-inducing intrauterine crowding that occurs toward the end of a term pregnancy (see Chapter 9). Infants who are sick also exhibit decreased muscle tone because of motoric and physiologic instability or sedation (see Chapter 8). Infants with Down syndrome, Prader-Willi syndrome, spina bifida, or myotonic dystrophy also may have significantly decreased muscle tone. Limited mobility and the pull of gravity on their hypotonic bodies lead these infants to adopt flattened postures against the supporting surface, whether lying supine or prone (Downs, Edwards, McCromick, Roth, & Stewart, 1991; Hallsworth, 1995). Prolonged exposure to static flattened postures may lead to the development of numerous deformities that interfere with functional performance, even in the absence of neurologic abnormalities (Bellefeuille-Reid & Jakubek, 1989; Fay, 1988; Hallsworth, 1995; Updike et al., 1986; Vohr et al., 1999).

ELBW preterm infants sometimes have an atypical skull shape, dolichocephaly (also spelled *dolicocephaly*), which is a bilateral flattening of the parietal bones of the skull, resulting in an elongated, narrow head shape (see Figure 30). Dolichocephaly is a type of plagiocephaly that occurs when preterm infants have to be positioned with the head to one side or the other, whether the infants are prone or supine, particularly in infants with low tone. In some nurseries, gel pads are used to distribute the weight of the head more evenly and reduce this effect; however, studies are inconclusive as to the benefit of these pads. NICU therapists are responsible for monitoring infant positioning and for making recommendations to prevent skull flattening whenever possible. Alternating an infant's head position regularly and using head rests to keep the infant's head in midline once he or she has been extubated may prevent skull shaping. Supervised sidelying and prone positioning can be used

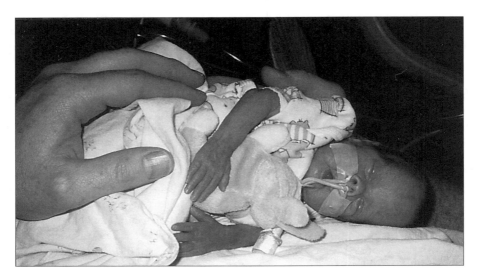

Figure 30. Lateral skull flattening is observed in this premature infant with dolichocephaly.

when the infant is awake. Allowing the infant to experience other positions, such as being held in semiupright positions with little or no pressure to the skull, may also be appropriate as the infant becomes more stable. Plagiocephaly interferes with head rotation in supine (Cartlidge & Rutter, 1998; Hemingway & Oliver, 1991; Peitsch et al., 2002; Rutter, Hinchliffe; & Cartlidge, 1993; Updike et al., 1986) and is more common in preterm infants.

Various maladaptive postures result from neonatal hypotonia. Frog-lying is one of the most common postural deformities in these infants. In supine or prone positions, infants with low tone are able to use the gravity-eliminated plane of the supporting surface to flex the externally rotated hips and the knees. They keep their hips widely abducted because of their inability to adduct the hips and elevate the pelvis against gravity (Figure 31). This posture may shorten the iliopsoas muscles and potentially interfere with weight bearing (Downs et al., 1991; Updike et al., 1986). In children born prematurely, remnants of frog-lying postures—excessive hip abduction and external rotation—can persist to 4½ years of age (Davis, Robinson, Harris, & Cartlidge, 1993). Another maladaptive posture—the W position of the shoulders (scapular retraction, adduction, and elevation; shoulder abduction, extension, and external rotation; and

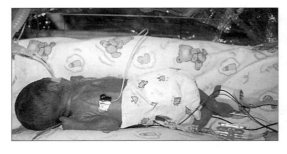
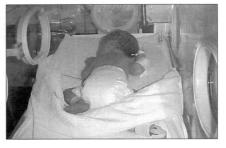

Figure 31. Illustrations of prone positioning. An infant in prone with arms in the W position, hips in wide abduction, and legs crossed (left photo). An infant in the frog-lying position with arms in the W position (right photo).

elbow flexion)—is the upper extremity counterpart of the frog-lying posture of the legs. It interferes with scapular protraction and midline hand activities (Updike et al., 1986) (Figure 32). The total-extension posture (hips and knees extended and ankles plantar-flexed) may shorten the hip adductors and extensors and the gastrocnemius and soleus muscles, potentially inducing toe walking and scissoring gait (Fay, 1988). The maladaptive posture of neck and trunk hyperextension is characterized by an arching, shortened neck and trunk and flexor overstretching. This postural pattern inhibits active neck and trunk flexion, preventing coactivation of the neck musculature from developing. This posture may contribute to an asymmetrical, unstable posture in which the child relies on a pattern of shoulder elevation and retraction (called *blocking* or *fixing*) to maintain an upright head position. Such hyperextension patterns occur more frequently in infants who are intubated and mechanically ventilated (Vohr et al., 1999) because they are likely to have been sedated or immobilized for long periods of time in prone or supine, with the neck in hyperextension to accommodate the endotracheal tube or CPAP apparatus (see Chapter 5). Infants who have to undergo ECMO intervention experience even more severe postural restrictions (see Chapter 2).

Disorganized, uncontrolled motor activity also may interfere with appropriate positioning. Wide range, random movements typically result from neurologic immaturity involving poor modulation of movements and/or states of arousal. Disorganized motor activity interferes with adoption of sustained flexor postures and with an infant's ability to bring his or her hands to the face, mouth, or midline for self-regulation (Vergara, 1993). Infants who do not remain for long in any given position may become distressed as they waste energy in needless movements, but they are not likely to develop postural deformities while in the NICU unless the NICU stay is excessively prolonged. However, without adequate positioning support, unregulated motor activity may induce dangerous physiologic instability. If persistent, it may eventually lead

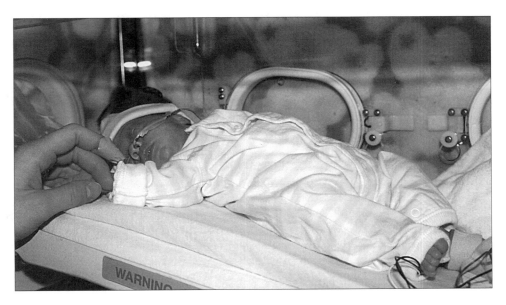

Figure 32. This premature infant's low tone and lack of nesting support in the supine position has led her to adopt an extended posture with shoulder girdle and lower extremity abduction.

to compensatory postural fixing patterns as the infant struggles to prevent purposeless motor activity. The prone position offers the most contact with the supporting surface and is most effective for reducing purposeless motor activity, including startles (Lynch, 1997; Vohr et al., 1999). Random, extraneous motor activity may be reduced through external containment or nesting (i.e., placing boundaries around the infant to simulate a nest), along with the use of a variety of positioning aids.

Medical and postsurgical management of numerous neonatal conditions (e.g., myelomeningocele, hydrocephalus, pneumothorax, certain cardiac and respiratory disorders, gastroschisis, tracheoesophageal fistula, congenital or perinatal fractures, hip dislocations, arthrogryposis, osteogenesis imperfecta) may initially prevent NICU infants from being positioned with adequate postural support. During the initial stages of care, such infants may have very specific positioning requirements to optimize the functioning of their central nervous and organ systems. Critically ill infants may have to be positioned in supine to facilitate access to anterior body structures. Contraindications at this stage include the use of boundaries, swaddling, or other positioning aids that may limit access to the infant. Moreover, infants receiving phototherapy for hyperbillirubinemia and those with chest or abdominal tubes, central arterial lines, or ventral (thoracic or abdominal) surgery or abnormalities are often restricted to supine, extended positions. Some orthopedic disorders may also require specialized care that interferes with ideal positioning. Semiupright (tilted), head elevated positioning may be prescribed for infants with conditions such as aspiration, absent gag reflex, gastroesophageal reflux, certain respiratory disorders, and IVH (Fay, 1988). Increased extensor tone and lower-extremity searching for boundaries may occur if infants feel insecure in the tilted position. These postural patterns may become more permanent if tilted positioning is prolonged without providing adequate postural support. Under these types of circumstances, however, the infant's medical well-being must always supersede developmental concerns.

Some infants occasionally exhibit intolerance to certain postures. Common behaviors that suggest postural intolerance are trunk arching, squirming, arm and leg thrusting, and fussing or crying. Postural tolerance and preferences should be respected and distressing postures should be avoided as much as possible to guard against undue stress and to preserve the infant's physiologic stability. When avoiding a distressing posture is not possible, the infant should be given the necessary external support to prevent loss of physiologic and motor stability.

In full-term infants with short-term illnesses, maladaptive postures are usually temporary and resolve spontaneously without long-term consequences. The effects of poor positioning and flattened postures on preterm infants, however, can persist well beyond term age (Davis et al., 1993; Konishi et al., 1994). The prevalence of extensor patterns, along with the difficulty in contracting low-tone muscles against the strong influence of gravity, can delay achievement of the balanced flexion and extension control necessary for a normal progression through early motor milestones; it also can limit the infant's engagement in age-appropriate, family-expected activities (Hallsworth, 1995). Adaptive positioning is an effective, preventive measure for facilitating flexion to counterbalance the effects of atypical extensor posturing, whether it is the result of increased extensor tone or is induced by a sustained flattened posture (Bellefeuille-Reid & Jakubek, 1989; Fay, 1988; Hallsworth, 1995; Updike et al., 1986; Vohr et al., 1999). Flexor containment and other strategies to enhance physiologic and motor stability should be introduced as soon as possible, especially once an infant's condition has stabilized, to prevent prolonged exposure to inadequate postural patterns.

ADAPTIVE POSITIONING

General Principles

Adaptive positioning is a nonintrusive form of intervention that enables infants to develop adaptive responses similar to those of healthy full-term infants through proper positioning. The infant's positioning environment is prearranged through the use of positioning aids, such as rolled blankets or diapers, stuffed toys, Bendy Bumpers (foam-covered, bendable wire positioners that are available from Children's Medical Ventures, http://www.childmed.com), and custom-designed positioners. Using these aids fulfills the following goals (adapted from Hunter, 1996, & Vergara, 1993):

1. Provide containment and a sense of security for a smoother adjustment to the extrauterine environment.

2. Discourage extension and promote flexion to achieve postural and movement patterns that resemble those of healthy full-term infants.

3. Optimize physiologic stability and neurobehavioral organization to enhance self regulation.

4. Promote hand-to-mouth activity to enhance the infant's ability to self-calm.

5. Maintain proper body alignment to prevent postural asymmetries.

6. Expose the infant to a variety of postures to prevent the development of fixed postural patterns.

7. Maintain skin integrity and prevent skin breakdown.

8. Maximize the infant's developmental potential and engagement in family-expected age-appropriate occupations.

The best posture to achieve these goals concurrently is symmetric physiologic flexion with the neck in slight flexion (less than 30°), the shoulders protracted, the pelvis elevated, and the hands close to the face in midline. Infants should be assisted to achieve this posture in all positions—prone, sidelying, or supine.

To enable early acquisition of kinesthetic and proprioceptive memory of proper postural patterns, adaptive positioning should be initiated as soon as an infant is no longer in a critical state. Routine positioning is usually determined by the infant's primary nurse or, in some institutions, by the developmental personnel. Well-regulated infants proprioceptively explore new positions and respond with procuring signals (e.g., arching, fussing, molding) that indicate their comfort in and tolerance of the position. A sensitive caregiver will respond to an infant's cues and adapt the position accordingly to promote comfort, prevent stress, and prevent loss of physiologic and motor stability. Infants with less clear behavioral procuring signals who are exposed to a position change need to be closely observed for possible life-threatening physiologic alterations, such as decreased or increased heart or respiration rates (apnea, bradycardia, tachycardia, or tachypnea) or decreased oxygen saturation. Although general positioning guidelines (i.e., promoting flexion, weight bearing, body alignment, and containment) are useful for routine positioning, infant individuality and stability must be the deciding factor in designing adaptive positioning arrangements for NICU infants. Positioning decisions for infants with specialized needs (e.g., intolerance to positions, medical or surgical issues) should be made by the nursing, medical, and the developmental team members and the family on the basis of the infant's preferences, presenting problems, and physiologic status.

Infants should be exposed to a variety of positions throughout their NICU stay to enrich their sensorimotor experiences and prevent the development of fixed postural patterns (Vergara, 1993; Vohr et al., 1999). For example, when an infant has been positioned in extension for prolonged periods, he or she may tend to resist the flexed postures. A few minutes of manual containment offered periodically, if the infant's condition permits, may allow the infant to reorganize and "mold" into the flexed position, thereby preventing the development of fixed extended patterns. Some positions are more effective than others in promoting the ideal neonatal flexor posture; however, with some creativity and the use of positioning aids, caregivers may vary the position of the infant while maintaining the ideal postural patterns. Prone and sidelying with nesting support are the preferred positions, particularly for sleeping (Grenier et al., 2003). The nested supine position is most often used in the NICU for caregiving procedures and when the infant's condition requires it.

Unless their well-being is at risk, sleeping infants should not be disturbed between feeding and care periods, lest they lose their ideal positioning. Minor positioning readjustments to tidy the bed or make an infant look more comfortable should always be avoided to prevent disturbing the infant's quiet rest (Appleton, 1997; Brandon et al., 1999; Symon, 1995). If an infant needs to be moved during a caregiving procedure, then he or she may be repositioned, assuming that the new position offers the necessary postural support. Postural support should be firm and consistent, but should enable the infants to stretch and move in and out of positions.

Prone Positioning

Most of the literature regards prone as the position of choice in the NICU. Although prone positioning of healthy infants is strongly discouraged because of a greater risk for SIDS (refer to the previous discussion in this chapter), its use in the NICU is considered safe as long as infants are closely monitored. The calming and sleep-inducing benefits of positioning newborns in prone have been recognized by caregivers for ages. Decades of preterm infant research have identified benefits of prone positioning over supine positioning (Monterosso, Kristianson, & Cole, 2002). (Few studies have compared prone to sidelying.) The following subsections present some immediate benefits and disadvantages of prone positioning documented in the literature.

Physiologic Benefits

Preterm infants in the prone position display fewer stress responses of startles, tremors, and twitches (Chang, Anderson, & Lin, 2002). Another physiologic benefit is increased thoracoabdominal synchrony and rib cage motion. Pressure from the infant's weight against the supporting surface is believed to enhance stability of the chest wall, allowing greater excursion of the diaphragm and ultimately resulting in mechanical advantage for breathing (Fox, Viscardi, Taciak, Niknafs, & Cinoman, 1993; Martin et al., 1995; Wolfson, Greenspan, Deoras, Allen, & Shaffer, 1992). In addition, preterm infants with tachypnea have lower respiratory rates when in the prone position (Sconyers, Ogden, & Goldberg, 1987; Martin et al., 1995; see also Chapter 6). Furthermore, fewer central and mixed apneas occur when this positioning is used (Kurlak, Ruggins, & Stephenson, 1994; McEvoy et al., 1997; see also Chapter 6). The benefits of improved oxygenation and ventilation (Baird, Paton, & Fisher, 1992; Bjornson et al., 1992; Chang, Anderson, Dowling, & Lin, 2002; Dimitriou et al., 2002; Fox & Molesky, 1990; Mendoza, Roberts, & Cook, 1991), lower oxygen consumption (Martin, Herrell,

Rubin, & Fanaroff, 1979; Martin et al., 1995), and greater heart rate regularity (Goto et al., 1999) also are evident. Finally, preterm infants in the prone position have improved cerebral venous return and lower intracranial pressure (Emery & Peabody, 1983; Goldberg, Joshis, Moscoso, & Castillo, 1983).

State of Arousal Benefits

Using the prone position with preterm infants increases time in quiet sleep (especially after feeding) and decreases time spent crying or in active sleep (Chang, Anderson, & Lin, 2002; Sahni et al., 2002), or it decreases the time spent awake, with no significant difference in time spent in active sleep. This suggests that improvements in quiet sleep occur at the expense of a decrease in awake time (Masterson, Zucker, & Schulze, 1987; Myers et al., 1998). Another state of arousal benefit is that the first postfeeding quiet sleep epoch is longer, with total sleep and percentage of time spent in each state remaining unchanged (Goto et al., 1999). The use of prone positioning also results in fewer awakenings (arousals longer than 60 seconds) (Goto et al., 1999) and lower energy expenditure (Masterson et al., 1987).

Neuromotor Benefits

The most important neuromotor benefit of prone positioning is longer duration of postures (i.e., fewer position changes), probably because of decreased motor activity (Chang, Anderson, Dowling, & Lin, 2002; Konishi et al., 1994). Another benefit in one study was that preterm infants who slept in prone were found to have better head control at 56 weeks of gestation than those who slept in supine, but no global developmental benefits of prone positioning were found (Ratliff-Schaub et al., 2001). Other neuromotor advantages of prone positioning, such as increased flexor tone and hand-to-mouth behaviors (Hunter, 1996), may depend on the provision of postural support to facilitate shoulder and pelvic girdle elevation, scapular protraction, and hip and knee flexion. Although the tonic labyrinthine reflex in prone is believed to facilitate passive flexor tone, its influence is often insufficient to overcome the effects of gravity on the weak muscles of very preterm and sick infants, unless positional support is provided. This may explain in part the higher prevalence of some infants to display frog-lying postures in prone (Downs et al., 1991; Konishi et al., 1994).

Other Benefits

Other advantages of prone positioning reported in the literature include being the "best position to expose diaper rash to air or heat lamp" (Hunter, 1996, p. 600) and improving GER (Blumenthal & Lealman, 1982; Vandenplas, Belli, Dupont, Kneepkens, & Heymans, 1997). Although the benefits of prone positioning (especially 30° elevated) for reducing GER have been extensively documented in the literature, some institutions no longer recommend it after discharge from the NICU because of parental anxiety associated with the increased risk of SIDS in prone (Vandenplas et al., 1997).

Overall Benefits and Disadvantages

The effects of positioning preterm infants in prone can be summarized into improved breathing and sleep, lower use of energy, and better overall physiologic status. Prone positioning also affords increased contact with the support surface, which has been associated with decreased incidence of startles and extraneous movements (Chang, Anderson, & Lin, 2002; Vohr et al., 1999). The advantages of prone positioning are accentuated when infants are cared for in head-elevated tilted (20°–30°) positions (Sconyers et al., 1987). The most dramatic effect of prone positioning with the head elevated (15°) is a reduction of hypoxemic episodes (Jenni et al., 1997). The short-term benefits of prone positioning, therefore, potentially lead to greater weight gain, overall well-being, and mechanical advantage for participating in newborn occupations and achieving early motor milestones.

Asymmetric head posturing is a notable disadvantage of prone positioning (Konishi et al., 1994). In particular, asymmetric head posturing is more severe in prone-positioned preterm infants whose head movements are restricted by mechanical ventilation or ECMO therapy (Vohr et al., 1999). Head flattening occurs more often in prone preterm infants as a result of the sustained lateral asymmetric pressure on the infant's soft skull. Head flattening can be reduced through the use of positioning aids and strategies.

It should be mentioned that the majority of the studies yielding these benefits were conducted with healthy preterm infants; thus, great caution should be used in extrapolating these findings to positioning the preterm or full-term infants who are sick.

Positioning Support in Prone

Postural development in prone can be improved significantly through the use of trunk and hip supports (Downs et al., 1991; Monfort & Case-Smith, 1997; Monterosso, Coenen, Percival, & Evans, 1995; Updike et al., 1986). Support is usually placed underneath the major weight-bearing areas (e.g., shoulders, trunk, and/or pelvis) to lift an infant's body off the supporting surface. Trunk and pelvic supports free the extremities from the effects of gravity, thereby facilitating the infant's ability to adopt a tuck (physiologic) posture. Support should only be sufficiently high to allow the infant to bring the extremities closer to midline in a flexion/adduction pattern; postural insecurity is observed when the support is too high. In turn, tucked postures promote newborn-appropriate weight bearing on the knees and elbows and enhance the infant's motor stability and ability to self-regulate (Figure 33).

Positioning support may be provided in different ways. The most common adaptive positioning aids used in prone are

- Rolled blankets, diapers, or washcloths
- Bendy Bumpers from Children's Medical Ventures
- Gel cushions, wedges, or pads (e.g., Gel-E Donuts from Children's Medical Ventures)
- Disposable or cotton/polyester buntings (e.g., SnuggleUps from Children's Medical Ventures)
- Custom-made foam devices
- Stuffed toys
- Swaddling blankets
- Huggel Buntings from Tarry Manufacturing (http://www.tarrymfg.com)

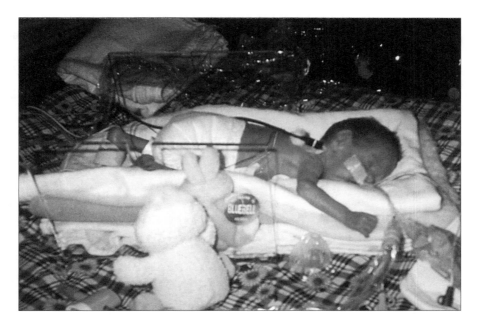

Figure 33. Use of postural support under the hips and right shoulder has enabled this infant to maintain a more adequate flexed posture in prone.

- Small beanbags (e.g., Fredrick T. Frog from Children's Medical Ventures), which should only be used under close monitoring

Positioning materials should be soft and smooth to prevent skin abrasions. The ears—often disregarded—are common site of skin breakdown. When an infant attempts to move his or her head, pressure and friction against the supporting surface irritate the soft skin of the ears (Vohr et al., 1999). Friction from foam or plastic-covered positioning aids should be avoided by using soft blanket covers to preserve skin integrity. Sheepskin (natural or synthetic) can also be used beneath tender skin.

Positioning support can be offered in prone through various arrangements. U-shaped support involves the creation of boundaries (a nest) around the infant to discourage extraneous movements, W postures, and hip and knee extension (see Figure 34). Bendy Bumpers offer the most stable form of nesting parallel to and around the legs. Rolled blankets, dense foam, egg-crate foam, stuffed toys, and beanbags are also frequently used for boundaries.

T-shaped support can be achieved through a custom-made foam positioner device or by placing thinly rolled blankets perpendicular to each other in the shape of a "T" (Figure 35). The top of the T provides head support, and the longitudinal section provides bolster-type trunk and pelvic support (Vohr et al., 1999). Raising the trunk and pelvis facilitates arm and leg flexion; the bolster piece encourages horizontal adduction and clinging. To prevent hip abduction, this type of support should not extend between the legs. The T-shaped arrangement works best when used in combination with U-shaped support.

I-shaped support is a modification of T-shaped support. The bolster piece in this arrangement is shorter, providing support only to the infant's upper trunk. The lower bar of the "I" provides support across the pelvis, elevating it while allowing

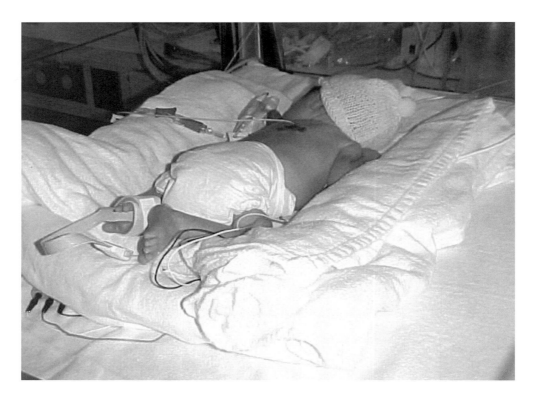

Figure 34. Blanket rolls can be used in a variety of ways to enhance comfort and to provide postural support in prone. These blanket supports have been shaped to bring the hips and ankles into a neutral position. Additional support beneath the chest would improve this infant's posture by allowing the shoulders to come forward into horizontal adduction.

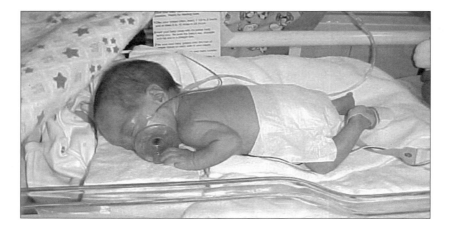

Figure 35. This infant is able to maintain a flexed posture in prone through the use of "T" support under his trunk. A narrower trunk support would have promoted shoulder horizontal adduction.

full hip adduction. This positioning arrangement works best with a one-piece, custom-made positioning device, but rolled blankets may also be used. It should also be used with nesting containment.

Monfort and Case-Smith (1997) designed a one-piece, custom-made foam positioner that is shaped like a vest and extends from the shoulder to the hips. With this vest-shaped arrangement, the upper trunk support is $1^1/2''$ thick, wedging down to $1''$ thickness at the pelvic level. The shoulder areas are cut off, resembling the upper part of a sleeveless vest, to encourage shoulder horizontal adduction. Use of lateral support may further enhance horizontal shoulder adduction postures. This device can be used with a thin gel-pad cushion to decrease pressure on the skull and prevent excessive neck flexion.

Vergara (1993) designed a one-piece positioning device that combines elements of trunk and pelvis support and lateral containment. The device is made from a rectangular piece of medium density, egg-crate foam. A rectangular hole is cut at hip level, $1''$ longer than the length of the infant's lower legs and $2''$ wider than the distance between the infant's hips. The trunk support area keeps the pelvis elevated, whereas the cut-off space facilitates leg tucking. The infant's legs are maintained in position by the walls of the hole. The egg-crate prongs at the level of the upper arms are shaved to create a depression for encouraging shoulder tucking (Figure 36). Draping a blanket around the infant while he or she is on the positioning device decreases random movements and postural changes and further enhances tuck flexion. The device is more effective for lower extremity than upper extremity positioning.

In the prone position, it is a challenge to position the infant's feet (to avoid excessive plantar flexion) and to maintain an appropriate amount of hip abduction. One solution is to use a narrow foam piece shaped as an inverted "T." The vertical

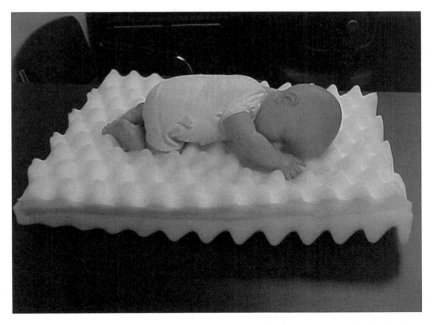

Figure 36. This positioning device is made of eggcrate foam. The foam has been cut away at the hip level to enable the infant to fully flex the legs in prone. Carved areas immediately lateral to the face and upper trunk promote arm flexion and adduction.

segment of the T is placed between the legs to promote neutral hip abduction. The horizontal segment forms a bar that provides support to the dorsal aspects of the feet. The entire device is then encircled with a strip of neoprene or a blanket strip to keep the infant's feet and legs in position (Vohr et al., 1999). A simpler alternative is to use a properly sized diaper to promote neutral hip abduction. For ankle support, a thin diaper can be rolled, soft side outward, and taped to maintain its shape. The diaper is placed under the dorsum of the infant's ankles, inside the "bumper" or boundary at the feet, to raise the feet slightly. This allows the infant's feet to hook over the roll, preventing eversion and plantar flexion.

Other prone positioning devices, such as support pillows (Downs et al., 1991) and postural support "nappies" (Monterosso et al., 1995), are described in the literature. Tarry Manufacturing's Huggel Buntings are described under the Sidelying Positioning heading.

Trunk and hip supports generally work well with infants who have hypotonia. Infants who are hypermobile and irritable, however, may need additional lateral support to maintain proper positioning. Positioning aids should be stabilized on the supporting surface to ensure consistency of positioning throughout an interfeeding period. Use of unstable supports may cause extraneous motor activity, loss of proper positioning, increased stress, and, possibly, loss of stability. Blanket rolls and other movable supports work best when placed under the infant's cover. Infant covers should be used cautiously because they delay access to the infant in emergency situations.

Swaddling is frequently used as an effective, practical, and stable complement to prone positioning; it provides flexor containment and enhancing neuromuscular development in VLBW infants (Short et al., 1996). Swaddling must be used with great caution with sick or very preterm infants because it also restricts access in emergency situations. Swaddling and the use of covers are considered safe NICU techniques for stable infants (Short et al., 1996).

The use of foam pressure-dispersing pads (Morris & Burns, 1994), gel pads (Vohr et al., 1999), and air-filled mattresses (Cartlidge & Rutter, 1988) decreases head flattening slightly in preterm infants. Head positioning aids can be used with other devices to improve cranial molding in prone-positioned infants. The effectiveness of waterbeds on head flattening has been studied but remains unclear (Hemingway & Oliver, 1991).

Some infants, especially those with temperament disorders and severe irritability, cannot tolerate the prone position. They may exhibit extreme arching or squirming when placed in prone (Figure 37). Tuck-flexion promoting positioning devices may

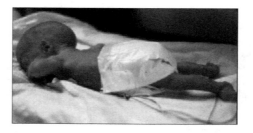

Figure 37.   This infant reacted to the stress he experienced when he was positioned in prone by arching his trunk excessively.

be calming for some of these infants. Infants with strong hyperextension patterns may require additional binding with blanket coverings to gently hold them in the tuck-flexion posture until the hyperextension pattern is inhibited and the infants adapt to the new flexor pattern. A few infants resist the prone position even when extra support is provided, and prone positioning should not be forced. In such cases, the use of alternative positioning arrangements is highly recommended until the infants gradually develop tolerance to and readiness for the prone position.

Prone positioning, especially when positioning aids are used, should be limited to infants who are under strict supervision and monitoring because of the increased risk of SIDS in prone. Prone positioning devices can increase an infant's exposure to dangerous levels of carbon dioxide. Therefore, upon discharge from the NICU, infants should *never* be sent home with positioning devices. AAP (1996) guidelines recommend sidelying or supine nesting positioning for infants making the NICU–home transition.

Sidelying Positioning

Sidelying is the best alternative to prone positioning in the NICU, particularly once an infant's condition has stabilized somewhat after birth. Sidelying is one of the positions recommended by the AAP because it is safer than prone, although not as safe as supine (Spieker & Brannen, 1996). In the NICU, sidelying is frequently recommended to bring the extremities toward midline and to expose infants to postures other than prone. It is one of the preferred positions for infants receiving mechanical ventilation (Bozynski, Naglie, Nicks, Burpee, & Johnson, 1988).

The goals for sidelying positioning are similar to those for prone: to facilitate neonatal flexion patterns and to prevent the development of abnormal postures. A stable sidelying position encourages flexion, symmetry, and hand-to-mouth behaviors (Hallsworth, 1995). The pull of gravity on the limbs of sidelying infants promotes shoulder and hip horizontal adduction and enhances neutral alignment and midline activities (Vohr et al., 1999). However, sidelying tends to be more unstable than prone or supine, especially for infants who have low tone or are weak, because of the narrower weight-bearing surface that it affords. Distress in the unsupported sidelying position is most commonly expressed as asymmetric shoulder retraction, neck hyperextension, and trunk arching (Fay, 1988; Hallsworth, 1995). Neck hyperextension patterns are particularly more common in infants who are intubated or spend prolonged periods in sidelying. Hyperextension patterns may be an adaptive response of intubated infants to enhance airflow by placing their CPAP prongs or endotracheal tube in a position of mechanical advantage (Vohr et al., 1999) (Figure 38).

Several strategies can be used to increase postural stability and decrease hyperextension in sidelying:

- Flexing the supporting extremities prevents spontaneous rolling to prone.
- Providing posterior nesting support—through beanbags, rolled blankets, or Bendy Bumpers—prevents spontaneous rolling to supine (Hallsworth, 1995). Support should extend from the back of the head to the hips to control neck and trunk arching.
- Placing a long, thin, snake-shaped blanket roll under the infant's top limbs promotes flexion through clinging (Fay, 1988; Hallsworth, 1995) and provides more neutral alignment of the hips (i.e., slight hip abduction) (Vohr et al., 1999). The

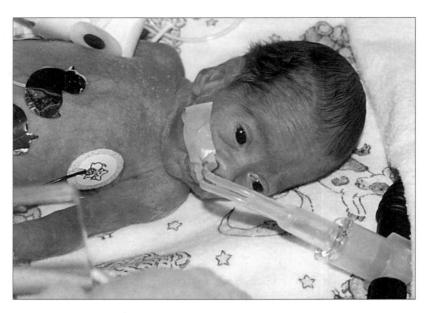

Figure 38. Note how the continuous positive airway pressure prongs and tubing may induce neck extension. This pulling force should be avoided or decreased to the extent possible to promote better neck positioning.

blanket can also be used in a pretzel arrangement, which is placed under the neck, then behind the back, between the legs (for abduction), and along the abdomen (for tucking the arms around).

• Covering the infant with a blanket that is tucked snugly under the mattress gives increased stability, enhances flexion, and discourages asymmetric postural patterns (Fay, 1988; Vergara, 1993).

• Placing a thinly folded diaper or small pad behind and under the infant's supporting hip minimizes arching and prevents rolling to supine (Fay, 1988).

• Nesting the legs in flexion facilitates overall flexor tone (Vohr et al., 1999).

• Simulating intrauterine containment can be achieved through the use of a Huggel Bunting or a SnuggleUp. Figure 39 illustrates the use of a SnuggleUp and a Bendy Bumper for support in the sidelying position.

Of the previously listed techniques, clinging to a soft roll is often the most effective for promoting flexion in sidelying. However, all of the techniques can be combined for greater effectiveness. For example, an infant can receive posterior support through a Bendy Bumper while he or she clings to a blanket roll and the supporting extremities are kept flexed (Figure 40).

Extreme care should be followed to avoid flexing the neck excessively when providing posterior support to infants who are intubated. Although neck flexion between 15° and 30° does not significantly interfere with airflow, neck flexion of 45° causes severe airflow obstruction and significantly interferes with pulmonary mechanics in preterm infants with respiratory disorders (Reiterer, Abbasi, & Bhutani, 1994). Reiterer and associates also found that 45° of hyperextension causes airflow interruption in some infants. As a precautionary measure, neck positioning in infants who are intubated should preferably be maintained within ±15° from neutral; it

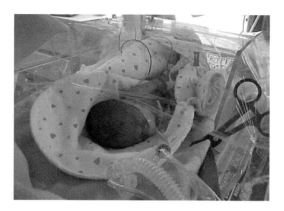

Figure 39. A SnuggleUp (available from Children's Medical Ventures, http://www.childmed.com) enables this infant to maintain an ideal posture while she sleeps on her side between feedings.

definitely should not exceed 30° of either flexion or extension. Breathing with the neck partly flexed, however, is a fundamental underlying capacity for important functional activities such as feeding and sitting in a car seat (Vohr et al., 1999). When an intubated infant is progressed to CPAP ventilation, for the initiation of functional activities, greater neck flexion (less than 45°) in sidelying should gradually be allowed to build up the infant's ability to breathe with the neck flexed.

When an infant is positioned on his or her side, the weight-bearing (supporting) side must be alternated once every feeding to prevent postural asymmetry, especially

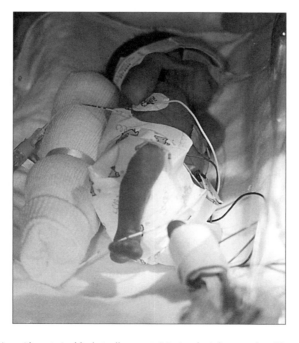

Figure 40. Infant sidelying with posterior blanket roll support. Bringing the infant onto her side, with ventral and posterior nesting support, would enhance flexion and improve comfort.

head flattening. If positioning devices are used, then they must be reversible to allow alternating sides.

Supine Positioning

Supine positioning is commonly discouraged in the NICU because it does not promote flexion and is stressful for many infants (Fay, 1988; Hallsworth, 1995; Hunter, 1996; Vohr et al., 1999). An important advantage of the supine position for infants who are not intubated is that head flattening can potentially be reduced, because the head can be maintained in midline with greater ease using lateral supports. Prolonged supine positioning, nonetheless, may contribute to increased extensor posturing and positional deformities, especially in infants receiving mechanical ventilation (Bellefeuille-Reid & Jakubek, 1989; Downs et al., 1991; Fay, 1988; Hallsworth, 1995; Hunter, 1996; Updike et al., 1986; Vergara, 1993; Vohr et al., 1999). Supine positioning also increases arousal, startles, and random movements (Amemiya et al, 1991; Fay, 1988; Franco et al., 1998; Hunter, 1996; Vohr et al., 1999) and decreases sleep (Hashimoto et al., 1983; Vergara, 1993). One study found that the supine position improved the strength of the respiratory musculature in preterm infants but that the infants' oxygenation was not enhanced by the superior respiratory strength (Dimitriou et al., 2002). Supine positioning in the NICU is crucial for a number of caregiving procedures, however, particularly during the acute phase of an infant's care. As discussed previously, it is most frequently used during the neonatal stabilization phase to facilitate access to the chest and abdomen and for infants with specific medical/surgical conditions that prohibit the prone and sidelying positions.

Supine positioning in the NICU is unavoidable for some infants. Any potentially detrimental effects can be ameliorated or prevented through the use of postural supports. As with the prone and sidelying positions, the general goal of adaptive positioning in supine is to promote flexor patterns and newborn-like sensorimotor experiences and to conserve energy by reducing unnecessary movements. This goal is best fulfilled in supine through the use of nesting supports. As noted previously, nesting involves creating a supporting arrangement that surrounds the infant under the neck, shoulders, and hips to promote slight neck flexion, shoulder protraction and horizontal adduction, pelvic elevation, and hip and knee flexion (Updike et al., 1986). Nesting should facilitate the infant's ability to bring his or her hands together and to the mouth (for self-calming and self-regulation) by reducing the effects of gravity on the arms through positioning. The incidence of random movements in supine may also be decreased through nesting. Nesting can be offered through the use of various techniques or positioning aids:

- Shaping a long, thin, snake-shaped roll of blankets into an elliptical "doughnut," over which the infant lays, promotes nesting. A similar alternative is to surround the infant by "walls of soft rolls" (Fay, 1988, p. 25), but the use of many rolls (versus one roll) makes it more difficult to maintain proper positioning. Cervical support should only be thick enough to achieve 15° of flexion (30° in infants who are not intubated). Support under the shoulders (laterally), pelvis, and legs should be as thick as needed to facilitate physiologic flexion.

- Bendy Bumpers are very useful and effective for providing lateral supports, but they are too thick to be used under the cervical region for positioning the neck. Thin gel pad cushions can be used to position the neck in combination with Bendy Bumpers for nesting (Vohr et al., 1999).

- Custom-making a foam positioner in the shape of a nest is another option (Updike et al., 1986).

- Partially filled waterbeds may also be used to promote flexion in supine. Fully filled waterbeds should not be used because they facilitate extension instead of flexion and may increase postural insecurity and stress (J. Angley, personal communication, July 2002). Research on the effectiveness of waterbeds is inconclusive (Vohr et al., 1999).

Beanbag-type positioning cushions were available commercially in the 1980s and early 1990s. These pillows were removed from the market because they were associated with increased incidences of SIDS when used in prone (Kemp & Thach, 1991), but some forms of beanbag cushions are still on the market. Although the safety of these pillows for supine positioning has not been questioned, their use is *strongly discouraged* to avoid the risk of caregivers mistakenly using them for prone positioning or in unsupervised situations.

Head Elevated Positioning

The head elevated (tilted) position is recommended for the care of many sick NICU infants. The most recommended position is prone with the head elevated 30°. Although most effectiveness studies on head elevation were conducted in the 1980s, the evidence consistently attributes several important benefits of head-elevated positions:

- Decreased intracranial pressure (Emery & Peabody, 1983; Goldberg et al., 1983; Urlesberger, Muller, Ritschl, & Reiterer, 1991)

- Decreased hypoxemia and bradycardia (Jenni et al., 1997)

- Fewer and shorter episodes of GER (Orenstein & Whitington, 1983; Vandenplas et al., 1997)

Intracranial pressure is also affected by head rotation, with the lowest pressure obtained with the head in the midline position (Emery & Peabody, 1983; Goldberg et al., 1983). The intracranial pressure decrease associated with head elevation and head position is believed to result from hydrostatic pressure changes and improvements in venous return (Goldberg et al., 1983).

Infants for whom elevated positioning is recommended are frequently very ill. When placed on a tilted surface, infants have a tendency to slide down because of the effects of gravity. They expend much energy searching for a base of security when tilted. An effective technique to prevent sliding is to use a rolled blanket as a sling (tucked under the mattress and around the infant's buttocks) keeping the infant's hips flexed and the pelvis elevated (Vohr et al., 1999). Commercially available devices such as the Tucker Sling (Children's Medical Ventures) may also be used with infants weighing more than 2 pounds (see Figure 41).

Head elevated positioning can be accomplished more naturally through kangaroo care (see Chapter 2). Kangaroo, or skin-to-skin, care is used in many NICUs to keep an infant warm when he or she is outside the incubator. The infant is placed upright against the caregiver's chest, preferably with skin-to-skin contact. Coverings are used to enclose both the infant and the caregiver, providing enough binding to maintain the infant in flexion without sliding. Research has found kangaroo care to be beneficial for the infant as well as the mother (Bohnhorst, Heyne, Peter, & Poets, 2001; Engler et al., 2002). One such benefit may be less positional skull flattening. Although the

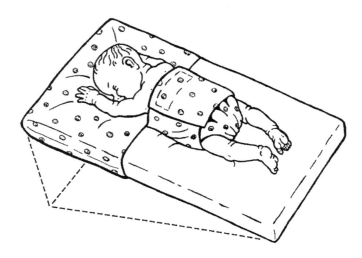

Figure 41. Infant with gastroesophageal reflux using a Tucker Sling (available from Children's Medical Ventures, http://www.childmed.com).

benefits of kangaroo care cannot necessarily be attributed to positioning alone, this form of care is an ideal alternative for infants who require head elevated positioning.

Alternative Positions

Infants who remain in the NICU beyond term age should be provided with a broader range of positioning options. Car seats or infant swings are frequently used as alternative positioning arrangements in the NICU (Figure 42). Upright positioning is often recommended for older infants because it expands exploration and social interaction opportunities. Prior to recommending upright or sitting positioning, an infant's neck control and the effects of neck flexion in the sitting position must be carefully evaluated. Neck flexion in sitting can obstruct airflow, especially in infants with respiratory disorders (Reiterer et al., 1994; Vohr et al., 1999). Straight upright sitting should be avoided for infants with weak neck control. Reclined sitting in an infant seat can be attempted for brief periods if adequate head support is provided. Upright wind-up swings are too challenging for infants with neck control problems and should be avoided.

It is important to note that a study of full-term and preterm infants revealed that infants placed in an appropriate-for-size car seat with head support provided through blanket rolls exhibited respiratory instability within 60 minutes (Merchant, Worwa, Porter, Coleman, & deRegnier, 2001). Oxygen saturation declined on average by 6% in both the full-term and the preterm infants. Three (6%) preterm infants and four (8%) full-term infants had oxygen saturation levels of less than 90% for more than 20 minutes, and eight (12%) preterm infants had apneic or bradycardic episodes while in their car seats. This study suggests that car seats should be used with great care,

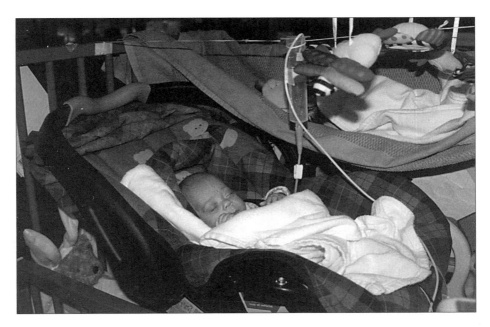

Figure 42. Use of an infant seat gives this infant the opportunity to explore alternative postural patterns as she grows in the NICU.

and only for short periods of time, with any infant, particularly infants with poor neck control or respiratory difficulties (Merchant et al., 2001). As recommended by the AAP, most NICUs require a "car-seat challenge" prior to discharge of preterm infants or infants with airway complications. This test entails placing an infant in his or her car seat for a 90-minute period, during which time he or she is connected to cardiorespiratory and oxygen saturation monitors. If the infant experiences oxygen desaturation, then modifications may need to be made to his or her seating or the infant may need to be discharged in a car bed (e.g., Cherish Car Bed by Graco, http://www.graco.co.uk; Ultra Dream Ride Infant Car Seat by Cosco, http://www.coscoinc.com/mainpg.html), which allows the infant to be strapped in while lying flat. The car bed may be more expensive than a typical car seat, but it can be converted to a typical semiupright car seat when the infant is ready for upright positioning.

Positioning During Handling

Caregivers must exercise great caution in adhering to the basic principles of positioning when handling or moving infants. To the extent possible, support must be provided, preferably in the form of manual containment or swaddling, to maintain extremities flexed and near midline during handling. Uniform and stable support must be provided when infants are moved slowly to decrease the likelihood of stress reactions, especially in infants who are physiologically unstable. Although swaddling provides the most consistent form of support, its use during handling may be impractical or impossible, particularly when an infant needs to be uncovered or undressed while being handled. The neck must be supported in neutral position or in slight flexion (less than 30°). Extreme care must be taken to prevent accidental extubation when handling intubated infants.

Cobedding

Cobedding is a positioning alternative that is gaining rapid popularity in response to the increased rate of multiple gestation births since the 1990s. Although several anecdotal articles in the literature address the potential benefits of cobedding, research on this topic is scarce. An observational study reported an increase in coregulatory activities between preterm twins—including touching, holding, hugging, rooting, sucking on each other, smiling, and being awake at the same time—and a decreased need for external temperature support (Nyqvist & Lutes, 1998). Another study compared the sleep patterns of healthy preterm twins (i.e., those without arterial lines or ventilator requirement) during a 24-hour period, 12 hours before and 12 hours during cobedding (Touch, Epstein, Pohl, & Greenspan, 2002). The authors found no adverse effects of cobedding; however, the risk of transmitting infection is greater. Of the many physiologic parameters examined, the only significant difference found in this study was a greater number of episodes of central apnea before cobedding. The authors hypothesized that the lower incidence of apnea during cobedding may have resulted from the proximity of the twins promoting more frequent arousal in both infants. Cobedding of healthy multiple gestation infants is strongly recommended, provided that there is close monitoring for potential infections (Figure 43).

Additional Considerations

Cosmetic appearance of the infant's positioning arrangements is an important consideration. Although promoting proper postural patterns and preserving physiologic and motor stability are the most important concerns regarding infant positioning, attention should also be given to how the infant looks. The infant's appearance projects the quality of care received and the infant's comfort and well-being. Efforts should be

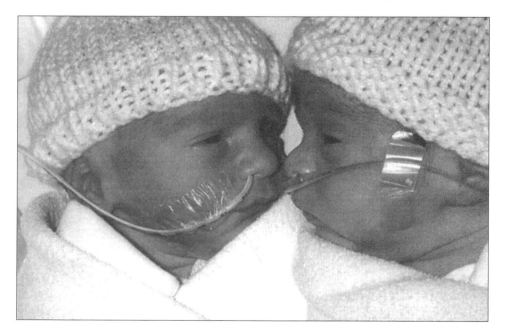

Figure 43.   Cobedding enables these twin infants to maintain physical contact with each other after birth.

made to provide postural support that is neat in appearance and will continue to support the infant between care periods, obviating the need for additional handling and repositioning during the infant's rest.

Other issues that must be considered when positioning infants in the NICU are the cleanliness and safety of the materials used. Certain materials, such as sheep skin and porous foams, accumulate dust mites and allergens that can be detrimental to an infant's health (Sawyer et al., 1998). Materials that cannot be laundered according to infectious control guidelines should not be used. The materials used must be washable, heat resistant, and fire retardant. Difficult-to-clean positioning equipment should be avoided or covered with washable bedding for better cleanliness and infection control.

CONCLUSION

Long-term positioning effectiveness studies are scarce. Monterosso and associates (2002) conducted a review of the few long-term studies of scientific rigor. One conclusion that they reached was that the prone position may lead to short- and long-term postural and associated developmental problems unless the proper support is provided. They recommended "empirically tested postural interventions" to prevent such problems (p. 138). Another review conducted by Downs and associates (1991) found that preterm infants who received positioning (hip) support had significantly greater stability in sidelying, smaller angles of hip rotation, and more appropriate weight bearing on the anterior aspect of the knee by term age than a control group of infants. These findings suggest that proper positioning may enable infants to achieve postural patterns similar to those of healthy newborns. It could be argued, however, that some of the effects achieved through positioning may not necessarily be advantages. For example, the potential impact that improved weight bearing on the knees could have on the developing hips of preterm infants is uncertain. Other studies cited in this chapter report gains in quiet sleep associated with prone positioning in preterm infants. Such findings are often interpreted as advantages; in reality, there is still much to learn about which type of sleep is most beneficial for developing infants (Goto et al., 1999). Therapists should stay abreast of emerging research to ensure that they are providing the most up-to-date, evidence-based positioning recommendations.

13

Ongoing Feeding
Evaluation and Intervention

OVERVIEW

This chapter begins with an overview of the role of the therapist in facilitating feeding performance in NICU infants. Feeding intervention is presented from two perspectives: 1) facilitating feeding competency of the infant (infant centered) and 2) promoting caregiver–infant interaction during feeding (infant–caregiver centered). The importance of the environmental context—human (e.g., caregiver sensitivity, psychosocial support) as well as nonhuman (e.g., noise, lights, temperature)—in supporting feeding performance in the infants is underscored throughout the chapter. Special emphasis is given to the benefits and constraints typically associated with breast feeding and the importance of supporting mothers in their efforts to breast feed their sick or preterm infants.

Feeding evaluation is described as a multifactorial, integrative, ongoing process that begins prior to nipple feeding and continues after nipple feeding has been well established. The underlying capacities that support nipple feeding and the factors and medical conditions that may contribute to the development of feeding problems are thoroughly discussed. Various feeding evaluation models are presented, based on the work of well-recognized theorists. These include problem-driven models, component-based models, and infant–caregiver interaction models. The chapter lays the foundation for evaluating and intervening with different aspects of feeding by applying elements from the various models.

A step-by-step sequence of the feeding evaluation process is presented. The sequence involves collecting preliminary data and conducting a prefeeding evaluation, setting the stage for evaluation, conducting the evaluation, preparing the feeding evaluation summary, and conducting ongoing reevaluation. Other elements of the feeding evaluation, such as positioning and monitoring of physiologic stability, are described. The chapter concludes with a thorough discussion of nipple selection and indications, specific feeding interventions, and breast feeding consultation. The principles, theories, and techniques discussed throughout the chapter are illustrated in two case examples.

OBJECTIVES

- Identify the major reasons for which newborns are referred to the NICU therapist for feeding evaluation and intervention

- Recognize that feeding success depends on a complex interaction among medical, anatomic, physiologic, motor, sensory, organizational, and relational elements
- Identify the main factors, including medical or neurologic conditions, that may contribute to the development of feeding difficulties in infants
- Describe the three common feeding evaluation models: problem-driven, component-based, and infant–caregiver interaction
- Describe the elements that should be reviewed during preliminary data gathering and the prefeeding phases of a feeding evaluation to determine readiness for feeding
- Identify the steps that should be taken to set the stage for a feeding evaluation, as well as the main elements of a feeding evaluation
- Recognize the role of the caregiver and the importance of his or her participation during the feeding evaluation of a NICU infant
- Describe the basic capacities that support feeding in NICU infants: neuromotor functions, sensory functions, and physiologic stability
- Identify clinical signs that may indicate that an infant is experiencing aspiration, reflux, or airway obstruction during a feeding
- Identify the nipples most commonly used in the NICU and their indications or uses
- Identify the typical presentation of the most common problems and medical conditions associated with feeding problems in infants, as well as recommendations for intervention
- Describe the role of the NICU therapist in providing breast feeding consultation

FEEDING IN THE NICU

Feeding is one of the most basic, albeit complex, human occupations. Efficient feeding involves a delicate balancing of neuromotor, sensory, and physiologic capacities. An infant's comfort and safety can be severely compromised when one or more of these capacities is impeded by immaturity, illness, or impairment.

Therapists working in the NICU are consulted more often for feeding problems than for any other matter. Regardless of the reason for an infant's stay in the NICU, feeding has a primary role as a management issue. Adequate nutrition is a vital aspect of growth and recovery from illness, whether the patient is a sick full-term infant or a "micropreemie." The early transition from parenteral (IV) feedings to enteral (gastrointestinal) tube feedings is a goal for most infants in the NICU. There are limits to the amount of time that an infant can be maintained on total parenteral nutrition (TPN) before he or she begins to experience serious complications, such as liver failure. Moreover, an earlier transition to gavage feeding is associated with improved physiologic functioning and growth for infants with widely varying conditions. Enteral feedings by gavage are usually introduced slowly, with gradually increasing volumes of either breast milk or formula. They can be given in combination with parenteral feedings while the infant is slowly weaned off the IV. There is no specific weight or gestation at which this process is initiated. Enteral feeding is initiated as early as the infant is able to tolerate it.

Once an infant has demonstrated a tolerance for bolus feedings by gavage and has reached a point (behaviorally and developmentally) at which nipple feedings are an option, the infant usually begins taking some feedings or portions of feedings by nipple. Parents may become more active participants in caring for their infant at this point. They begin to see their infant as a competent being with the capacity to interact with others and to signal his or her own needs and wants. The process of assisting the infant to take nipple feedings has a profound effect on the parent–infant interaction. Because successful feeding is one of several criteria for discharge, parents are able to assist in the process of preparing their infant for the transition home. They become more integral members of the team at this time, often providing daily input into the plan of care.

Breast milk is far superior to formula for its immunity properties as well as for its digestibility (Schanler, Hurst, & Lau, 1999), so mothers are strongly encouraged to provide pumped breast milk until the infant is ready to nipple feed exclusively from the breast. At the time of discharge from the NICU, most preterm infants require some supplementation to their breast feeding, thus requiring the mother to continue pumping after the infant has been brought home. Skin-to-skin (kangaroo) care is also encouraged to promote breast feeding of premature infants. It may begin as soon as the infant is stable and breathing spontaneously, with CPAP or nasal cannula, as early as 27 weeks (Bauer, Pyper, Sperling, Uhrig, & Versmold, 1998). Occasionally, skin-to-skin care is used with infants on ventilators (Moran et al., 1999), as shown in Figure 44. Mothers who provide skin-to-skin care while their infants are still being fed by IV and/or tube are more likely to follow through with breast feeding after discharge (Bier et al., 1996). The breast milk of a mother who delivers prematurely may need to be fortified with additional human milk factors to enhance its nutritional value for the infant's optimal growth (Schanler et al., 1999).

The NICU therapist may be asked to assist with many aspects of feeding to facilitate competency of the infant and/or the interaction between the infant and his or her caregivers. Indications for a feeding referral can be broadly categorized as *infant centered* or *infant–caregiver centered*. Infant-centered concerns are focused on the infant's feeding performance. Some infants have difficulty maintaining an alert state for feeding, require gavage to complete the full volume of their feeding, are physiologically unstable during feedings, or exhibit defensive responses to stimuli around the mouth. Many have difficulty learning to coordinate breathing with sucking and swallowing or simply expend too much energy attempting to nipple feed. Some require simple modifications to their feeding routine or to the ways in which they are handled during feeding; others need to await further maturation and/or improved airway management before they can nipple- or breast-feed. Whether the presenting problem is slow feeding, the transition to nipple feeds from IV or gavage, or physiologic distress associated with feedings, the NICU therapist has much to offer in evaluating the infant's capacity and readiness to take the breast or bottle. Rarely, the solution to the problem can be addressed solely by modifying some aspect of the infant's feeding regimen—for example, by reducing the volume taken per feeding to reduce reflux or by changing the schedule from every 3 to every 4 hours to provide a longer rest period between feedings. More often, the intervention needs to address a combination of infant-centered and infant–caregiver centered issues.

Most feeding evaluations need to account for the interaction between the infant and the caregiver because feeding by either breast or bottle is a nurturing and social activity. Caregiver sensitivity is an important component of feeding a high-risk infant and is an area in which NICU therapists may need to intervene. Parents who receive additional psychosocial support and opportunities to care for and feed their infant

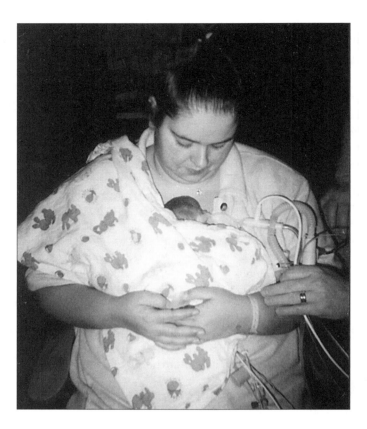

Figure 44. This intubated infant is able to spend prolonged periods outside the incubator through his mother's provision of skin-to-skin care and is able to explore the breast in preparation for future breast-feeding.

experience significantly less stress during their infant's NICU stay. These parents also have improved feeding interactions with their infant, and have a lower incidence of depression following the infant's discharge from the NICU (Meyer et al., 1994).

Feeding cannot be adequately evaluated without also considering the existent environmental context. Some infants require careful attention to the physical environment to enhance their feeding—for example, dimming lights to sustain visual alertness. Others need to be handled and positioned carefully to prevent obstruction of the airway. Most require vigilant attention to their color and behavioral cues to reduce the stress associated with feeding (see Figure 45). Thus, feeding is a clear example of why a contextual frame of reference is needed for assessment and intervention. The therapist responding to a referral for poor feeding can anticipate the need to evaluate and recommend interventions for the infant within the total NICU context, which includes infant–caregiver interactions and the physical environment. The remainder of this chapter presents a contextual model for feeding evaluation and intervention, as well as an overview of specific interventions.

FEEDING EVALUATION

Feeding evaluation requires a wealth of knowledge and experience, strong problem-solving skills, and sensitivity to both the infant and the caregiver. Assisting parents

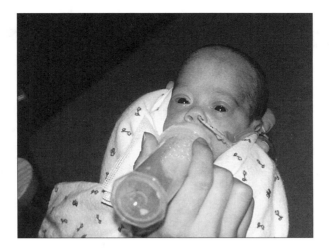

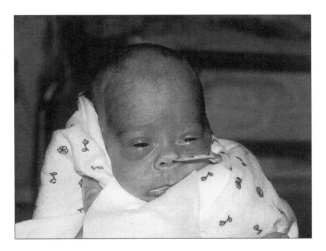

Figure 45. This infant is initially nipple-feeding without distress (top photo). Observe the changes in skin coloration and facial expression as her oxygen saturation decreases during a feeding evaluation (bottom photo).

to feed their sick or preterm infant is one of the most emotion-laden elements of NICU practice because feeding is a basic nurturing experience that every parent expects to be able to offer his or her infant. For this same reason, having a role in optimizing the feeding experience for an infant and caregiver is one of the most satisfying aspects of practice for a NICU therapist.

Feeding evaluation continues to have primary importance even after nipple feeding becomes a routine part of an infant's care plan. A number of feeding problems may present after nipple feeding has been initiated. Potential sources of these feeding problems may range widely, from simple mechanical issues to highly complex dysfunction in the infant's neurophysiologic interactions.

The majority of referrals for feeding evaluation and intervention in the NICU are made for one of the following reasons: slow feeding or inability to complete a feeding (i.e., inability to take the full volume of feeding by nipple within 20–30 minutes), physiologic instability during feeding (e.g., apnea, bradycardia, oxygen desaturation), inadequate weight gain when nipple feeding, and refusal to accept feedings by nipple. Many factors may contribute to the development of such types of feeding problems:

- Poor infant–caregiver interaction during feeding
- Limited caregiver knowledge or skill
- Poor regulation of states of arousal (heightened irritability or decreased alertness)
- Poor endurance
- Excessive work of breathing
- Poor self-pacing of suck-swallow with breathing, leading to gulping, choking, coughing, or apnea
- Weak suck-swallow or inability to sustain a suck-swallow rhythm
- Oral hypo- or hypersensitivity
- Inadequate nipple compression
- Inability to generate adequate intraoral negative pressure to express the liquid
- Irregular or delayed timing of swallowing in association with the suck (pooling of liquid in the pharyngeal spaces)
- Atypical lip, tongue, or jaw movement
- Hyper- or hypoactive oral/pharyngeal reflexes
- Heightened or decreased postural and oral muscle tone

The previously listed factors may directly result from a variety of medical and neurological conditions. They may also be part of a complex interaction between a variety of conditions, such as

- GER and delayed gastric emptying
- Decreased functional lung capacity (FLC) (e.g., severe chronic lung disease/bronchopulmonary dysplasia or hypoplastic lungs)
- Congenital heart disease
- Neuromuscular disease
- Hypoxic ischemic encephalopathy
- Paralysis of the epiglottis and/or the vocal folds
- Congenital anomalies (e.g., cleft lip, cleft palate, retracted jaw [retrognathia], retracted tongue, tracheoesophageal fistula)
- Structural limitations in lip, tongue, or jaw movement (e.g., arthrogryposis)
- Syndromes and sequences (e.g., CHARGE association, Down syndrome, Moebius syndrome, Pierre Robin sequence)
- Side effects of medications

Feeding Evaluation Models

Successful feeding in the NICU is multifactorial and integrative in nature. It is the result of a complex interaction among medical, anatomic, physiologic, motor, sensory, organizational, and infant–caregiver components (Wolf & Glass, 1992). For this reason, there is no single best approach to feeding evaluation and intervention in the

NICU. Rather, feeding evaluation and intervention demand a meticulous approach to information gathering. The NICU therapist must have a flexible framework from which to generate hypotheses about the nature of a particular feeding problem and its possible causes. This framework is constructed from a number of working models for evaluation and intervention. Moreover, to propose interventions that are safe and effective, the therapist must be able to integrate all of the information and resources available in the NICU to test hypotheses and identify possible solutions.

Problem-Driven Models

Wolf and Glass (1992) made an important contribution to evaluation of feeding and swallowing in infants through their comprehensive text. The authors summarized their multidisciplinary approach to assessment and intervention for the more common presenting problems through four "problem-driven models": 1) feeding-related apnea, 2) feeding problem, 3) respiratory compromise, and 4) poor weight gain.

The basic premise for these four models is that systematically investigating the underlying cause of the feeding difficulty will most likely lead to the best possible solution. These models provide a critical path for initial evaluation, obtaining further diagnostic information when needed, and intervention, and they can be useful tools for therapists in the NICU. The first three models are immediately applicable to the NICU, whereas the poor weight gain model is more useful in neonatal follow-up programs. Readers are referred to the original source (Wolf & Glass, 1992) for a detailed explanation of the evaluation components, including medical diagnostic tests and their use for feeding evaluation, and case examples of each model. These models emphasize the infant's occupational performance during feeding—that is, whether the infant is meeting expectations for feeding. By articulating the specific problem that the infant is experiencing rather than listing the medical conditions or diagnosis (e.g., bradycardia associated with feeding versus prematurity, obstruction of the airway during feeding versus Pierre Robin sequence), the evaluation focuses on function.

Therapists should communicate closely with the medical team in their individual NICU prior to recommending a particular diagnostic test (e.g., pneumogram with pH probe, radiographic and barium swallow studies, videofluoroscopy), as teams vary in their use of these tests. Thorough history taking, meticulous attention to detail during feeding observations, and cautious evidence-based hypothesis formation— along with good communication skills—ensure optimal team evaluation and management of the infant's presenting feeding problems.

Component-Based Models

Another approach to evaluation relates specifically to the oral-motor components of feeding and to their possible origins in the infant's processing of sensory or motor information within the nervous system. The Neonatal Oral-Motor Assessment Scale (NOMAS) provides a useful format for the motor aspects of the feeding evaluation (Braun & Palmer, 1985; Palmer, Crawley, & Blanco, 1993). Palmer and Heyman (1993) proposed a framework for intervening with sensory and/or motor-based problems once the feeding evaluation is complete.

The following elements are observed during a NOMAS evaluation of the functional motor components of feeding:

- Posture of the lips, tongue, and jaw at rest, as well as their movement during nonnutritive sucking (NNS) and nutritive sucking (NS)
- Duration and rhythmicity of sucking bursts and degree of jaw excursion
- Degree of success in expressing the liquid
- Coordination of sucking, swallowing, and breathing
- Ability to sustain a sucking rhythm

An interesting feature of this assessment is its comparison of NNS bursts with NS bursts, as typically developing infants adapt their sucking pattern to a slower burst/pause ratio during NS to accommodate the need to swallow the bolus of liquid. The NOMAS is very appropriate for the NICU because of its brevity and focus on aspects of feeding that are relevant to premature and full-term infants. The overall pattern of feeding is judged to be *normal* (as present in typical infants), *disorganized* (as seen in immature preterm infants or in full-term infants with sensory processing difficulties), or *dysfunctional* (as seen in infants with central or peripheral nervous system involvement). However, the NOMAS is by no means comprehensive. It is meant to be used within a framework that considers a number of interrelated factors, including environmental, postural, mechanical, sensory, and psychosocial elements.

Infant–Caregiver Interaction Models

A third approach to feeding evaluation focuses on the infant–caregiver interaction. Models that take this approach are based on the premise that an infant's behavior provides essential cues to the caregiver regarding the infant's ability to be engaged in the feeding process. There are three commonly used caregiver–infant interaction assessment instruments. Wolf and Glass (1992) presented an outline for interviewing caregivers about their infants' feeding problems. The outline includes questions that are relevant for feeding evaluation in the NICU and in follow-up. The questions are simple and direct and designed to reveal the sensitivity of the caregiver to infant cues. For example, the therapist might ask the caregiver, "What does the baby act like when you first give the bottle/breast?" and "How do you know the feeding is over?" Another assessment tool, the Nursing Care Assessment Feeding Scale (NCAFS) (Barnard, 1978), can be used in the NICU and during follow-up to evaluate parental responsiveness to infant cues, signs of distress, and social interaction opportunities during the feeding process.

The Feeding Scale developed by Chatoor and colleagues (1997) is designed for infants between 1 month beyond term age and 3 years, particularly those who live at home and are referred for evaluation of failure to thrive. It provides a detailed format for evaluating parent–infant/toddler interactions during feeding. A 20-minute observation is used to rate the infant/toddler and parent in the following areas:

- Dyadic reciprocity
- Dyadic conflict
- Talk and distraction
- Struggle for control
- Parental noncontingency

The Feeding Scale differentiates three clinically defined groups of feeding interaction disorders: homeostasis, attachment, and separation. A study of 46 infants/toddlers with a diagnosis of failure to thrive and their mothers demonstrated the reliability and validity of the scale, as well as its accuracy in correctly classifying "four out of five infants with and without feeding disorders" (Chatoor et al., 1997). Because of the strong psychosocial orientation of this tool and the necessity of designing clinical interventions for the conditions identified, administration by a team of professionals that includes a clinical psychologist and/or psychiatrist is recommended. The scale can be learned in an average of 10 hours of intensive training.

Preliminary Data Gathering

NICUs vary in the ways that therapists receive and respond to feeding referrals. Some NICUs have a "blanket referral" through which the therapist is free to assist patients as needs are identified by the therapist, parents, or other NICU staff. More often, the therapist's work is done on a referral basis, by which requests for evaluation, consultation, and intervention are made in the form of a medical order. The physician or nurse practitioner may discuss the presenting problem with the therapist, or the therapist may receive a generic order, such as "therapy evaluation for slow feeding." Occasionally, the infant and family are already receiving therapy services when the referral for feeding evaluation is made. However, if the infant and family are new to the therapist, it is important to learn everything possible about the infant and the nature of the problem at hand before making contact with the infant and his or her family.

A careful review of the infant's medical record provides vital information about his or her history and hospital course, as well as details about the family that may influence the feeding evaluation (see Chapter 10 for a summary of the information that is needed prior to any feeding evaluation). Some of the most important information may also be obtained from the bedside chart and through direct communication with referring members of the medical team, the infant's parents, and the bedside nurse.

When checking in at the infant's bedside for a feeding evaluation, it is important to obtain the infant's current weight and rate of gain during the past few days. In addition, the following information must be obtained if nipple feeding has been initiated:

- Current mode of feeding (e.g., nipple, breast, gavage [bolus versus continuous], IV, combinations)
- Schedule for feedings (e.g., every 3 hours, on demand)
- Current frequency of nippling attempts
- Amount given per feeding (e.g., minimum and maximum volume in cubic centimeters [cc] to be given per feeding, ad lib) and the amount typically taken via each modality (e.g., how much by gavage versus by nipple and/or breast)
- Type of nipple currently used, as well as what has been tried to date and with what results
- Level of parental involvement to date and the parents' degree of competency and comfort with skin-to-skin care or feeding, if applicable (may not be available in the bedside record and may need to be obtained directly from nurses, social workers, or from a medical team member)
- Typical range of physiologic parameters (i.e., heart rate, respiratory rate, oxygen saturation, peripheral carbon dioxide) at rest and during feeding

- Current need for oxygen supplementation at rest and during feeding
- Frequency of apneas, bradycardias, and oxygen desaturations during or soon after feeding (including how much stimulation was required, if any, to revive the infant; whether the infant requires additional oxygen supplementation with feedings; and whether standby oxygen is to be given by nasal cannula or blow by)
- Nurses' notes and observations regarding feeding

Chart review should be followed by a brief discussion with the bedside nurse to clarify or obtain additional pertinent information. Components of this discussion include the nurse's perception of the problem, what has been tried to ameliorate it, and how successful those attempts have been. The bedside nurse knows the next appropriate time to evaluate feeding and whether a nurse will be available to assist, if needed. In addition, the bedside nurse may be able to indicate whether the parents will be available to participate in the evaluation.

Prior to the evaluation, the therapist also should ascertain whether all of the necessary supports are available at the infant's bedside. For example, if standby oxygen is needed, does the equipment need to be obtained from respiratory services? If the need for a Haberman Feeder (available from Medela; http://www.medela.com) or other specialized feeder is anticipated, is one available?

Readiness for Nipple Feeding by Breast or Bottle

An infant's physiologic stability and state of arousal are crucial components of feeding success because he or she must be an active participant in the feeding process. Therefore, an important part of any feeding evaluation in the NICU is the prefeeding evaluation—that is, determining whether it is appropriate to attempt feeding at that particular time in the infant's development.

Prefeeding Evaluation

A number of infant-related components or underlying capacities should be considered when evaluating readiness to nipple-feed infants by breast or bottle (Shaker, 1999; VandenBerg, 1990; Wolf & Glass, 1992):

- Physiologic stability: structural maintenance of the airway, potential for cardiorespiratory compromise during feeding, work of breathing, autonomic and cardiorespiratory signs of fatigue, temperature regulation
- Regulation of states of arousal: ability to achieve and sustain an alert state, and to be soothed
- Responsiveness to sensory and social stimuli
- Integrity of the oral structures: degree to which the infant's lips, palate, tongue, and pharynx are available to support the various components of feeding
- Presence of protective oral/pharyngeal reflexes: NNS/swallowing, tongue lateralization, gag, cough
- Ability to handle oral secretions independently: need and frequency of oral/pharyngeal suctioning, thickness of secretions
- Ability to handle NNS/swallowing without physiologic distress
- Adequacy of overall body posture and tone to support the infant's efforts to feed
- Experience with skin-to-skin care and NNS on the breast

The feeding evaluation should never proceed without verifying the infant's status and readiness for feeding.

Setting the Stage for Feeding Evaluation

For several reasons, it is preferable to conduct the evaluation at the infant's bedside. First, the infant's nurse will be in close proximity. This facilitates joint observation and problem solving throughout the evaluation. In addition, the infant's monitoring equipment can be used throughout the evaluation. For some infants, it is absolutely necessary to continue monitoring heart rate, respiration, and oxygen saturation throughout the evaluation for safety and information-gathering purposes. Finally, the infant is going to be fed at the bedside on a regular basis; therefore, it is important to observe the infant's current feeding status within his or her actual caregiving environment.

Before beginning the evaluation, the therapist should ensure that the infant has received a temperature check, a diaper change, and other needed nursing care to avoid unnecessary distress and handling after feeding. Doing so also optimizes the benefit of the calories ingested. In some nurseries, the therapist may be expected to check the infant's temperature, change the diaper, and prepare the bottle before proceeding with feeding; *however*, taking vital signs and administering any medications should be the responsibility of the infant's nurse.

The therapist should note the infant's state of arousal, color, heart rate, respiratory rate, oxygen saturation, and carbon dioxide levels prior to removing the infant from his or her bed for a feeding. This makes it possible to assess the infant's physiologic responses to handling, positioning, and feeding procedures as they occur. Some infants may find the bedside environment overstimulating, and their nipple feedings may need to be conducted in a quiet space to optimize success.

Caregiver Participation During the Feeding Evaluation

The bedside nurses and the infant's parents are the primary caregivers in the NICU and will be carrying out recommended interventions. Invariably, NICU nurses have a wealth of knowledge about the feeding process and can make important contributions to the assessment. For an infant who is less physiologically stable, nurses may also be very helpful, assisting the therapist in recognizing any physiologic distress that the infant may be experiencing and offering support to the infant, if necessary. Thus, whenever possible, it is important to include nurses and parents in prefeeding and feeding evaluations.

Some therapists avoid having parents present for the initial assessment out of concern that potentially witnessing a temporary loss of physiologic stability might increase parental anxiety. In most cases, however, parents are already acutely aware of their infant's tendency to desaturate ("desat") or experience a bradycardic spell ("brady") during a feeding, and their chief concern is in learning to take part in the problem-solving process. When the therapist has adequately prepared the parents for what will or might occur, the parents will have enough confidence in the therapist to participate without experiencing undue anxiety or distress (Thoyre, 2000).

Other Important Elements of a Feeding Evaluation

The complexity and integrative nature of the feeding process cannot be underestimated. This complexity and the risks associated with feeding demand closer attention to underlying capacities than do most other areas of occupational performance. Feeding success is not possible until the underlying capacities are adequately developed and contextual support is offered to optimize function. In many instances, however, an apparent immaturity of an underlying capacity actually may be the result of a poor fit between the environment (physical or social) and the infant's capacities. Therefore, it should be understood that no feeding evaluation is complete without thorough consideration and documentation of all of the following elements:

- The physical environment and the infant's response to environmental stressors
- The infant's initial state of arousal and ability to achieve and maintain a calm, alert, or semialert state
- Adequacy of the infant's posture and containment required to support feeding
- The infant's physiologic stability initially and during feeding
- Integrity of the oral-motor mechanisms
- The infant's sensory response to the nipple or breast
- The infant's active engagement in sucking, first nonnutritively and then nutritively, as appropriate
- Characteristics of the infant's tongue, lip, and jaw position and movement
- Infant's coordination of the sucking, swallowing, and breathing triad (self-pacing of the feeding versus the need for external pacing)
- Characteristics of the nipple, the thickness of the liquid, and the infant's response to these factors
- Rate of nipple flow, resistance to compression, passive flow (e.g., with the Haberman Feeder)
- Adequate shape and size of the nipple for enhancing lip and tongue action
- The need for facilitation to support rhythm, suction, or compression (e.g., pressure to palate, cheek and/or jaw support)
- Desensitization procedures, if needed, to engage the infant actively in feeding
- Caregiver competency and sensitivity to the infant's behavioral cues
- The length of time needed to complete the feeding
- The necessity of supplemental feeding by gavage

Underlying Capacities for Feeding and Specific Considerations for Evaluation

Sensory

Infants diagnosed with conditions affecting central nervous system functioning such as hypoxic-ischemic encephalopathy, IVH, or Moebius syndrome may demonstrate atypical movements of the lips, tongue, and jaw during the feeding evaluation that can be related to overall motor impairment. More often, NICU infants have feeding patterns that can be described as disorganized rather than dysfunctional.

Many preterm infants display disorganized feeding patterns because of the demands of the extrauterine environment on neurologic and physiologic systems that are still immature. These infants tend to demonstrate continued progress over time if provided with individualized approaches to their care and modulation of sensory experiences within the feeding environment.

For some infants, however, the experience of feeding is intertwined with uncomfortable, even painful, past experiences: infants who have undergone surgeries, prolonged intubation, and total parenteral nutrition (e.g., after ECMO, necrotizing enterocolitis, gastroschisis, tracheoesophageal fistula, esophageal atresia, diaphragmatic hernia, cardiac surgeries). When oral feedings are finally initiated, many of these infants may have the capacity to suck and swallow normally, but they are unable to feed because they perceive feeding to be an aversive experience. Typically, these infants accept NNS eagerly but reject nutritive feeding. The sensations associated with introducing liquids into the mouth may be perceived as abnormally unpleasant. These infants may gag at the introduction of liquid into the mouth and may retract and elevate their tongue to avoid contact with the nipple. They may have difficulty engaging the nipple, moving their head from side to side in an unsuccessful "searching" pattern, or they may spit out the nipple after only a few sucks, despite a typically eager sucking pattern on the pacifier.

The sensory aspects of feeding seem to be the source of these infants' feeding problems, and feeding evaluation and intervention need to address their specific preferences and aversions in a systematic fashion. Once the specific barriers to nipple feeding have been identified, the therapist may recommend the use of perioral and intraoral desensitization techniques in conjunction with a slow, graded progression of feeding experiences. Sensory-based feeding difficulties need to be managed in a sensitive manner, with consistency across all caregivers. This is another situation in which the family and the NICU team need to work closely together in planning the infant's care for optimal results. In some cases, the progress to total nipple feeding will require an extensive period of time, during which the infant may require supplemental gavage feedings or placement of a gastronomy tube for adequate nutrition. In these instances, tube feedings should be viewed as an interim feeding strategy that is necessary to maintain nutrition while oral experiences are offered in a graded manner. Palmer and Heyman (1993) suggested an "Oral Sensory Protocol" that has proven to be helpful in assisting infants to make the transition from tube feedings to oral feedings by nipple and/or cup and spoon. This protocol systematically records the type of food (e.g., liquid versus strained), the amount offered, the amount swallowed, the placement of the food, and the amount given by tube for each meal throughout the day. Systematic record keeping is often the best way to track progress (or lack of it) when very small changes are being made.

Neuromotor

Evaluation of the infant's posture and tone (particularly with respect to the head, neck, trunk, face, and mouth) is necessary because these may have an impact on feeding. Infants who are tense or hypertonic may require inhibitory handling and positioning in preparation for feeding. Infants who are hypotonic may need added postural support throughout feeding. Swaddling can be used as a source of neutral warmth and containment for an agitated and/or hypertonic infant. Swaddling may also be useful for hypotonic infants to provide secure containment of floppy limbs and some support to the neck and trunk. Swaddling also makes it easier to keep the infant in a stable position for feeding evaluation and intervention. Wrappings should be avoided for infants who tend to be overly warm or who are drowsy.

Positioning

Positioning is an important neuromotor aspect of feeding in which a minor change can produce immediate positive or negative consequences for the infant. When evaluating feeding, the infant's position must be continuously monitored, as it is easy for the caregiver to shift either his or her own position or the infant's position in subtle ways that can result in discomfort, distress, or mechanical disadvantage, and, ultimately, feeding inefficiency (see Chapter 12). Preterm infants usually require added postural support during feeding because they have not developed the neck and trunk control or the flexion present in full-term newborns. Swaddling and holding the infant facing the caregiver, with one hand behind the infant's head and neck, usually provides adequate support (see Figure 46). Furthermore, preterm infants continue to have soft cartilage until they are close to term age, placing them at higher risk for obstructive apnea when their necks are ventroflexed. Holding the infant's head in the crook of the caregiver's elbow rather than on the hand can sometimes contribute to obstruction

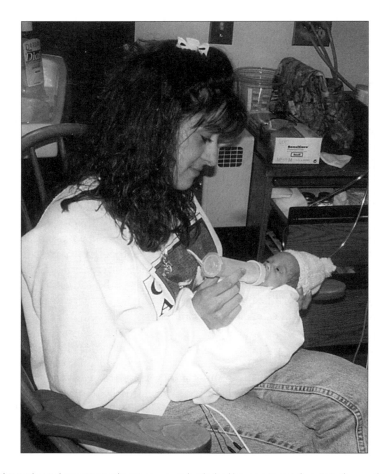

Figure 46.   This mother is demonstrating the proper way to bottle-feed her premature infant. Note the way that she supports the infant's neck as she feeds her in the en face position.

of breathing, as the infant may tend to slip down into a hyperflexed position. Conversely, sucking and swallowing are predominantly flexor activities, and excessive neck and shoulder extension can contribute to difficulty with these aspects of feeding. In addition, when the neck is extended and the scapulae are adducted, the airway is less protected, making aspiration of liquids more likely. Supporting the infant in an upright-sitting position over the caregiver's hand, propping the infant's head with the hand that is holding the bottle, and placing two fingers under the infant's jaw help maintain regular respirations and allow easy monitoring of the infant's color. This position is also useful when an infant needs to be assisted to breathe after a desaturation or bradycardic spell.

The infant's position during burping is another issue of concern. When burping, the infant can be placed on the caregiver's shoulder, but it is more difficult to monitor the infant's color in this position. The previously described upright position on the caregiver's lap may also be useful for burping the infant by tilting the infant's body forward while supporting his or her head.

Physiologic Stability

The infant's physiologic stability is a primary consideration in evaluating feeding in the NICU. Feeding imposes stresses on the infant from a variety of sources. For a sick infant, just maintaining a calm, alert state requires effort and places demands on the physiologic regulatory capacities (see Chapters 8 and 9). To become competent at feeding, the infant must be able to demonstrate reactivity and self-regulation. That is, the infant must be able to increase his or her arousal in response to a challenge and react to stress with appropriate changes in heart rate and respiration, then recover from such perturbations by returning to physiologic homeostasis without external assistance (i.e., self-regulation). Reactivity is a function of the sympathetic branch of the autonomic nervous system, and regulation is a function of the parasympathetic branch. The synchronous actions of both of these systems are needed for the infant's safety and comfort during feeding.

The coordination of sucking, swallowing, and breathing can be an enormous challenge for a preterm or sick infant. Periodic breathing, apneas, and bradycardias may occur at random in infants who were born prematurely, particularly at less than 35 weeks of gestation. The work of breathing may increase significantly during feeding, leading to oxygen desaturation, and, eventually, to apnea and/or bradycardia. Experiencing such a "spell" during the feeding process saps precious energy and makes it more difficult for the infant to proceed with the feeding (see Figure 40). Therefore, during a feeding evaluation, it is vital to be alert for behavioral signs of distress and for signs of increased work of breathing, such as nasal flaring, increased respiratory rate and shallow breathing, and circumoral or periocular cyanosis (i.e., discoloration of the skin around the mouth or between the eyes). At the first indication of increased work of breathing, the therapist should begin considering how to ease the infant's work load, perhaps by removing the nipple to allow a rest or by changing the nipple flow. Depending on the characteristics of the infant's suck, the nipple may flow too quickly or not easily enough, and either extreme can result in increased work for the infant. Characteristics of various nipples and the indications for their use are provided later in this chapter.

Reflux, Aspiration, and Airway Obstruction

Reflux

Other factors have the potential to contribute to an infant's stress during feeding, including GER. All infants experience some degree of GER, which is regurgitation of the acidic stomach contents into the esophagus, often accompanied by spitting up small amounts of undigested milk or formula. Infants who experience GER may require treatment when there is choking, frequent spitting up, or vomiting during or shortly after feedings or when these events are associated with a vagal response involving a rapid drop in heart rate. During a feeding evaluation, GER should be suspected when any or all of the previously listed symptoms are observed. The acidic nature of the regurgitated contents can result in significant discomfort for the infant and, with prolonged exposure, can cause inflammation of the esophagus, epiglottis, and vocal folds. Thus, GER may also be suspected when an infant feeds eagerly for the first portion of the feeding and then refuses the nipple, has difficulty burping and then vomits with the burp, or demonstrates a raspy cry during or after feeding. Some infants begin to fuss when placed in a horizontal position and are relieved when moved to a semiupright position—another potential sign of GER. Aspiration of the refluxed material is a danger at any time, particularly when the infant is lying in bed, when the infant has immature suck-swallow organization, or when the infant has oral/pharyngeal dysfunction (as with central nervous system or cranial nerve abnormalities). Thus, while further testing is being pursued, reflux precautions are usually implemented immediately for infants who are suspected of having GER. Reflux precautions include positioning the infant with his or her head above the body at an angle of approximately 30° or greater and keeping the infant in a semiupright position for 20–30 minutes after each feeding. Medical treatment for reflux is discussed in Chapter 5.

Aspiration

Aspiration of liquids during feeding is a serious complication that may present in infants with the following problems:

- Incomplete innervation of the oral/pharyngeal area
- Immature sucking/swallowing/breathing coordination
- Paralysis of one or both vocal folds and/or of the epiglottis
- Delayed swallowing with pooling of liquid in the pharyngeal spaces secondary to immature or atypical swallowing coordination
- Central nervous system depression, including inhibition of the gag and cough reflex

Aspiration of liquids can be immediately life threatening. It can lead to aspiration pneumonia, a serious condition, particularly for infants in the NICU whose health is already compromised. When evaluating feeding in small or sick infants, the therapist must always be aware of the risk of aspiration.

Infants are at higher risk for aspiration when there is frequent facial grimacing, gagging, coughing or choking, upper airway congestion, or stridor (a high-pitched sound on inspiration) associated with nipple feeding. Cyanosis, oxygen desaturation, apnea, and bradycardia are other possible signs of aspiration that should be taken seriously. Infants who consistently display more than one of these signs during nipple or gavage feeding should be referred for specialized testing. Oral feeding should be discontinued until aspiration is ruled out.

For the infant's comfort and safety and for optimal feeding, suspected aspiration and/or GER should be confirmed medically through radiographic examination and/ or a pneumogram with pH probe. Evidence of GER can be seen on abdominal ultrasound if the infant has been fed sweetened water just before the test. Aspiration and GER can also be detected through videofluoroscopy and barium swallow. The pneumogram with pH probe can be helpful because it provides a printout of physiologic events as they occur in real time, showing whether reflux events trigger obstructive apnea and/or bradycardia.

Airway Obstruction

One of the most common airway obstructive conditions is caused by severe jaw retraction, or retrognathia, as seen in Pierre Robin sequence. Retrognathia brings the tongue into an extreme posterior position directly over, and in some cases occluding, the trachea. The infant's airway may be opened further simply by bringing him or her into a prone or forward sitting position. Many infants, however, require an oral airway instrument (a curved tube placed in the mouth and over the tongue to keep the airway clear) or intubation for maintenance of air exchange. This is particularly important when relaxed or asleep, as the tongue tends to slip back over the trachea.

In addition to problems with inspiration, a serious side effect of this type of airway obstruction is difficulty in completely moving air out of the lungs, leading to carbon dioxide retention. Prolonged carbon dioxide retention leads to drowsiness, apnea, and eventually, metabolic acidosis and central nervous system damage. Thus, the NICU therapist needs to be thorough in evaluating not only the oral motor capacities of infants with retrognathia but also their capacity for efficient air exchange. These evaluations are usually conducted jointly with other knowledgeable members of the medical team. Some infants with retrognathia learn to protract their tongue sufficiently over the course of several days, when stimulation of NNS is given with a firm pacifier or gloved finger and when an oral airway instrument is provided during sleep (see Figure 47). Other infants with more significant anatomic anomalies require tracheostomy or glossopexy (suturing of the tongue to the floor of the mouth and to the lower lip) for airway maintenance. Once the airway has been established, the infants are usually able to take nipple feedings using a passive feeder such as the Haberman Feeder (see Figure 48) or an inverted orthodontic nipple, depending on the presence and severity of a cleft palate.

Interactions and Interventions with Caregivers

Successful feeding interventions with infants require close interaction and cooperation with the infants' caregivers. When the NICU therapist consistently involves an infant's primary caregivers in the feeding evaluation, the family members and nurses are more likely to understand the intervention goals. Taking part in the problem-solving process makes them more likely to follow through with the plan of care, to problem solve on their own, and to request further assistance from the therapist as the infant's feeding patterns change.

Throughout evaluation and intervention, the NICU therapist has the opportunity to form alliances with the infant's caregivers, which ultimately benefits all concerned.

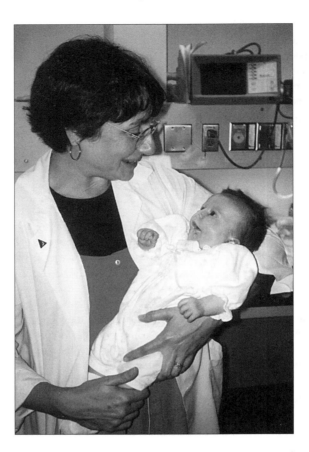

Figure 47. This infant has the small and retracted jaw characteristic of infants with retrognathia. A lip–tongue adhesion procedure has been performed to provide her with a more stable airway.

This approach is consistent with the philosophies of relationship-based and family-centered care (see Chapter 6) because it underscores the primacy of the family in feeding, an intimate element of the infant's life. It acknowledges the psychosocial aspects of feeding an infant, which should always be part of the evaluation and intervention plan. Finally, this approach prepares the family members for their continuing roles as problem solvers and nurturers for their infant.

Nipple Selection

Evaluation of NNS prior to the feeding evaluation provides vital information for determining the size, shape, and flow of nipple that may be most appropriate for each infant. The NICU staff often uses trial and error to determine the best nipple for a particular infant. A more direct approach matches the characteristics of the nipple with the purpose for which the nipple will be used—for example, to compensate for a problem with some element of sucking or to stimulate a more efficient sucking pattern.

The most appropriate nipple for any infant is the one that requires the least effort to express an adequate amount of liquid into the mouth, thereby helping maintain physiologic stability. Nipples come in a variety of sizes, shapes, and degrees

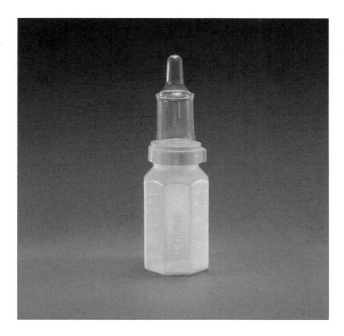

Figure 48.   Haberman Feeder (available from Medela; http://www.medela.com).

of firmness. Table 14 describes the nipples most commonly used in NICUs, as well as the indications for their use.

Regular Nipples

Bottle feeding requires compression of the nipple and cupping of the tongue to move the bolus of liquid to the pharyngeal area for swallowing. The standard yellow nipple is appropriate for most neonates. It requires compression, some cupping and stripping action of the tongue, and the ability to stabilize the nipple in the mouth, thereby generating sufficient negative pressure to express formula from it. The yellow cross-cut nipple with a yellow-colored rim can be used with neonates who require the addition of thickening substances to their formula or breast milk to improve caloric intake or to reduce GER. The cross-cut allows thicker liquid to be expressed without clogging.

The yellow orthodontic nipple is similar in shape to the NUK brand nipple sold in stores, but it is softer and therefore faster-flowing than a store-bought NUK. It also differs from the store-bought NUK in that the hole for expression of the liquid is located directly on the tip of the nipple rather than on the top. The liquid is expressed directly into the pharyngeal area rather than deflected first to the palate, bypassing the need to move the bolus toward the back of the mouth and speeding the feeding process. This nipple is appropriate for larger infants with good coordination of sucking and swallowing. It may also be useful for infants who have difficulty cupping the tongue and stabilizing the nipple in the mouth because its flat shape facilitates stability on a flat tongue or when the tongue is held in a bunched, rounded shape. This nipple flows with minimal compression. (The Ross Products orthodontic nipple is the only one discussed that is made of latex. Its use with any infant predisposed to

Table 14. Manufacturer information, characteristics, and indications for the use of various nipple types

Nipple type	Manufacturer	Characteristics	Indications for use
Standard yellow	Ross Products (http://www.ross.com) Mead Johnson & Company (http://www.meadjohnson.com)	Straight, firm nipple Moderate flow	Typical newborn capabilities Good cupping and stripping action Tongue retraction or jaw retraction (retrognathia)
Cross-cut yellow	Mead Johnson & Company	Straight, firm nipple Fast flow	Formula with cereal or other thickening additives
Red preterm	Ross Products	Straight, soft nipple Moderate to fast flow	Weak suck
Peach preterm	Ross Products	Small nipple Fast flow	Small oral cavity Weak suck
Blue-rimmed yellow preterm	Mead Johnson & Company	Small nipple Moderate flow	Small oral cavity Moderate suck Strong gag reaction
Orthodontic yellow	Ross Products	Flat nipple Moderate to fast flow Hole on end of nipple	Weak lip closure Weak compression Weak negative pressure (incomplete cleft palate) Strong gag reaction Poor cupping and stripping action
NUK	Gerber (http://www.gerber.com) Ross Products	Flat nipple Slow, moderate, or fast flow Hole on top of nipple	Poor cupping and stripping action Strong gag reaction Oxygen desaturation and/or bradycardia with feeding
Nipple Brights Healthflow Slow Flow	Gerber Munchkin (http://www.munchkininc.com)	Straight, firm nipple Slow flow	Oxygen desaturation and/or bradycardia with feeding Excessive dribbling
Clear silicone dome nipple	Avent (http://www.avent-baby.com) Gerber Munchkin	Dome shape Firm, small nipple with wide, soft bulb to simulate breast feeding	Supplementation for breast feeding
Haberman Feeder	Medela (http://www.medela.com)	Clear, straight nipple Adjustable flow Active and passive action	Weak or absent negative pressure (cleft palate) Severe retrognathia Poor sucking endurance (cardiac involvement)

latex allergy [e.g., an infant with myelomeningocele] should first be approved by the attending physician.)

Preterm Nipples

The red preterm nipple is a softer version of the standard nipple and can be used with infants who have weak compression. Once the suck has strengthened, most preterm infants need to progress to the yellow nipple to prevent excess expression, which may lead to an increase in the speed of sucking bursts, choking, oxygen desaturation, and bradycardia. The blue-rimmed yellow preterm nipple is shorter, but its flow is similar to that of the red preterm nipple. The small peach-colored preterm nipple is approximately the same size as the blue-rimmed yellow preterm nipple, but it is stiffer and provides a faster, steadier flow. Some infants in the NICU require the smaller nipples, especially infants with IUGR who have reached an appropriate age for nipple feeding. Of the two, the blue-rimmed nipple is often preferred because of its more moderate flow.

The previously discussed nipples are commonly stocked in most NICUs. Other nipples may be necessary to meet special requirements. Slower flowing nipples may be needed for some preterm or full-term infants who have strong NS but poor coordination of swallowing and breathing. A slower flow enables these infants to regulate the speed of their sucking bursts and begin to self-pace breathing pauses.

Slow-Flow Nipples

There are a number of nipples on the market labeled as "slow flow," however, these vary considerably in their firmness and flow. There are many commercially available brands of standard yellow nipples, most of which are slightly firmer and slower flowing than the yellow nipple available in the NICU. The Munchkin (http://www.munchkininc.com) Healthflow Slow Flow nipple is a silicone nipple that also is slightly firmer than the standard yellow nipple. The Gerber (http://www.gerber.com) Nipple Brights nipple is firmer than Munchkin's Healthflow Slow Flow, but Gerber's Slow Flow is the firmest of the three. Most of the commercial nipples also come in medium and faster flows (i.e., flows for older infants).

Nurser-Type Nipples

The Playtex Nurser nipple is not recommended for preterm infants because the "pulling" sucking action requires more energy expenditure than a standard compression nipple. There are other more desirable options for families who want to use disposable bag-type bottles with preterm infants. Avent, Munchkin, and Gerber make dome-shaped silicone nipples that incorporate a firm nipple with a soft bulb, approximating the action used when breast-feeding. These nipples come in various flow rates and have been used successfully by some families of preterm infants, particularly families that are supplementing breast feedings with bottle feedings during their infant's transition home.

Other Nipples

The Haberman Feeder (see Figure 48) is unique for infants with an inability to generate negative pressure for expression of liquid—for example, infants with cleft palate or severe retrognathia. It consists of a squeezable nipple with a one-way valve. The nipple has a cut on the end to adjust the flow rates, depending on the position of the nipple in the mouth in relation to three markings on the nipple. Unlike other passive squeeze-type bottles, its most important feature is the one-way valve, which makes it possible for the infant to feed actively, using only compression, or to be fed passively by squeezing. In addition, the valve prevents backflow of the liquid, making it easier to express the same amount of liquid with each squeeze.

The names and characteristics of particular nipples on the market, and their manufacturers, continually change. NICU therapists should be familiar with the different types of nipples and how to obtain them because parents may ask for recommendations not only while their infant is in the NICU but also during the transition home and beyond.

CASE EXAMPLES

Specific intervention techniques are beyond the scope of this book. However, any recommendations generated from the feeding evaluation with regard to nipple selection, positioning and handling for breast and bottle feeding, energy conservation and modification of the environment, and enhancement of caregiver–infant interaction provide potent contextual elements that may be considered intervention strategies. The following case examples illustrate many of the principles presented in this chapter. The first case summarizes the evaluation process to determine an infant's readiness for nipple feeding from an infant-centered perspective, and it offers recommendations for enhancing the infant's feeding readiness and participation in the feeding process. The second case discusses the transition from gavage to nipple feeding for a preterm infant who has respiratory distress and requires initial intubation and subsequent oxygen supplementation.

Full-Term Infant with Asphyxia

Suzanne was a full-term infant who was born to a 40-year-old gravida 2 (a woman in her second pregnancy), para 2 (second live birth) mother by emergency cesarean section secondary to a posterior rupture of the uterus. Suzanne required resuscitation at birth, with Apgar scores of 1, 3, and 6. She experienced seizures immediately after birth, for which she was given phenobarbital. She also required mechanical ventilation for the first 2 days after birth.

Assessment of Nipple Feeding Readiness

Suzanne was referred for an evaluation of her readiness for nipple feeding at 10 days of age, when her seizures had ceased and she had been weaned off her seizure medication. She was receiving supplemental oxygen at 25%–30% by nasal cannula, having her oral secretions suctioned, and being gavage fed. Her neurological assessment revealed some jitteriness and mixed hypo- and hyperreflexia. A repeat electroencephalogram (EEG) and magnetic resonance imaging (MRI) were pending, and she had received a working diagnosis of presumed hypoxic-ischemic encephalopathy.

Both parents were at the infant's bedside for the consultation. Suzanne was in a quiet alert state in an open crib. Her eyes remained open, although focusing on faces or objects could not be elicited. Suzanne responded to increased noise and activity around her bedside by squirming and becoming restless, but she did not startle to loud sounds. She turned to localize her mother's voice on the right side. Overall tone was mixed—there was noticeable extensor tightness in her pelvis and lower extremities, but her neck and trunk were floppy, and her arms moved actively toward her face and mouth with fingers loosely fisted. Some cortical thumb posturing could be seen intermittently. Suzanne's movements were poorly graded, with clonus elicited at the end of the range in all four extremities. Upper and lower extremity reflex responses such as the Babinski sign, palmar and plantar grasps, and proprioceptive placing could be described as weakly present.

It had been 3 hours since Suzanne's last gavage feeding. Her nurse reported that she had required suctioning of her oral secretions once during that 3-hour period and at the time of her gavage feeding. Suzanne was wrapped in a receiving blanket and brought to a semiflexed, semiupright position for examination of her oral structure and function. Visual inspection of the oral cavity was difficult to initiate because Suzanne clamped her jaw tightly. Containment through swaddling and gentle facial massage relaxed her enough to proceed with the exam. Suzanne's oral cavity appeared normal, with the exception of strong retraction and tongue elevation. She engaged in occasional lip smacking in response to perioral stimulation, but a rooting response was not elicited laterally or vertically. Suzanne had no lateral tongue movement, no cough, and no gag in response to intraoral stimulation to her tongue, gums, or hard and soft palate. When her posterior pharyngeal wall was touched, however, she had a gag reflex. To engage the tongue, the therapist had to place her gloved finger into the side of Suzanne's mouth and carefully scoop the tongue away from the pharyngeal wall, giving gentle downward pressure to bring it forward. Once the tongue was brought forward, Suzanne produced a few arrhythmic sucks on the finger. This sucking response was obtained several times, with repeated downward/forward strokes on the tongue. NS was not attempted at the time. Suzanne remained calm throughout the evaluation, and her physiologic measures were stable and within normal limits for a full-term newborn.

Suzanne's parents were appropriately concerned about her lack of visual responsiveness. The therapist discussed this observation, along with the rest of the exam, with them in the context of an infant who is recovering from a traumatic birth. The therapist explained that some of the atypical neuromotor findings would likely become less apparent over the next few weeks, as Suzanne's recovery continued, but that some others may linger or even strengthen over time. The next few weeks were to be a period of ongoing assessment for Suzanne. In the interim, the parental role as Suzanne's nurturers was emphasized, as was the importance of providing a restful, soothing sensory environment as Suzanne learned to feed. It was recommended that whenever possible, feedings be done in the NICU's quieter family room rather than in the incubator bay to optimize Suzanne's participation in prefeeding activities and family interactions.

Nipple feeding was not recommended on the basis of the evaluation. Suzanne required suctioning of her oral secretions; had no protective cough; and her gag response was weak, inconsistent, and deep in the pharyngeal area. It was determined that she would not be able to protect her airway from aspiration of the liquid at this time. However, Suzanne was able to press her lips together and to suck nonnutritively with facilitation—strengths that were to be encouraged.

Recommendations to Promote Feeding Readiness

NNS was recommended as a way to stimulate Suzanne's suck-swallow reflex. It was hoped that this would also lead to further development of her cough and gag responses because sucking, swallowing, gagging, and coughing share common sources of innervation. A long, firm, straight-nippled pacifier—in this case, the Playtex (http://www.playtexbaby.com) pacifier with a butterfly-shaped lip mold— was suggested because it was long enough to reach her retracted tongue and could be gently used to stimulate tongue protraction.

Initial Plan

The initial feeding plan was established after discussing the recommendations with the medical team. The following instructions were posted at Suzanne's bedside:

- Foster relaxation and optimal responsiveness by keeping Suzanne's bedspace as quiet as possible. Gently massage her extremities and adhere to specific positioning recommendations to encourage flexion while she is lying in her crib or when she is held. Swaddle Suzanne in flexion prior to gavage feeding.

- Take Suzanne to a quieter space for gavage feeding and social interaction with her family.

- Offer a Playtex pacifier (long, firm nipple) when she is awake, especially during gavage feeding, to encourage NNS and suck-swallow coordination for active clearing of oral secretions and to begin an association between sucking and feeding.

- Give Suzanne gentle downward pressure strokes with the pacifier or a gloved finger to bring her tongue forward and encourage cupping of the tongue around the nipple.

Suzanne's parents were eager to participate in her feeding process. Suzanne was to be reassessed on an ongoing basis. During these daily visits, the therapist would monitor her progress and assist her nurses and parents in providing positioning and handling for the reduction of extensor tightness in her lower extremities.

Reevaluation

Suzanne repeatedly demonstrated a protective gag reflex on her 15th day after birth; with the attending physician's permission, nipple feeding was initiated. She *required help in getting her tongue forward for nipple placement but had good lip closure over the nipple, and once it was placed on her tongue, she engaged it with some cupping action. Suzanne had a rhythmic suck, but her sucking bursts were of short duration—one or two sucks, followed by a long pause. Some upper airway congestion could be felt and heard as Suzanne was being fed, suggesting that she needed additional time for swallowing to clear the liquid from her pharyngeal area. Once she had swallowed the liquid, she required intermittent facilitation to continue sucking. This consisted of stroking her tongue forward with the nipple once or twice, then pausing for her to begin sucking again. With this type of support, Suzanne was able to take 5 cc of sterile water from a standard yellow nipple without distress.*

Feeding Progression

At the next feeding, expressed breast milk was given, and Suzanne took 10 cc in 5 minutes with some facilitation, then became drowsy and fell asleep. The remaining 25 cc of her feeding was gavaged through a thin Silastic gavage tube, which remained in place for several days at a time. The plan was to nipple feed whatever Suzanne could comfortably take within a half hour using a standard nipple, which would provide the appropriate length and firmness for facilitating her sucking bursts. The milk that remained in the bottle was to be gavaged.

With each experience, Suzanne showed longer sustained sucking bursts, demonstrated better coordination of sucking and swallowing, and took greater total volumes of breast milk. A week later, she no longer required intermittent facilitation to reinitiate sucking. Her feeding competence had continued to progress. She was taking 40 cc by nipple every 4 hours. Her mother was instructed in gavage feeding, which enabled Suzanne to be discharged and to continue her nipple feeding progress at home with daily visiting nurse support.[3] Suzanne's eyes seemed to focus on faces at times, but it was still difficult to determine whether she could see because she did not track moving faces or objects. Although she responded with temporary relaxation to the massage and passive ranging provided at each care period, Suzanne continued to show signs of emerging spasticity in her lower back, pelvis, and lower extremities. To provide ongoing assistance with nipple feeding, positioning and handling, and developmentally appropriate sensory activities, her discharge plan included a visit by the NICU occupational therapist during the transition home. It also included referrals to the feeding team and to physical therapy specialists at the local hospital's pediatric rehabilitation department. This would allow uninterrupted service provision while Suzanne's referral to the local early intervention program was being processed.

In Suzanne's example, the most important considerations regarding readiness for nipple feeding were airway protection and the ability to coordinate sucking, swallowing, and breathing. Given these considerations, the evaluation revealed her initial

---

[3]Due to the high risk of aspiration during gavage feedings, this method of feeding is used at home only in exceptional cases and only when the medical team is absolutely confident about the parents' competence in gavaging their infant.

of readiness for nipple feeding. The evaluation also resulted in recommendations or intervention and a plan for monitoring and optimizing Suzanne's readiness. Nipple selection for both pacifier and NS were important factors in Suzanne's intervention plan. After 1 week of preparatory care and the selection of an adequate nipple, Suzanne was able to begin nipple feedings. The feeding support enabled Suzanne to gradually gain feeding competence over a period of 1 week, enabling her discharge from the NICU.

Preterm Infant Making the Transition to Nipple Feeding

Another common scenario for prefeeding evaluation and feeding intervention in the NICU is that of a preterm infant who has been gavage fed and is beginning to make the transition to nipple feedings. Neonatology textbooks and journal articles typically report that the earliest coordination within the sucking, swallowing, and breathing triad occurs between 32 and 34 weeks (Blackburn & Loper, 1992; Omari et al., 1999). Practical experience, however, suggests that some preterm infants have adequate coordination within this triad as early as 30 weeks. Depending upon their medical status, physiologic stability, and behavioral organization, many preterm infants in the NICU are introduced to nipple feeding between 30 and 34 weeks (Kinneer & Beachy, 1994). The trend toward earlier discharges has contributed to earlier introduction of feeding (Raddish & Merritt, 1998). Many preterm infants are discharged from the NICU at 32–34 weeks, as long as they have reached the minimum discharge criteria (i.e., maintenance of body temperature outside the Isolette, absence of life-threatening apneas or bradycardias, and the ability to take full feedings by nipple and/or breast) (Kinneer & Beachy, 1994). Thus, weight and GA are no longer the primary considerations for initiating nipple feeds. More important factors in making discharge decisions are the infant's physiologic stability, regulation of states of arousal, and organization of oral-motor/pharyngeal functions. For these reasons, the feeding assessment cannot be confined to the infant's oral structures and mechanics. A thorough feeding evaluation should also encompass the infant's physiologic, motor, and behavioral organization; the types of caregiver support that are needed; and environmental modifications that may need to be made to optimize the infant's participation. This case example illustrates a rather typical progression of the feeding program to help a preterm infant make the transition from gavage to nipple feedings.

Matthew was a tiny preterm infant with IUGR; he was born at 28 weeks of gestation, weighing only 600 g. His mother's pregnancy history revealed no obvious complications except for Matthew's slow growth, which had been followed closely by the obstetrician. A specialized ultrasound had revealed no congenital anomalies. Premature rupture of membranes occurred at 26 weeks, and Matthew's mother remained on bed rest for 2 weeks before it was decided that he should be delivered by cesarean section. During that time, the antenatal steroid betamethasone was administered several times to enhance Matthew's lung growth. He was delivered without incident, initially breathing on his own, but required intubation and ventilatory assistance within an hour of his delivery. Matthew remained on mechanical ventilation for a week before he was weaned to CPAP and, eventually, to nasal cannula oxygen at 31 weeks. At 32 weeks, he was small but very active, weighing just 1,280 g and, according to his nurses, sucking vigorously on his fists and clothing. Matthew tolerated gavage feedings well and had used a pacifier since his first days on the ventilator. He was referred for evaluation of his potential to begin nipple feeding because his nurses felt he was consuming precious calories being active in his crib and that nipple feeding might soothe him. They requested a formal assessment prior to attempting to feed Matthew because in their NICU, he was smaller by size and weight than most infants who are typically started on nipple feeding.

Assessment

Matthew was in a light sleep state when the therapist approached his Isolette but came to active alertness when his mother lifted the blanket covering the Isolette. His movements were quick and of wide excursion, and his posture was symmetrical. His overall tone was appropriate for an infant of 32 weeks, with greater tone in the lower extremities than in the trunk and upper extremities. Palmar and plantar grasp reflexes were easily elicited. He made crawling movements in prone, attempting to turn his head to clear his nose. He made an effort to right his head when brought to supported sitting and seemed particularly responsive to his mother's voice, attempting unsuccessfully to turn his head toward her. He was visually alert throughout handling and demonstrated some signs of distress when his position was changed—splaying his fingers, saluting, and attempting to brace his feet against the sides of the Isolette. When contained and held in flexion, he easily brought his hand to his mouth and inserted his thumb, something that his mother reported he had been doing for some time.

The oral exam was unremarkable. Matthew had a strong, rhythmic NNS with good cupping and stripping action of the tongue. Rooting, tongue lateralization, and gag reflex were present. The therapist offered to feed Matthew (to evaluate his capacity to handle liquids) while his mother watched. Matthew's mother was happy to be the observer at this time; she had expressed anxiety about feeding Matthew because he was so small. Matthew's NS was rhythmic, with sustained sucking bursts of more than 8 sucks without pausing to breathe. Using a red preterm nipple, he seemed to be able to express an adequate amount per suck but with some dribbling and choking. Arm salutes, paleness around the eyes and mouth, and a drop in oxygen saturation signaled Matthew's need for a break. A change to the yellow standard nipple resulted in less dribbling and choking, but sustained sucking without pausing to breathe and oxygen desaturation continued. External pacing (i.e., removing or tipping the nipple to stop the flow of liquid every six to eight sucks) was necessary to elicit a breath from Matthew with each sucking burst. Desaturation stopped with external pacing, but Matthew continued to appear fatigued and began to have difficulty expressing the breast milk from the bottle. His respiratory rate increased, and nasal flaring was observed during his pauses to breathe. Even though his nurse increased his oxygen, Matthew began to require some facilitation to reinitiate sucking. He became drowsy and *refused to feed any further after taking approximately 15 cc in 10 minutes. Mat-thew's mother was excited to see his ability to feed, but she was concerned about learning to feed him without oxygen desaturations.*

Impressions and Recommendations

Matthew was a small infant of only 32 weeks with appropriate reflexes and muscle tone. He had a good rhythmic suck, and had some difficulty coordinating the swallowing and breathing components of feeding, resulting in behavioral and physiologic distress. A slower flowing nipple reduced dribbling and choking and allowed Matthew's swallowing to keep pace with the flow of liquid, but he also required assistance in pacing his breathing. For this, the nipple needed to be removed from his mouth or tipped to stop the flow of liquid, enabling him to take a breath. In addition, feeding obviously increased his work of breathing, and he eventually fatigued into a drowsy state of arousal, perhaps as an adaptive means of ending his participation in this stressful activity.

Matthew's many strengths were emphasized to his mother. His initial energy and competence at bringing his hand to his mouth and at NNS were good preparations for nutritive feeding. However, he required oxygen supplementation at all times, especially during feeding. He also demonstrated increased work of breathing with the effort of NS, even when provided with external pacing to promote regular breathing. His regulation of states of arousal was an additional strength because he used this capacity adaptively to end his participation in feeding once he became fatigued. Emphasizing external pacing and framing Matthew's fatigue in this way made it seem less frightening to his mother, and she expressed eagerness to learn to recognize his behavioral cues and to externally pace his feeding.

Matthew was ready to be gradually introduced to nipple feeding. He would require a slower flowing nipple to accommodate his strong suck but immature suck-swallow organization. He also would require external pacing to ensure that he takes regular breaths. The following recommendations were posted at his bedside:

- *Offer nipple feedings only a few times a day to conserve his energy, ideally at times when Matthew's mother is present.*

- *Nipple feed with the nasogastric tube in place to gavage feed whatever Matthew is unable to take by nipple.*

- *Use the yellow standard nipple to obtain a moderate flow of liquid and thereby accommodate his immature suck-swallow organization.*

- *Attend to Matthew's behavioral cues and color changes as signs that he may require a break or an increase in supplemental oxygen.*

- *Provide external pacing, leaving the nipple in Matthew's mouth to avoid dis-rupting the sensory experience of nipple feeding but tipping it to stop the flow of liquid until he has taken a breath.*

The plan was to meet with Matthew's mother on a regular basis to assist her in learning to read his cues and to pace his feedings. The therapist would continue to evaluate Matthew's progress and change the bedside recommendations as needed. Within 2 weeks, Matthew began to pace his own breathing and to take all his feedings by nipple. During the next 2 weeks, ongoing evaluation of feeding indicated that his feeding volumes continued to increase, and he had adequate weight gain, demonstrating that he was not expending energy excessively during feedings. He was discharged 1 month after his initial feeding evaluation, using the standard yellow nipple. As shown in this example, Matthew had demonstrated the ability to sustain NNS without distress but needed to gain further control over his physiologic functions before he could nipple an entire feeding and before nipple feedings could become a regular part of his care.

BREAST FEEDING CONSULTATION

Having an infant in the NICU can be a major barrier to breast feeding for many infants and their mothers. Whether the infant is extremely premature or sick, many factors interfere with breast feeding in the first days and weeks of life for infants in the NICU. Many women with a sick newborn in the NICU have experienced a difficult labor and delivery and often are ill. They may not be well enough to begin pumping their breast milk immediately after their infant's delivery, or they may be on medications that prohibit use of the breast milk.

The most common barrier to breast feeding, nevertheless, is the status of the infant. Breast milk is the preferred infant food, and mothers are encouraged to bring expressed milk for their infant whenever possible. However, it can be weeks or even months before a sick or extremely premature infant is stable enough to begin feeding from the breast. The lactation consultant and the bedside nurses have important roles in assisting mothers to stimulate an adequate milk supply and encouraging them to continue pumping throughout this long wait. The stresses of having a sick infant in addition to all of the other demands of daily life often result in mothers becoming tired and discouraged during this time and, in turn, abandoning their pumping regimen (Furman, Minich, & Hack, 1998). Other mothers are given little encouragement or instruction in placing the small infant to the breast (see Figure 49) and give up trying once the infant is home. Still others place their concern for the infant's weight gain before their desire to breast feed and will discontinue trying to breast feed if the infant seems to be getting all that he or she requires from the bottle.

Some myths about breast feeding preterm infants are being dispelled by research. The first myth is that breast feeding is more physiologically demanding than bottle feeding and is therefore to be avoided with infants who have a tendency toward physiologic instability. In fact, infants whose physiologic responses were measured alternately on the breast and on the bottle consistently showed higher oxygen saturation on the breast and no problems maintaining temperature (Bier et al., 1993). Although these infants expressed less liquid from the breast than from the bottle, indicating their continuing need for a supplementary feeding, they were not stressed by breast feeding per se. Oxygen desaturation occurred more frequently during bottle feeding than during breast feeding, presumably because the bottle flows more quickly, resulting in gulping and occasional choking, whereas the flow of breast milk responds to the infant's demand, according to the strength of his or her sucking.

Another myth is that supplementing with bottle feeding results in "nipple confusion," making infants lose interest in breast feeding. The notion of nipple confusion

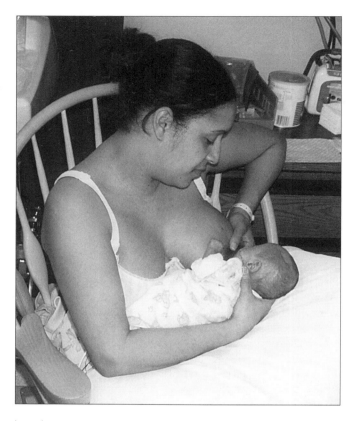

Figure 49. This mother is demonstrating one of the most effective positioning arrangements for postural support of a preterm infant during breast feeding.

has not been studied, but anecdotal accounts in the literature as well as the clinical experience of this book's authors suggest that there is little basis to the claim that supplementation with a bottle dooms a mother's breast-feeding efforts to failure. Furman (1995) gave examples of mothers who successfully incorporated the bottle and breast with preterm infants, including mothers of "multiples."

One important way to assist mothers and infants in preparing for the breast feeding experience is to offer skin-to-skin care (kangaroo care). Skin-to-skin care provides the tactile and proprioceptive experiences of breast feeding when an infant is too fragile or too encumbered by ventilatory equipment to attempt sucking on the breast. As the infant becomes more stable and active, he or she can be encouraged to nuzzle and to begin NNS on the mother's breast. When used in combination with gavage feeding, this becomes a natural entrée to breast feeding because it enables the infant to begin associating sucking on the breast with a feeling of satiety. Another alternative for infants who are able to coordinate sucking and swallowing but unable to express milk from the breast is to provide breast milk via a supplemental nursing system. A thin tube is taped to the mother's breast so that when the infant nibbles on the breast, milk is delivered passively through the tube, which is connected to a syringe held by the mother or hung around her neck with a lanyard. The Supplemental Nursing System (available from Medela; http://www.medela.com; see Figure 50) obviates the need for placement of an oral or nasal gavage tube and is therefore a more comfortable alternative to passive feeding than gavage. Through both of these

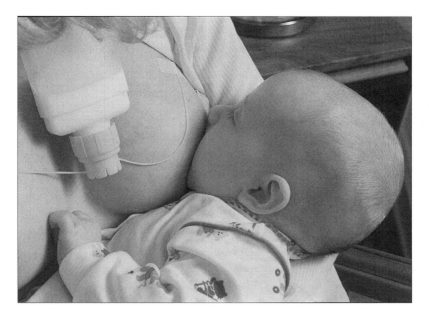

Figure 50. The Supplemental Nursing System (available from Medela; http://www.medela.com).

approaches, the infant learns to latch on to the breast in a natural, nurturing context and is gradually prepared for active breast feeding (Kliethermes, Cross, Lanese, Johnson, & Simon, 1999).

For the mother, benefits of skin-to-skin care and the infant's early exposure to the breast include the closeness that she experiences with her infant, the familiarity that she gains with placing the infant to the breast, and increased milk production compared with women who have not engaged in skin-to-skin care (Bier et al., 1996). Moreover, Bier and colleagues (1996) found that experience with skin-to-skin care and putting the infant to suck nonnutritively on the breast was predictive of a mother's increased success in breast feeding after the infant's discharge. Thus, it seems important to provide such experiences as early as possible in the NICU stay to enhance the infant's familiarity with the breast and the mother's comfort with and sensitivity to her infant's efforts to breast-feed. The therapist has an important role in facilitating breast feeding and infant–caregiver attachment by encouraging skin-to-skin care and early breast feeding for infants in the NICU; by evaluating the infant's capacity to participate in breast feeding; and by providing recommendations for sensory, motor, and positioning accommodations to enhance the infant's participation. For optimal timing and infant safety, the mother's decision to initiate skin-to-skin care needs to be made jointly between the therapist and the medical team.

Specific Feeding Interventions Applicable to Infants in the NICU

A thorough initial evaluation is the first intervention step for an infant with feeding problems. The evaluation usually identifies specific problems that interfere with the infant's ability to feed. Some problems identified in the evaluation may require further evaluation by the medical team and specific medical and/or pharmaceutical interventions (e.g., anemia, GER, hyperbilirubinemia, poor gas exchange, withdrawal/abstinence from prenatal or postnatal drug exposures, worsening cardiac status, worsening congestion in the lung). Other types of problems may be responsive to neonatal therapy interventions.

Practical suggestions for enhancing an infant's feeding skills through proper preparation include

- Keep feedings within scheduled times, especially with preterm infants who do not wake up for feedings.
- Eliminate or minimize unnecessary stimuli.
- Select a quiet place in the nursery, particularly when feeding an infant who is irritable or hypersensitive.
- Secure a comfortable chair with armrests (the infant will relax more easily when the caregiver is comfortable).
- Position the chair to allow enough slack on any wires or tubing.
- Have a pacifier available to enable NNS prior to feeding, if necessary.
- Change the diaper before starting to minimize handling after feeding.
- Swaddle the infant to facilitate flexion and provide external postural support.
- Arouse the infant gently prior to feeding (mild upright positioning facilitates quiet alertness).
- Position the infant in a semiupright position, with his or her head and neck in neutral, shoulders protracted, and arms and legs flexed toward the midline of his or her body. Maintaining the neck in neutral is essential: Ventroflexion can result in obstruction of the airway, whereas hyperextension can contribute to tongue retraction and aspiration.
- Keep the infant well supported and contained throughout the feeding.

The appendix at the end of this chapter lists some common problems that interfere with feeding, as well as typical recommendations to address each problem. As mentioned previously, each problem could be related to a medical condition that requires further medical evaluation and/or pharmaceutical management. However, for simplicity's sake, the appendix includes only practical recommendations. This list is by no means comprehensive and is meant only to give the reader a general overview of the kinds of interventions that may be appropriate in the NICU. For success in feeding intervention, each infant must be evaluated individually and on an ongoing basis. Most infants exhibit a combination of feeding problems. Feeding intervention should incorporate a number of methods to address the various feeding needs. The intervention plan should reflect the unique behavioral, neuromotor, physiologic and psychosocial needs of that infant and his or her caregivers.

CONCLUSION

Feeding intervention is a specialized and complex area of care. Therapists must establish the necessary competencies to independently engage in feeding intervention to ensure infant safety and best practice in the NICU.

Appendix

Common Feeding Problems and Solutions

Presenting problem/ condition and potential causes (listed in descending order of frequency of occurrence)	Typical presentation	Recommendations
Low arousal		
Immature regulation of states of arousal	The infant is unable to complete a nipple or breast feeding.	Feed infant in a semi-upright position.
Hyperbilirubinemia	The infant falls asleep or becomes too drowsy to eat.	Use an en face (facing the caregiver) versus an in-arm hold.
Anemia		Dress/wrap the infant lightly.
Fatigue after stressful procedures		Reduce or block lighting and noise.
Seizure medication		Burp the infant sitting up versus over the shoulder.
		Avoid rhythmic stimuli (rocking, singing, music).
		Provide intermittent stimuli (touch, voice, movement).
		Review the care schedule for adequacy of rest between feedings.
		Suggest every (q) 4° if infant is being awakened for feedings q 3°.

(continued)

(continued)

Fatigue/increased work of breathing

Exposure to stressful procedures	The infant is initially alert but has a weak suck-swallow.	Determine whether the infant requires increased oxygen with feeding (for infants receiving oxygen by nasal cannula).
Recent weaning off CPAP or a ventilator	Oxygen desaturation occurs during feeding.	Check nipple flow; the infant may require a faster flowing nipple for less work.
Inadequate rest	The infant's respiratory rate increases.	
Worsening pulmonary or cardiac status	The infant has chest retractions.	Review the care schedule for adequacy of rest between feedings.
Evolving sepsis	The infant shows nasal flaring.	Suggest q 4° if infant is being awakened for feedings q 3°.
	There is a color change (flushed, pale, cyanotic).	Limit nipple feeding to 30 minutes with the remainder gavaged, if necessary. (Suggest using a thin, Silastic, indwelling nasogastric tube to reduce airway obstruction and interference with swallowing.)
	The infant has limp posture.	
	The infant is drowsy.	

Poor coordination of swallowing with sucking

Immature suck-swallow organization	The infant initially has an eager, strong, rhythmic suck.	Check the position of the infant's neck and head for adequacy of airway during sucking and swallowing.
GER	There is dribbling or choking.	Check the adequacy of the infant's pharyngeal reflexes to protect the airway.
Vocal fold paralysis	There is gagging with NS but not with NNS.	
Central nervous system involvement	The infant has bradycardia with quick self-recovery or bradycardia with slow recovery and associated oxygen desaturation.	Check for excessive ventroflexion, lateral flexion, or rotation of the neck, which may interfere with swallowing.
Cranial nerve involvement		Check nipple flow; the infant may require a slower flowing nipple.
	There are behavioral signs of stress (e.g., pulling away from the nipple, grimacing, saluting, finger splaying).	Provide external pacing: Remove or tip the nipple q 5–8 sucks to allow time for swallowing.
	There is a color change (pale, cyanotic).	Encourage use of a pacifier between feedings and during gavage feedings to reinforce suck-swallow.

Poor coordination of breathing with suck-swallow		
Immature suck-swallow-breathing organization Mouth breathing (e.g., after prolonged intubation) Temporary depression of suck-swallow-breathing (e.g., after labor with anesthesia)	The infant initially has an eager, rhythmic suck-swallow. Respiratory rate decreases while the infant is sucking. Oxygen desaturation occurs while the infant is sucking. There are behavioral signs of stress (e.g., grimacing, saluting, finger splaying). There is an immediate recovery of respiration rate and oxygen saturation with the removal of the nipple.	Check the nipple flow; the infant may require a slower flowing nipple to allow time for breathing. Provide external pacing: Remove or tip the nipple q 5–8 sucks to allow time for breathing. Encourage the use of a pacifier between feedings and during gavage feedings to reinforce breathing while sucking.
Weak suck and/or hypotonicity		
Central nervous system involvement Syndrome (e.g., Down, Prader-Willi) Hypoglycemia Anemia Hyperbilirubinemia	There is minimal expression of liquid from the nipple. The infant has a normal, flat, or bunched tongue. There is poor cupping and/or stripping action of the tongue. There is weak tongue elevation and/or a tendency for the tongue to flop back and obstruct the airway. The infant has poor lip closure.	Swaddle or contain the infant for optimal stability. Ensure that the neck and head are in the neutral position. Position the infant semi-upright (more forward if the infant's tongue flops back to obstruct the airway). Choose a nipple shape that fits the infant's tongue movement (e.g., a flat nipple for a flat or bunched tongue). Use a soft, steady-flowing nipple. Provide gentle external support to cheeks in a downward and forward direction or provide a steady upward pressure to the lower jaw, just behind the chin. Stimulate sucking by pressing the nipple against the infant's palate.

(continued)

(continued)

Limited tongue and jaw mobility and/or hypertonicity		
Central nervous system involvement Arthrogryposis	There is limited jaw movement with sucking, or there is phasic biting. There is tongue retraction and elevation. There is trunk and neck extension. Stiffness is evident in the extremities.	Prepare the infant for feeding by providing a relaxing massage, particularly of the face, temples, and mandible. Check posture for neutral neck alignment and adequate flexion of the hips and knees. Swaddle the infant for neutral warmth, flexion, and containment. Provide support to the back of the neck and head, avoiding pressure to the occipital protuberance (which stimulates increased head extension). Facilitate palmar grasp reflex (using the therapist's finger), and use eye contact to promote flexion and chin tuck. Ensure that the nipple is on top of the infant's tongue. Stimulate sucking by using the nipple to give a few gentle, rhythmic presses to the infant's tongue, then pause for a response from the infant.
Oral hypersensitivity		
Status: post-ECMO; surgery for tracheal, esophageal, or cardiac conditions involving prolonged intubation with sedation Minimal positive oral experiences	There is an overactive gag reflex, elicited on the anterior half of the tongue or at the gums. There are behavioral signs of stress during attempts to feed (arching away, grimacing, fussing, arm waving, spitting the nipple out). Choking and gagging occur with NS but not with NNS.	Prepare the infant for touch by providing gentle sustained touch to the trunk, shoulders, head, and face. Give sustained presses (with a gloved finger) to the outer lips, laterally to medially. Give several firm lateral swipes to the palate, just behind the alveolar ridge (P. Wilbarger, personal communication, July 1997).

Give some firm, rhythmic presses to the tongue, using a downward, forward motion.

Encourage hand-to-mouth exploration.

Provide NNS experiences, particularly during gavage feedings, by using a pacifier and then progressing to other objects with differing textures and shapes.

Monitor signs of distress and proceed only according to the infant's tolerance.

Irritability

Central nervous system irritability

Drug withdrawal or abstinence

GER

Swallowing dysfunction

Airway obstruction

Stressful environment

Uncomfortable positioning/handling

The infant fusses before and during feeding.

The infant fusses only during feeding.

The infant fusses or refuses to feed midway through the feeding.

Assess for swallowing difficulty and/or airway obstruction during NS to rule out sources of distress.

Check nipple flow; it may be too slow or too fast for the infant.

Review the care schedule for adequacy of rest between feedings.

Prepare the infant for feeding with inhibitory activities involving neutral warmth, containment, soothing, and rhythmic stimuli.

Provide a calm environment, as free from irritating stimuli as possible.

Handle the infant with minimum touching and positioning changes.

Keep social interaction to a minimum.

Consider GER as a problem if fussing occurs after feeding has been progressing.

(continued)

(continued)

Poor lip closure		
Cleft lip	There is dribbling.	Try breast feeding, which may be easier than bottle feeding because there is a larger surface for stability.
Low tone oral musculature	The infant is unable to sustain a seal on the nipple.	
Facial paralysis (usually unilateral facial droop)	The infant has weak intraoral suction.	Provide cheek and/or jaw support.
		Use a soft, steady-flowing nipple or a Haberman Feeder (Medela).

Inadequate intra-oral suction		
Cleft palate	The infant has rhythmic sucking but is unable to express liquid from the breast or bottle.	Recognize that breast feeding usually is not possible in this case due to the infant's inability to generate sufficient negative pressure for expression.
Retrognathia	The infant has nasal reflux.	Provide a fast, steady-flowing nipple, such as the Ross Products orthodontic nipple used in the inverted position, or use a passive flow nipple, such as the Haberman Feeder.
	The infant has excessive gas (secondary to inefficient sucking).	
	The infant shows early fatigue.	Deliver liquid in a steady, rhythmic manner to help the infant anticipate when the next mouthful will be given.
		Feed the infant in the upright position to reduce nasal reflux.
		Burp the infant frequently.
		Give occasional pauses to allow extra time for swallowing and, in turn, to clear the pharynx.
		Allow extra time for feeding.
		Recognize that the infant may require a different feeding method after being fitted for palatal appliance and after surgeries for lip and palate repair.

14

Issues Related to the Transition Home and Prolonged NICU Stays

OVERVIEW

Discharge from the NICU is an exciting yet stressful event for most families. Many infants, especially those who are discharged early or dependent on technology, continue to require intervention services beyond discharge. Adequate family support in preparation for discharge is required to make the transition as smooth as possible for both the infant and the family and to minimize disruption of intervention services. Infants who experience complications during the neonatal period or who have complex medical conditions, such as prolonged ventilatory dependence or congenital anomalies requiring medical or surgical and post surgical management, often need to remain in the NICU for an extended period. Although the main focus of NICU care for these infants is to preserve and promote their medical stability and well-being, the infants' developmental and behavioral needs also require attention to prevent sensory deprivation and potential developmental delays. Including the family in the infant's intervention may be more challenging as time goes by because the family's ability to visit the infant may become increasingly limited. Provision of developmental and behavioral intervention for older infants who are sick is often a challenge because any intervention strategy must protect an infant's medical and physiologic integrity while promoting his or her development and well-being.

This chapter discusses the major issues faced by NICU infants and their families under two different situations: 1) making the transition from the NICU to the home or 2) staying in the NICU for a prolonged period of time. The first section addresses the intervention and support needs of both the infant and the family in preparation for discharge and after discharge from the NICU. Particular emphasis is given to infants discharged early or sent home on technological support. The second section discusses important considerations for the behavior and development of infants whose stay in the NICU extends beyond the neonatal period, including issues related to family-centered care. This information is presented through case examples.

OBJECTIVES

- Identify the major issues of families preparing to take their infants home and as they assume the responsibility for their infants' care at home, particularly for families with infants who are discharged early or dependent on technology

- Recall information and sources of support that may help families with the transition home and minimize the disruption of intervention services
- Identify common medical conditions, complications, and other factors that may require infants to remain in the NICU beyond their expected due dates; issues that are specific to growing, older infants in the NICU; and the types of intervention commonly used to safely address the specific issues
- Identify the multiplicity of contextual factors that may influence the development of growing NICU infants, which must be considered when providing intervention services from a family-centered perspective
- Describe strategies that should be used in providing intervention services during the various stages of older infants' illness and recovery (e.g., observation and positioning during critical stages; more comprehensive, developmental intervention during periods of greater stability)
- Recognize the need to employ and adapt preventive strategies as infants grow in the NICU to optimize their long-term outcomes (e.g., positioning to prevent or minimize postural deformities, environmental enrichment to promote sensory processing and sensorimotor development)
- Recognize the need to work with the team, particularly the bedside nurse, the parents, and social services staff to ensure consistent follow-through of therapy recommendations.
- Identify the assessment instruments that are available to determine infants' needs as the infants grow in the NICU

GROWING AT HOME AFTER THE NICU

Most expectant parents plan a joyful homecoming for their newborn baby. The homecoming represents the culmination of the pregnancy and the new addition to the family. It is usually a time of great excitement and pride—a time to be shared with family and friends. However, the homecoming of an infant who has had a prolonged NICU stay is often in sharp contrast with this scenario. Since birth, the infant has been primarily cared for by professionals. Opportunities to engage in parenting occupations have been severely restricted. Weeks or even months may have passed before the parents were able to provide some basic care for their infant. Moreover, most interactions with their infant have taken place in an environment that is stressful and lacks privacy. There has been little opportunity to share the experience of parenting with friends and family.

Following such an experience, the day of NICU discharge certainly can be joyful for the family. For many infants who have been cared for in the NICU, however, the discharge represents a gradual progression to a lower level of care rather than a declaration of health. Thus, in addition to preparing a cozy space for their infant at home, parents may have to install additional electrical outlets and make space for monitors, oxygen tanks, and medical supplies (Figure 51).

Instead of spending the first days and nights admiring their baby and learning to accommodate his or her routines, parents may be lying awake listening to the sound of monitors, and leaping up at every hint of trouble. They may be kept busy coordinating their work and at-home schedules with visiting nurses and therapists,

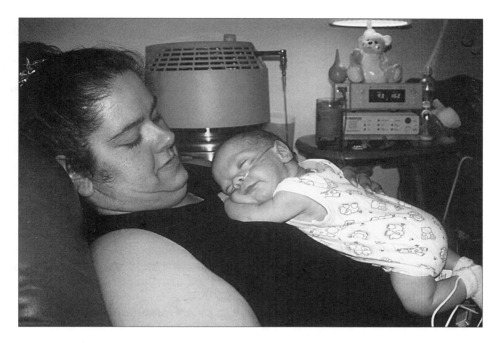

Figure 51. The discharge plan for this extremely low birth weight infant included supplemental oxygen by cannula, pulse oximetry, and heart rate monitoring, as well as visiting nurse support. Equipment is visible in the photo's background.

telephoning equipment vendors, and shuttling the infant to follow-up visits with a succession of specialists. In addition, instead of finally being able to share their infant with friends and family, they may be asking loved ones to keep their distance to protect the infant from respiratory and gastrointestinal viruses.

Family Preparation and Support

This book emphasizes family participation in the care of NICU infants. This is especially true for interventions surrounding the infant's discharge and the transition home. A recurrent theme during this transition is the family members' recognition that they are now totally responsible for their infant's care, every day and every night. After having an infant with a prolonged stay in the NICU, this is sometimes a difficult concept to absorb. Altering their perception of their infant, from one who is extremely fragile to one who is healthy and ready for the experiences of daily life is another challenging task for many parents. In most cases, the infant is ready for typical newborn care. Ideally, during the first days at home, a nurse will visit to check the infant's health status and weight gain and to reinforce appropriate care. However, parents of premature infants or full-term infants who have spent more than a few days in the NICU need to be aware of some of the behavioral difficulties that their infant may experience in making the transition home. Parents must also be cognizant of the psychosocial aspects of their own adjustment to taking their infant home. Predischarge classes for parents and family members are an excellent means of communicating some of this information to families. Printed handouts and videotapes can be very helpful for educating the family as well. Information that is particularly helpful includes the following:

- Suggestions for "caring for the caregivers"
- Recommendations for reducing exposure to respiratory and gastrointestinal viruses
- Guidelines for breast and bottle feeding of preterm infants or full-term infants with feeding difficulties
- Suggestions for enhancing sleep for an infant who has been exposed to constant noise and light for a period of time
- Information about reading and responding to infant cues
- Suggestions for enhancing social and play interactions with infants who must conserve energy and stability for continued growth (see the sample handout in the appendix at the end of this chapter)

Postdischarge Intervention

Ideally, the therapist who provided assessment and intervention in the NICU environment makes a home visit during the transition home. The main purpose of the visit is to enhance aspects of infant care such as feeding, care routines, social interaction, play, and energy conservation. Parents often relate their profound relief when they have encountered a problem—large or small—during the transition home and have been able to collaborate with the therapist in finding a solution. For example, a small, fragile preterm infant who awakens after sleeping for brief (half-hour) periods of time may benefit from a bedtime routine of nesting for containment, using a night-light, and playing a half-hour lullaby tape to help him make the transition in states of arousal from drowsiness to quiet sleep. An infant who gulps and dribbles during feeding and then refuses to take more food may benefit from a slower-flowing nipple to help her to pace her swallowing and breathing. A full-term infant with low postural tone may benefit from suggestions for positioning and handling to enhance body symmetry and play activities to promote mid-line activity and head control. A mother whose preterm infant receives breast feeding and supplemental bottle feedings may benefit from assistance in planning her breast pumping around the infant's nap and feeding schedule, thereby conserving her infant's and her own energy.

Therapy services during the transition home provide a natural bridge to community-based developmental services and are usually discontinued when community services are initiated. Communication between the NICU therapist and the receiving early intervention program ensures continuity of care and reassures the family that their infant will continue to receive quality care.

Infants Dependent on Technology

Families of infants who depend on technology and are discharged home with block nursing services (or even around-the-clock nursing care) must become experts in their infant's care. NICUs offer training in cardiopulmonary resuscitation and in use of the monitors and other equipment that may accompany the infant home. The parents of infants who go home with tracheostomies or gastrostomy or nasogastric tube feedings require extensive supervised opportunities at the NICU bedside to learn about their infants' care. Clinical pathways help staff and parents predict the time required to learn particular aspects of an infant's care (Vecchi, Vasquez, Radin, & Johnson, 1996). Bedside teaching tools are charts that list the necessary skills that must be learned prior to discharge. These charts are useful for recording the parents' progress in learning to provide the necessary care. These tools also provide all staff involved in discharge planning with a realistic appraisal of the parents' caregiving competencies in the necessary areas (e.g., giving gavage or gastrostomy feedings, suctioning and changing a tracheostomy, monitoring oxygen saturation and HR, putting splints on hands, giving passive range of motion and massages, positioning for comfort and physiologic stability). Opportunities for rooming alone with the infant for long blocks of time (e.g., 8-hour blocks, overnight) are ideal for helping families gain confidence and competence in caring for their infant.

Parents of infants with complex care and/or technology dependency must also learn to be managers of their infant's care. Prior to discharge, setting up adequate communication and follow-up with the infant's primary care pediatrician is a must because the pediatrician will assume ultimate responsibility for medical aspects of care. An achievement with regard to safety is the establishment of PEDI-STAT programs in many communities. These programs augment the local 911 emergency system, providing it with important facts about every high-risk infant who is discharged home (i.e., medical diagnoses and active medical issues and potential risks that may be associated with responding to an emergency call, as well as specific directions to the home). Infants who are prone to seizures, apnea, or bradycardia; infants with tracheostomies; and/or infants who are on mechanical ventilation at home particularly need such programs.

Transition to Follow-Up Programs

Another important aspect of a smooth transition home is referral to the appropriate medical specialists for follow-up and to community-based programs that provide family support and early intervention. Programs that assist families in care coordination can ease the transition home and prevent or reduce rehospitalizations (Berger, Holt-Turner, Cupoli, Mass, & Hageman, 1998; Gamblian, Hess, & Kenner, 1998). Choosing the programs that best fit the family's needs is an important but often overlooked aspect of discharge planning. Optimally, the family participates in choosing the programs and services that are likely to provide the greatest benefits to them and to their infant. Predischarge family–team meetings are an appropriate opportunity for parents to meet with professionals from these programs. Having a prior acquaintance with some of the individuals who will assist in coordinating their baby's care, particularly those who will make home visits, greatly enhances a family's comfort level during this stressful time.

Early Discharge

Early discharge is a growing trend in the United States (Gamblian et al., 1998; Raddish & Merritt, 1998), but how *early discharge* is defined varies considerably from one region to another. In some parts of the country, it refers to infants being discharged while still requiring medications such as methylxanthines to reduce the risk of apnea and bradycardia, nasal cannula oxygen, and supplementation of nipple feedings with gavage. In other regions, *early discharge* refers to sending stable infants, who are younger than 35 weeks of gestation and weigh less than 2,000 g, home to *feed and grow*. Increasingly, the criteria for discharge relates more to an infant's medical stability, particularly regarding the absence of "spells" (e.g., apnea, bradycardia, oxygen desaturation), than to GA or weight.

A typical set of criteria for early discharge includes the ability to 1) maintain body temperature in an open crib, 2) take full feedings by breast and/or bottle, and 3) remain free of spells for a minimum of 5 days prior to discharge. Beyond these basic criteria, Merritt and Raddish (1998) acknowledged that many medically related issues must be considered in preparing an infant for early discharge from the NICU. One of the most daunting is the variability in competencies among families and among professional care providers in the community. This issue is not exclusive to early discharges. The adequacy of both sources of caregiving support must be evaluated prior to any discharge from the NICU. Some families require minimal professional support to adequately care for their infant after the NICU discharge. Other families initially require daily contact with certain professionals (Ritchie, 2002). To provide additional support to families during the transition home and to enable some infants to be discharged earlier, some NICUs offer integrated home-care programs. These programs utilize NICU nurses and therapists to provide home-based services, including family support during the transition home. These services can be particularly helpful for families with infants sent home on supplemental gavage feedings or with oxygen (Evanochko et al., 1996; Kotagal, Perlstein, Gamblian, Donovan, & Atherton, 1995). Additional benefits of these programs are that the family knows and trusts the integrated home-care staff and that with the family's permission, the home-care staff may share the family's home transition experiences with NICU-based staff. This communication can increase staff sensitivity to the potential difficulties encountered during the transition home and improve their understanding of how to prepare future NICU "graduates" and their families for early discharge (Swanson & Naber, 1997).

GROWING IN THE NICU

Most premature infants are able to leave the NICU near their expected due date, and most full-term infants with transient conditions usually go home a few days or weeks after birth. Infants who have life-threatening complications, have conditions requiring extended care, or are waiting to be adopted or placed in foster care may need to remain in the NICU for a longer period. These infants may require intervention approaches that differ from those of infants who continue intervention at home.

The NICU is, by definition, an environment for sick neonates. However, many infants require treatment in the NICU far beyond the neonatal period. In the case of preterm infants, the smallest and most fragile infants—born between 23 and 26 weeks of gestation and weighing less than 1,000 g—require a NICU stay of at least 3–4 months. Complications such as sepsis, chronic lung disease, NEC, or IVH with hydrocephalus can extend a preterm infant's stay to his or her original due date and beyond. Full-term infants with complex conditions such as meconium aspiration syndrome, diaphragmatic hernia, or PPHN sometimes require a prolonged recovery period as they are weaned from sedation and prolonged ventilation and are started on oral feedings. Infants with congenital anomalies requiring a series of surgical interventions also may remain in the NICU for extended periods of time. The developmental and behavioral needs of these infants change as their condition progresses from a critical, physiologically unstable status to convalescence. Sometimes these infants can be transferred to a pediatric intensive care unit or a subacute pediatric rehabilitation hospital, but in many cases, the NICU is the only care environment for the infants and their families.

Case Examples

The following case examples illustrate the developmental and therapeutic interventions provided to infants whose NICU stay extended well after the neonatal period. These examples also demonstrate important issues that needed to be considered in providing the infants' therapy services.

Julia

Neonatal History

Julia was the firstborn of Pam, a young, single mother who had been working and going to school until 27 weeks of gestation, when premature rupture of membranes required her to be hospitalized. Two weeks later, tocolysis failed, and Julia was born by emergency cesarean section, secondary to a weak fetal tracing. Her birth weight was 950 g. Julia initially responded well to a high-frequency oscillation ventilator and progressed to nasal CPAP by the time she weighed 1,000 g. However, at 32 weeks, her respiratory status worsened and her head circumference began to increase rapidly. A cranial ultrasound revealed a grade-III IVH, bilaterally, with hydrocephalus. She received a ventricular-peritoneal shunt, the shunt failed several days later, and the surgeons opted to place an exterior shunt. Drainage of the external shunt required Julia to be positioned at a precise angle for most of the time, limiting options for positioning and handling. During this time, several attempts to wean Julia to CPAP ventilation failed. Her lung disease worsened, and she was generally agitated, necessitating sedation. The external shunt became infected, and she was treated aggressively with antibiotics.

Pam lived 35 minutes from the hospital, and transportation was a problem because she did not have a car. Julia's father visited infrequently at nights. With the help of family and friends, however, Pam initially visited daily to spend time at Julia's bedside providing gentle containment and softly reading poems and stories. In light of Julia's unstable condition, Pam was not able to hold her daughter. In fact, due to heavy sedation, Julia often lay very still on an open warmer. Her position rarely varied. Surgeons could not allow pressure on the external shunt site, which was in the right occipital area. The fact that Julia required ventilatory support further limited options for positioning; thus, her head was consistently turned toward the left for several months. Although a gel cushion was used to distribute pressure, Julia developed a significant plagiocephaly. During these months, the NICU therapists were available to assist with positioning but were not able to institute hands-on therapy because of Julia's fragile condition. Whenever her sedation was reduced, Julia became agitated, flailing in the bed and risking self-extubation. This was a difficult time for Julia's family. Pam became depressed about her daughter's condition. She reduced her visits from daily to only a few times weekly, and she came late in the evening, when support staff was not available. Pam did not return calls from the NICU social worker, but the social worker left supportive messages on Pam's answering machine, encouraging Pam to visit Julia whenever she could. Taxi vouchers were provided to make it easier for Pam to come in during the day, when she could meet with the social worker.

Julia's lung disease eventually stabilized, and the infection resolved by 3 months' corrected age, allowing surgery for another ventricular peritoneal shunt. She recovered quickly after surgery and began the slow progression from continuous nasogastric feeds to bolus feedings, with oxygen provided by nasal cannula. It was at this stage that Julia's family resumed more frequent visits. Two weeks after the surgery, the NICU therapist was able to become more involved in Julia's care.

Intervention Process

Julia had excessive tightness in the shoulder adductors, back and pelvis, and, along with plagiocephaly, a pronounced asymmetry with shortening of the neck musculature on her left side. Her strengths were that she was visually alert and socially responsive and was motivated toward antigravity movement, pushing her head and shoulders up when placed in prone and attempting to right her head in supported sitting. Julia had been given opportunities to suck nonnutritively throughout her NICU stay. She had a rhythmic suck with appropriate compression but weak tongue cupping and stripping action. Feeding assessment revealed that she was eager to suck nonnutritively and could handle swallowing her own secretions well. When presented with nutritive feedings of fortified breast milk, however, Julia resisted the nipple, turning her head from side to side and arching her back. The NICU therapist advised a slow introduction to nippling, making Julia's body posture a focal point for intervention. To prepare her for feeding, Julia was provided with neutral warmth, gentle massage and range of motion, and gentle elongation of the neck and trunk muscles, with flexion and rotation at the shoulders and pelvis. Oral-motor preparation included providing some inhibitory input by giving firm touch pressure around the outside of Julia's mouth, followed by pressure to her gums and, finally, to her tongue to facilitate cupping and stripping action. A slow-flowing nipple was used to introduce very small amounts of liquid at a time. When Julia exhibited distress by arching or resisting the nipple, these cues were respected and the nipple was removed. Touch pressure was repeated, and the nipple was reintroduced. If Julia persisted in resisting or if her oxygen requirement increased, the feeding session was terminated and the remainder was fed by gavage. These intervention strategies were demonstrated to the nursing staff and posted at Julia's bedside. The strategies were to be used by nursing staff at each care period, as time permitted, and by the NICU therapist on a daily basis. Pam was educated about the interventions as well, allowing her to provide them at each visit. She began to plan for daytime visits so that she could work with the therapist, and she became quite adept at positioning Julia optimally and providing massage, range of motion, and oral-motor preparation. During this time, Pam also became more attuned to Julia's cues and more patient regarding the slow progression to nipple feeding, as she could see small improvements daily.

Contextual Challenges

Julia's nurses were understandably anxious for her to take nutrition from a bottle, and there were times when the nursing staff would attempt to "feed through" her distress cues. Some of the nurses felt that Julia should be much further along, expressing comments such as "After all, she's a 6-month-old—my kids were crawling and pulling up at this age!" To address these concerns, the therapist worked with the team to emphasize that only Julia's corrected age of 3 months should be used. The therapist also noted that considering Julia's history of prolonged periods of inactivity and severe lung disease (a constant drain on her energy), she was not as delayed as one might expect. The nurse manager was consulted to request primary nurses for Julia, not only for the day shift but also for evening and night shifts. In this way, the primary nurses could be more easily included in Julia's care planning.

In addition, the Posture and Fine Motor Assessment of Infants (Case-Smith & Bigsby, 2000) was administered to evaluate Julia's posture and fine motor control. Pam and the daytime primary care nurse were present for the evaluation. They were able to observe Julia's interest in the stimulus toys as well as her obvious attempts to move against gravity in prone and supine and to reach for the toys in supported sitting. They were able to review the scoring with the therapist and to compare Julia's score with the scores of other infants of her corrected age. Julia scored in the "at risk" category for her age in posture and in the "delayed" category in fine motor skills. Nevertheless, Pam and the nurse were reassured by this assessment because they could see Julia's emerging skills in both domains. With the therapist, Pam and the nurse identified areas of concern and priorities for intervention. They began to see with greater clarity how Julia's posture may influence her feeding efforts and how her current lack of movement limited her ability to explore her environment and obtain appropriate sensory experiences. These insights were communicated to the primary nurses on evenings and nights, and the end result was greater follow-through with the bedside care recommendations.

Discharge Plans

Julia continued to make slow, steady progress. Three weeks after the assessment, she consistently took a little more than an ounce by nipple at each feeding. Her oxygen requirement stabilized, and she was not receiving any additional medical interventions. At that time, a team meeting was called, and the medical team decided that placement of a gastrostomy tube would enable Julia to continue working on feeding tolerance at home—an environment more conducive to her overall development. Pam was receptive to this idea because she was more than ready to take her baby home. Pam learned this additional aspect of Julia's care without difficulty, and Julia was discharged home at 4 months corrected age, on nipple feedings as tolerated (with gastrostomy feedings for the remainder) and with supplemental oxygen by nasal cannula.

A week after discharge, the NICU therapist made a follow-up home visit. Julia greeted her visitor with a bright, alert smile. Pam reported Julia had remained on her 4-hour feeding schedule during the transition home. The first night was restless, but with the aid of music, Julia was sleeping more soundly than she had in the NICU and waking on schedule to be fed. During the visit, Julia played on a blanket on the floor, tolerating handling by her mother and the therapist, reaching to mid-line with both arms while in supine, and, for the first time, attempting to roll from tummy to back with some dissociation of the trunk and pelvis. Then, Julia demonstrated her bottle-feeding prowess, taking 2 ounces without difficulty and remaining alert for some additional play. Oxygen administration by nasal cannula was at the minimal 1/8-liter setting, and there were no signs of fatigue or stress after all of this activity. Pam was more relaxed than she had ever been when Julia was hospitalized. Although she was definitely Julia's primary caregiver, Pam had been receiving help from her mother and from Julia's father. The appointment with Julia's pediatrician had gone well—he was delighted to see how well Julia looked considering her prolonged hospitalization and her numerous medical risks. She had follow-up visits scheduled with a number of services: pediatric surgery, neurosurgery, pediatric gastroenterology, and neonatal follow-up. She had also been enrolled in her local early intervention program. The early intervention providers had received copies of Julia's intervention plan from the NICU and were planning an initial home visit from nursing, nutrition, occupational therapy, and physical therapy professionals the following week. The NICU therapist was able to discharge Julia from the hospital's Infant Development Center program, reassuring Pam that she or Julia's other caregivers could call anytime for additional consultation.

Discussion

Julia's story provides opportunities to address a number of issues that may arise in the care of preterm infants with complications and prolonged NICU stays. Depression is a common experience among parents of infants in the NICU. Meyer et al. (1994) demonstrated that parents of preterm infants experienced clinically significant levels of depression, even when they had no previous history of depression. In their randomized controlled trial, Meyer and colleagues found that a family-based approach to developmental intervention for preterm infants resulted in significantly reduced levels of depression among the parents after the infant's discharge. As in Pam's case, parents may become weary of spending time at the bedside of an infant who is too sick to be held or who is unable to respond to social approaches. As discussed in Chapters 1 and 11, violated expectations for typical parental roles can derail the parent–infant attachment experience and interfere with parental involvement in care. Pam reestablished her involvement when Julia became more accessible, and her emotional connection with Julia did not appear to be jeopardized by the temporary distancing. This may not always be the case; thus, it is always important to include a qualified mental health professional on the NICU team.

Having primary nursing staff limits the number of caregivers, which is an important strategy for consistently carrying out the care plan. In this case, all of Julia's primary nurses performed an additional, vital role in focusing on Julia's changing strengths, identifying priorities for developmental aspects of Julia's ongoing care, and participating in her intervention plan.

Although Julia was a preterm infant, several issues in her case presentation are similar to those of full-term infants with prolonged NICU stays. Two such issues are oral aversion and atypical tongue movements. Another is atypical posturing with scapular adduction, trunk and neck extension, and, sometimes, asymmetry of neck musculature and plagiocephaly.

Full-term infants who have prolonged intubation and sedation (e.g., after surgery or ECMO) often present with these postural and oral-motor issues. Infants who have survived ECMO (i.e., received a heart–lung bypass—a rescue procedure for the sickest term neonates) are particularly vulnerable to these problems because they have to be immobilized for days, with the head turned to one side, to enable arterio-venous or veno-venous cannulation. Unlike preterm infants, who usually experience NNS even while intubated, these full-term infants have been completely immobilized, and organization of sucking and swallowing are put on hold from birth—often for several weeks. As the infants are weaned from sedatives, they usually experience symptoms of abstinence (i.e., withdrawal) and are given additional medications to assist the weaning process, such as deodorized tincture of opium. NNS during this time can be quite disorganized, with a predominance of phasic biting and compression. The tongue may remain elevated and retracted in the mouth. Efforts to engage these infants in NNS sucking may be unsuccessful because of inadequate contact between the nipple and the tongue and an overall aversive response to oral stimuli. As with Julia, it is necessary to focus intervention on oral-motor *and* postural issues because some oral-motor problems (e.g., retracted tongue) may be related to body posture.

Nat

Neonatal History

Nat's intervention is a good example of the previously described dual oral-motor approach. He was a full-term infant, delivered by emergency cesarean section at an outlying hospital and transported to the NICU by ambulance. He had respiratory failure, an enlarged liver, and ascites. He was given nitric oxide treatment and was transported to the specialized nursery for ECMO. Nat's condition was exacerbated by hemachromatosis (i.e., inability to metabolize iron). His liver became grossly enlarged, and he remained in the specialized nursery for 7 weeks before returning to the regular NICU. By that time, he had been weaned off ventilatory support, needing only oxygen by nasal cannula at 30%, and was judged ready for nipple feedings. However, the ear, nose, and throat (ENT) specialist had diagnosed a true left vocal cord paralysis. On the first day of Nat's admission to the NICU, the NICU therapist was consulted to begin Nat's nipple-feeding program.

Intervention Process

Nat's parents, Jane and Ron, reported that Nat had an alert expression and was very attentive to his surroundings. He had a torticollis and tightness in shoulder adductors and back extensors. His liver was enlarged to the extent that he was unable to be supported in sitting. Increased abdominal pressure interfered with his breathing unless he was positioned in supine. Through trial and error, Jane and Ron discovered that Nat's breathing improved when he could be reclined against the caregiver's chest, so that position was chosen for initial feedings. Due to his paralyzed vocal fold, feeding assessment was initiated with thickened formula. Nat was fed a special formula that was not fortified with iron and was thickened with Thick-It 2 (available from Precision Foods, http://www.precision foods.com), which is also iron free. NNS had been initiated when Nat returned to the conventional ventilator, so he accepted a pacifier eagerly but had difficulty bringing his tongue forward to engage in sucking. Because his suck was character- ized by rapid compressions, a broad, flat orthodontic nipple was tried. This nipple would accommodate the thickened consistency of the formula and would allow him to express liquid using only compression. When the formula was introduced, Nat initially choked but quickly learned to swallow when provided with external pacing. His position (lying across the therapist's reclined chest) was awkward, but Nat seemed to manage his swallows without distress. Some upper airway congestion could be felt after a few swallows. When the nipple was removed and he was allowed to "dry swallow" a few times, the congestion disappeared, suggesting some pooling in the pharyngeal area with eventual clearing. Nat appeared visually distracted by the activity in the bay; using a screen allowed him to focus on feeding and to improve his sucking organization.

In light of known vocal fold paralysis and suspected pooling, the therapist recommended a swallowing study (to ensure adequate handling of the liquid without an increased risk of aspiration) prior to initiating nipple feedings. In the interim, a long, firm pacifier was recommended to enhance tongue protraction and cupping, and therapeutic handling was initiated to begin addressing the torticollis and shortened postural musculature. To reduce visual distractions, it was recommended that Nat be fed in the family room or behind a screen. Ron commented that he, too, has a tendency to become distracted by the activity and the monitors in the bay. He anticipated that moving to the family room would improve his ability to focus on Nat and Nat's feeding.

The swallowing study verified a slight delay in the swallow, with some pooling in the valecular area; however, there were no signs of aspiration, so nipple feedings were begun. Nat seemed motivated to be fed by nipple but required careful positioning for his comfort during the process. He continued to require external pacing to allow him to clear the pharynx. This amounted to allowing him to take two to three swallows and then pause for a short break. During this time, he alternated some "catch-up breathing" with completion of his swallows. Using this technique, he progressed in a week's time to taking 25 cc, eventually learning to self-pace his breathing and swallowing. Nat reached a plateau at this volume, refusing to continue once he had taken this amount. He would vigorously turn his head from side to side and push the nipple out with his tongue. The nurses were concerned that this behavior was evidence of a feeding aversion, but because Nat sucked eagerly for the first part of his nipple feeding, that explanation did not seem likely. He was still receiving continuous feedings, night and day, by a nasogastric tube and pump. The therapist requested an hour-long break in Nat's feeding schedule, prior to each nipple feeding, which resulted in his being able to take 45 cc on his first try. His parents were overjoyed. With continual increases in the time between tube feedings, Nat progressed to full volume across a week's time. Nat's trunk flexibility improved slightly, and his abdominal swelling reduced as well, allowing for a small amount of trunk flexion during feeding. Jane continued to develop her expertise at positioning him optimally against her body. She was able to adapt her positioning as Nat's flexibility improved, and with these changes, improvements in swallowing were observed. At this point, he also demonstrated improved tongue protraction and cupping. Therefore, the nipple type was changed to a standard-shaped nipple with a single slit to enhance Nat's tongue action while allowing adequate flow. He was discharged on full nipple feedings and continued with this postural and feeding intervention plan through the transition into early intervention services, from which he received home-based physical therapy.

Discussion

Nat's feeding difficulties were multifactorial. Atypical posture exerted negative influences on his tongue action and his swallowing. The pressure of the enlarged liver on his diaphragm impeded his breathing. In addition, he had true vocal cord paralysis. As a result, thickened feeding for increased control and external pacing were necessary to prevent aspiration while he learned to coordinate his swallows. Nat required environmental modifications (i.e., reducing visual stimuli) to organize his feeding. He needed to experience hunger to progress to full feedings. Each issue had to be addressed for Nat to feed successfully and, in turn, be discharged home.

Older infants in the NICU often present with multifactorial intervention issues. In working with fragile preterm infants, the focus of NICU therapy generally is to provide an environment that protects the infants from stimuli that may be overwhelming. Older infants in the NICU may be at a stage of greater procurement. They may seek stimulation but be ill-prepared to accommodate these sensations. Work with older infants should focus on providing necessary sensory experiences while monitoring the infants' ability to process the stimulation. The next two case examples illustrate these concepts.

Emma

Neonatal History

Emma was a 26-week preterm infant with severe IUGR. Her birth weight was 480 g. She responded well to ventilatory assistance but could not be weaned to CPAP. After several failed attempts to do so, the ENT was consulted, and it was determined that Emma had a subglottic stenosis. Anti-inflammatory medications were recommended; however, it was decided that if her condition did not improve, a tracheostomy would be placed. When Emma was 32 weeks' corrected age, the NICU therapist was consulted to provide suggestions for positioning and for developmentally supportive care. Emma was expected to be ventilator dependent for a prolonged period.

Emma was a restless infant. She usually was irritable and difficult to settle once she awakened, and the nurses went to great lengths to assist her in staying asleep. Her open crib was draped with a heavy blanket to block the light, and a bedside sign designated her area as a "quiet zone." Her care was strictly clustered; pediatric residents and phlebotomists who sought to examine Emma or to draw her blood were briskly removed from the bedside and asked to return at her set care time. Despite these efforts, Emma remained fussy and hard to soothe, with poor weight gain. Her weight gain was of particular concern because she was too small for any of the available tracheostomy tubes. That is, she needed to grow before she could have her surgery.

Emma's family lived an hour's drive away and was not able to visit often. In addition, Emma had five older siblings at home, three of whom were younger than 4 years of age. As a result, Emma's mother, Leah, tended to visit in the late evenings, when all of her other children were settled for the night, and only once or twice per week, when she could obtain a babysitter. Emma's father was no longer involved with the family.

Intervention Process

The NICU therapist spent considerable time discussing Emma's response to care with Emma's primary nurse. She observed Emma prior to, during, and after care to become familiar with Emma's behavioral and physiologic responses to handling. Emma's oxygen saturation tended to drop alarmingly (to the 60s) when she was handled, and she recovered slowly, with postural containment and careful adjustment of her ventilator's settings. The therapist noted that Emma utilized foot bracing prior to settling down, and the primary nurse agreed that containment seemed to be beneficial. Nursing staff were already providing nesting, using blanket rolls for containment. To allow Emma to benefit from bracing her feet, the therapist suggested providing a positioning arrangement that was more consistent in shape and resistance than blanket rolls. A commercially available nest was provided for this purpose. Emma appeared to love this positioning assistance. It stayed in place better than the blanket rolls, and she was able to use this added support to brace her feet more effectively. The additional height of the nest prevented her feet from sliding over the top, which was a common problem with the blanket rolls.

Leah was updated by telephone and at occasional family meetings, for which she made special trips to visit Emma during daytime hours and to meet with the NICU team. Leah was delighted to learn that Emma had begun having extended periods of deep sleep. For her part, Leah made a point of laundering the nests and returning them to ensure that Emma always had a clean spare positioner.

For a time, the positioning assistance was the only intervention provided. Any attempt to provide visual, auditory, or tactile stimulation resulted in physiologic instability. Focus on faces or black-and-white designs could not be elicited. Emma merely averted her gaze or shut her eyes completely, so her nurses were beginning to question her functional visual status. As Emma began to sleep more deeply between care periods and to gain weight, however, her tolerance for handling increased and she began to open her eyes and gaze at her caregiver briefly, without losing physiologic stability. Within 2 weeks, she became more receptive to routine care, and she was able to begin a program of daily gentle massage and face-to-face interaction with her caregivers, including her mother and oldest sister. Emma also became receptive to NNS on a tiny pacifier that could be used along with the endotracheal tube, and she was able to bring her hand to her face to keep the pacifier in place.

Discharge Plans

Emma was 38 weeks' corrected age when her tracheostomy was placed. She began her nipple feedings a few days later and made rapid progress toward discharge. Her increased comfort with the removal of the endotracheal tube was apparent. From that point on, her care needs resembled those of any full-term infant, with the exception of needing tracheostomy care. She went home at 41 weeks' corrected age; block-nursing time was provided to assist the family with Emma's care. After discharge, Emma was to be followed by ENT, neonatal follow-up, and early intervention services to continue monitoring her feeding and her responses to sensory experiences.

Joshua

Neonatal History

Joshua's mother, Beth, arrived at the emergency room of the regional perinatal center by ambulance. She had a ruptured placenta and was hemorrhaging and in acute distress. Joshua's fetal tracings were poor. An emergency cesarean section was performed, and Joshua was born at 24 weeks of gestation, weighing only 510 g. He was intubated and rushed to the NICU. His temperature was dangerously low and he was difficult to stabilize on the ventilator.

Placenta abruptio is sometimes associated with cocaine use; therefore, Beth's urine was sent for toxicity screening. Joshua's meconium (his first stool) was also sent for screening. Both tests were positive for exposure to cocaine and opiates. Beth admitted to using cocaine and heroin prior to his delivery. She denied knowledge of this pregnancy. She explained that she was a heroin addict and was receiving methadone and counseling for substance abuse. However, she said that she had difficulty managing on methadone alone. She had recently left a residential treatment program against medical advice and had begun supplementing her methadone with street heroin. Beth did not have a steady boyfriend and had no idea who Joshua's father was. Her closest support person was her friend, Jerry, a former heroin addict who had been clean for a year. Beth requested that Jerry be allowed to visit her son in lieu of family members.

Joshua's first weeks were extremely difficult. He continued to be difficult to stabilize on the ventilator, moving from a conventional to an oscillating ventilator and remaining on the oscillator for weeks. He was small for his GA, and because he was experiencing neonatal abstinence from heroin and methadone, he required sedation to increase his tolerance to care. His skin was extremely fragile, and he was more sensitive to touch and handling than is typical for a 24-week preterm infant. Thus, he was placed in a Giraffe OmniBed Isolette (manufactured by Ohmeda Medical; http://www.ohmedamedical.com),[4] which provided optimal humidity for his skin while allowing him to remain on the oscillating ventilator. Another advantage was that this Isolette protected Joshua from the excessive NICU noise, to which he was reacting with oxygen desaturation, and from unnecessary care such as "tidying" (Appleton, 1997), particularly by his mother.

The NICU team had initially filed a report with the local department of children and families when the meconium toxicology screen revealed exposure to illegal substances in utero. The NICU social worker had been in constant communication with Beth, who was awaiting word from investigators on the status of her request to take Joshua home. Although Beth denied knowledge of the pregnancy, she embraced the idea of fully mothering Joshua.

At the NICU social worker's suggestion, Beth enrolled Joshua in a specialized program, which provides assessment of infants exposed to illegal substances in utero and assists parents in obtaining the necessary supports to successfully negotiate the legal system.[5] To bolster her case with investigators, Beth reapplied for residential treatment and was placed on a waiting list. In the interim, she made daily bedside visits and did all that she could to convince Joshua's caregivers of her devotion to him. However, Beth's visits were a constant source of concern to the nurses. She brought toys with every visit and insisted on placing them in his Isolette despite the nurses' admonitions that the toys were too stimulating for him. Beth talked to him and touched him throughout her visits, even when the nurses requested that she allow him to rest undisturbed. Her behavior always seemed extreme: either drowsy and nodding off to sleep at the bedside or loud and exuberant, proclaiming her determination to turn her life around for her child's sake. It was clear to the staff that Beth had very little impulse control and that her states of arousal were not well regulated on the methadone. Joshua would have

---

[4]The Giraffe looks like a conventional enclosed Isolette, with ports for entry. However, it has a top that rises at the touch of a pedal to enable complete access to the infant, as with an open warmer. Rather than using a plastic wrap cover to maintain humidity around the infant, the Giraffe offers graded humidity with special filters to prevent entry of the yeasts and bacteria that are common threats to ELBW infants.

[5]When parents accept counseling support and comply with all the stipulations made by the court, they may receive more favorable legal decisions. Support programs emphasize careful assessment of infant and parental needs and attempt to ensure that all avenues are explored for keeping families together. Staff of such programs usually attend court hearings to report on infant behavior and development, parental involvement in care and compliance with treatment, and overall parental competency. However, an infant's best interests are always the court's first consideration. If a parent is unable to meet the requirements for reunification despite receiving significant supports, then the infant is placed in foster care, and the process toward permanent adoption is begun.

benefited from primary nurses on each shift, but there were few nurses with the patience to work with his mother on a regular basis. The medical team sought assistance from the specialized support team.

Joshua's initial assessment was completed when he was 29 weeks' corrected age, still intubated and nested on his side in the Giraffe Isolette but on conventional ventilatory support. The NICU Network Neurobehavioral Scale (NNNS) was used because it evaluates neurodevelopmental integrity as well as behavioral organization and signs of neonatal abstinence. Items were modified or omitted to accommodate his young age, his limited handling options while on the ventilator, and his sensitivities. Beth attended the evaluation so that she could participate in and contribute to the observations.

Joshua needed to be awakened for care. He came to quiet alertness gradually, squinting in response to increased light when the Isolette cover was lifted and startling to his mother's voice. This provided the therapist with an opportunity to discuss Joshua's clear responses to light and sound as strengths and to make Beth aware that Joshua's sensitivity to louder voices could be accommodated by modulating her voice. Joshua complied with Beth's second, softer attempt to speak to him by opening his eyes and gazing at her face. He followed her face in a very short horizontal arc, then lost focus and closed his eyes. The therapist discussed how powerful the human face is as a stimulus and how interesting it can be for infants. She also explained that some of the toys at Joshua's bedside may be too stimulating at this time in his development and might be taken home until he is able to process such complex stimuli. Then the therapist removed Joshua's booties to reveal his feet and briefly assessed tone and reflex responses of his lower and upper extremities. During this process, it was necessary to pause several times to allow Joshua to reorganize his behavior. Gentle containment was a successful strategy for assisting him in this process, and Beth was happy to learn this alternative to stroking. The therapist asked her how Joshua usually responds to the stroking, and when she described his kicks and "high-fives," the therapist was able to explain how those jerky movements may actually be signs of stress. The therapist explained how immature Joshua's development is at this stage, how he may actually be signaling stress when he salutes, and how he may be attempting to organize himself when he brings his hands to his face or searches for a place to brace his feet. Beth was intrigued by this concept and provided some other examples of things that he did for self-calming—for example, tucking his legs up under him.

When the nurse began Joshua's care, the therapist remained to help Beth observe his clear physiologic and behavioral distress with certain procedures and to show her how the nurse adeptly assisted Joshua in returning to a comfortable position. The therapist pointed out that Joshua's breathing and color changes were additional cues to watch for when interacting with him. Finally, the therapist and Beth observed Joshua return to a peaceful sleep after his care, and they discussed the importance of rest and deep sleep for Joshua's healing and growth. Beth seemed very appreciative of this opportunity to observe his strengths and vulnerabilities in a new light. She also seemed exhausted by the experience. The therapist deferred writing up Joshua's developmental plan of care until the next day.

The following day, Beth was at Joshua's bedside, singing softly to him and cradling his legs with her hand. She had clearly taken in some of the assessment information and was ready to contribute her ideas to the care plan that would be posted on his Isolette (e.g., "My strengths are . . . ," "I become stressed when . . . ," "You can help me by . . . "). When Joshua was placed in Beth's arms, the therapist pointed out some of his physiologic and behavioral signs of stress. Beth adapted her approach accordingly, softening her voice and attempting to keep her hands very still. She still required some cues from the nurses or the NICU therapist to modulate her voice or movements, but she accepted these prompts without becoming angry, as she had in the past.

A week later, at 30 weeks' corrected age, Joshua was successfully weaned to CPAP, providing more frequent opportunities to be held outside the Isolette. The therapist met with Beth at Joshua's bedside to assist her in interpreting her son's behavior and in modifying her approach to optimize his responses.

At this time Beth was called to begin residential treatment. She would be unable to visit him for 6 weeks. However, if she succeeded in individual residential treatment, she would qualify for a special residential program for mothers who had abused drugs during their pregnancy, which allowed infants to live with their mothers while the mothers continued treatment. Joshua continued progressing to nasal cannula and having his behavioral and neuromotor status reevaluated while his mother was in treatment. Updates were typically telephoned to his mother. Unfortunately, Beth was unable to comply with the residential program and left against medical advice, as she had done in the past.

When Joshua was 34 weeks' corrected age and almost ready for discharge from the NICU, Beth returned to visit him in a very disorganized state, which had to be reported to the department of child and family services. Two days later, she was arrested for using heroin in an abandoned house. Beth had to reappear in court, and Joshua was permanently removed from her custody. The plan was for him to be discharged from the NICU to foster care and to eventually be adopted.

Joshua continued to demonstrate strengths in visual and auditory responsiveness and became quite accepting of social approaches. He fed well by nipple and made continued progress in tolerating various types of stimulation. When Joshua was 37 weeks' corrected age, he was discharged from the NICU and placed as a "boarder baby" in the normal newborn nursery, where he continued to be provided with appropriate developmental interventions while awaiting foster care placement. His care plan was routinely updated based on his reassessments. The nurses provided his care accordingly, and he was also visited regularly by volunteers who are specially trained to spend time with the boarding infants, holding and caring for them when the nurses are occupied with the newborns. The nurses and volunteers provided verbal and written feedback to developmental therapists on the specialized support staff, who modified Joshua's plan accordingly.

At the time of discharge from the hospital, Joshua, at 42 weeks' corrected age, had appropriate neuromotor and behavioral responses. Joshua's development was followed by the therapist through the transition to foster placement. He had no difficulty settling in with his foster parents, who were delighted with his bright alertness and the ease with which he adapted to their home. Beth was unable to remain in any sort of treatment program. She clearly loved Joshua and wanted to mother him. Some women who use drugs respond to the birth of a child by aggressively pursuing treatment to be able to care for their child. In this case, however, the strength of Beth's addiction prevented her from successfully discontinuing her drug use.

Joshua's foster parents eventually adopted him permanently. Although he was followed by early intervention professionals to monitor his development, he demonstrated no delays at 1 year corrected age.

CONCLUSION

This chapter has focused on issues related to infants who leave the NICU as well as infants who need to stay in the NICU for longer periods. It is clear that most, if not all, families need some form of support when taking home a NICU graduate. Preparing families for discharge when infants are sent home early or while still dependent on technology is more complex and requires the development of transitional intervention services to ensure adequate continuity of the infants' and the families' care. The chapter also has focused on some of the postural, feeding, and sensory issues inherent in a prolonged NICU stay. Whether a tiny preterm or a full-term infant, the types of interventions needed to sustain an infant's life can have a number of associated sequelae, affecting development of postural/motor, sensory, and feeding abilities (Bishop & Lobo, 1994; Davison, Karp, & Kanto, 1994; Jones, McMurray, & Englestad, 2002). Infants with prolonged ventilatory support present some unique issues, such as pain and discomfort, and need to be weaned from sedative medication, which further complicates their assessment and intervention (Anand, 2000). Finally, psychosocial aspects of a prolonged NICU stay that affect infants and their families also need to be addressed to provide appropriate care (Van Riper, 2001). The NICU therapist has the challenging opportunity to provide environmental modifications and interventions that improve function and reduce the risk of poor outcomes for infants who are sent home early or with complex needs or for infants with prolonged NICU stays. Although some NICU infants require extended care beyond term age, most go home from the NICU to lead normal lives (see Figure 52).

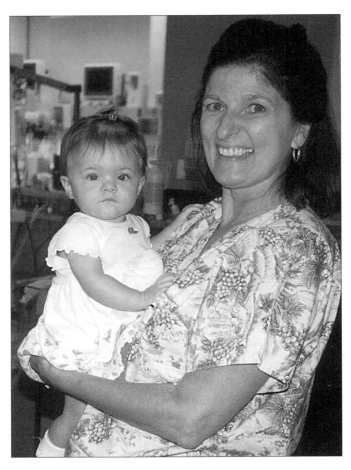

Figure 52.   This NICU graduate is shown at 7 months corrected age on a return visit to her primary nurse. Although she was born at 23 weeks, weighing only 380 g, her follow-up clinic evaluations indicate age-appropriate performance in all areas of development.

Appendix

Helping Your Preterm Infant Settle in at Home

Rosemarie Bigsby, Sc.D., OTR/L
Infant Development Center, Department of Pediatrics
Women & Infants' Hospital, Rhode Island

Your premature baby has been in the world, responding to the environment for weeks or even months. He or she has probably changed a lot during that time and

- Has graduated to an open crib
- Takes feedings by bottle or breast
- Responds to your face, voice, and touch in ways that are now familiar to you

However, your baby probably will be going home before his or her due date—the date on which he or she was supposed to be born. That means, developmentally, that your baby will be physically less mature than a full-term baby; he or she may

- Be smaller, thinner, and less energetic
- Need more head and body support during dressing and bathing
- Be more sensitive to changes in temperature

Your baby's behavior will also be less mature than that of a full-term baby; he or she may

- Startle to unexpected noises or movement
- Have less energy for crying
- Need more time to calm down once he or she becomes overstimulated

Premature babies need to go through a few more changes before they are able to do all of the things that full-term newborns do. So when you first take your baby home, you may notice that he or she is still a little bit different from full-term babies you have known.

Even once they reach term age, preterm infants may still need to take things at a slower pace so they can conserve extra energy for growth. Some preterms develop skills at a different rate than that of full-term babies. However, most preterm infants eventually achieve the important developmental milestones and grow to become healthy, active children.

During those first important weeks at home, there are a lot of things that you can do to help your baby settle in more easily while fostering development.

Read and respond to your baby's cues.*

Babies communicate with their caregivers through facial expressions and movements. Premature babies have their own special signals to let their parents know that they are feeling calm or playful or that they are becoming tired or stressed. Look for instances when your baby is quiet and alert—these are the ideal times for interacting with your baby. You can tell when your baby is feeling calm and ready to interact with you when he or she

- Has a soft, relaxed facial expression
- Keeps his or her arms and legs relaxed (but not floppy)
- Is able to stay calm while being touched, looking at your face and listening to your voice

It is easy for preterm infants to become overstimulated by all that is going on around them. You can tell that your baby is feeling tired or stressed when he or she

- Avoids looking at you directly
- Changes color (becomes pale or flushed)
- Frowns, grimaces, or looks worried
- Becomes limp or stiff
- Has startles or tremors

When you notice your baby becoming tired or stressed, stop whatever you were doing at that time. You can hold your baby quietly, bringing his or her arms and legs close to the body. Let your child grasp your finger. If you talk to your baby, do so quietly and watch for his or her response. Sometimes, just your face is enough stimulation for the baby.

Another option is to put your baby down for a rest, building a nest around him or her with blanket rolls, which provide boundaries to lean and press his or her feet against. *Any object in the crib can potentially suffocate. Blanket rolls and other positioners should be kept away from your baby's face.* Help your baby get his or her hand to the mouth or offer a pacifier—sucking is very soothing for babies and helps them conserve energy for feeding and interaction.

Establish routines that are comfortable for you and your baby.

Sleeping is important for energy and growth. After becoming accustomed to the continuous background noise and light in the hospital's special care nursery, premature infants often have difficulty settling down to sleep at night in a quiet home. Although they may startle to unexpected sounds, preterm infants often tune out continuous sounds and may even find that these sounds help them sleep.

Set the stage for sleeping.

- For the first few days or weeks after discharge, try playing a radio softly near your baby's crib to provide continuous sound. You can also try a fan (avoid drafts on your baby) or a clock that ticks loudly.

---

*The ideas of numerous professionals—especially Heidelise Als, Zack Boukydis, T. Berry Brazelton, Jean Cole, Barry Lester, and Ed Tronick—are included in this section.

- In the special care nursery, most premature infants sleep with blanket rolls against their backs and near their feet. It is a good idea to continue providing these boundaries for your baby at home. Babies like to press up against a support when they are sleeping, and they seem able to stay asleep longer when they have this support. *Again, any object in the crib can potentially suffocate. Blanket rolls and other positioners should be kept away from your baby's face.*

- Use a long blanket that can cover your baby and be tucked into the sides of the mattress. This gentle pressure helps reduce startling awake and increases quiet sleep.

- Avoid layers of blankets or pillows under your baby because these may be smothering.

- Help your baby establish a routine for going to sleep by putting him or her to bed with familiar sounds, such as a musical mobile.

- Do not be alarmed if the routine changes in several weeks. As your baby grows and develops, he or she will be awake for longer periods during the day, and sleeping patterns may change.

Remember that feeding provides energy for growth and development.

Parents of small babies should record intake and output. A therapist from the special care nursery may be able to provide a sample chart for doing so. During this time, a visiting nurse will conduct weight checks and ascertain the general health of your baby.

Set the stage for feeding.

- Become aware of your baby's level of stimulation and how it affects arousal and feeding.

- Position your baby properly during feeding.

- Make feeding an enjoyable experience for both you and your baby.

- Select nipples that are appropriate for your baby's feeding needs.

Encourage play and social interaction.

Read your baby's cues during play and social interactions. Try to find the amount of stimulation that is just right for your baby. Regarding toys and activities, find appropriate things to look at, listen to, and touch.

15

Follow-Up of High-Risk Infants

Betty R. Vohr and Michael E. Msall

OVERVIEW

This chapter presents a comprehensive review of the literature on follow-up assessment and intervention programs designed for NICU graduates. A historical overview of the evolution of these high-risk programs sets the tone for discussing the risk criteria on which follow-up programs may be based. Criteria discussed include weight, medical condition, psychosocial issues, dependency on technology, and research. Examples of follow-up assessment schedules are provided, along with the rationale for the adoption of a variety of schedules.

The enablement model of the *International Classification of Functioning, Disability and Health (ICF)* (World Health Organization, 2001) and its precursor, the *International Classification of Impairment, Disability, and Handicap (ICIDH)* (World Health Organization, 1980) have been proposed as frameworks for understanding the impact of health status and well-being on children's functioning and social participation. The ICF framework can help guide health professionals in identifying key areas of assessment that need attention and in making decisions about which assessment tools to use.

Numerous assessment instruments are reviewed in this chapter. Major areas discussed include the purpose of each assessment, its age appropriateness, and the statistical soundness of the instrument. The instruments are classified into 10 assessment categories: health/growth, neurologic/neurosensory, vision, hearing, developmental/cognitive/educational, behavior, speech/language/vocabulary, gross and fine motor, functional/adaptive status, and kindergarten readiness. The chapter concludes with a description of the teaching roles and responsibilities of neonatal follow-up programs and the importance of conducting evidence-based research as part of follow-up program activities.

OBJECTIVES

- Identify the main purposes of follow-up programs and the common risk criteria used by various types of follow-up programs

Partial support for the work contained in this chapter was provided by Maternal and Child Health Bureau Grant No. MCJ-449505-02-0.

- Identify common assessment schedules used by the different types of follow-up programs in the context of children and families served, severity of the infants' conditions, funding sources, and program objectives

- Explain the dimensions of the ICIDH and the ICF frameworks of disablement and enablement and how they can be used to understand the complexity of a child's condition and his or her need for follow-up

- Recall the major purposes and goals of neonatal high-risk follow-up assessment

- Identify the various categories of assessment that should be considered in providing follow-up services to NICU graduates

- Identify common assessment instruments used for monitoring the health and developmental progress and for optimizing the outcome of NICU graduates

- Recognize the importance of incorporating education and research components among the major activities of follow-up programs

HISTORICAL PERSPECTIVE

A French obstetrician, Pierre Budin, was the first physician to make progress in the care and follow-up of high-risk infants. He established a clinic for "nurslings" at La Charité Hospital in Paris in 1892 and later became the supervisor of a "special department for weaklings." His book *Le Nourisson* [The Nursling] covered issues related to the care of full-term and preterm infants after discharge (Budin, 1907). At the time, there was tremendous public interest in prematurely born infants, and Budin was instrumental in establishing an exhibit on premature infants in incubators at the Chicago Exhibition in 1914. Later, Dr. Julian Hess, a pediatrician at Michael Reese Hospital in Chicago, established the first premature center in the United States.

Early publications dedicated to high-risk infants and their follow-up began to appear in the German literature between 1919 and the early 1930s (Peiper, 1924, 1931; Ylippo, 1919). One of the first U.S. follow-up studies of a large cohort of premature infants was published in *Pediatrics*; Hess (1953) reported on the outcomes of 317 survivors who had birth weights between 605 and 1,260 g and were born between 1922 and 1950. The follow-up rate of 93% was excellent, and the "severely handicapped" rate was 15%. Another physician, Lula Lubchenco, was a forerunner of follow-up for premature infants. She and her colleagues conducted neonatal and follow-up studies at the premature center established at the University of Colorado in 1947 (Lubchenco, Delivoria-Papadopoulos, Butterfield, et al., 1972; Lubchenco, Delivoria-Papadopoulos, & Searls, 1972; Lubchenco et al., 1963; Lubchenco et al., 1974). In addition to providing care for high-risk infants, this center accepted maternal transports from outlying areas and developed a training program for physicians. In the 1960s and 1970s, other physicians in the United States and in Europe began to report that neonatal mortality could be reduced by the regionalization and coordination of maternal and neonatal services for high-risk pregnancies (Baird, 1969a, 1969b; Drillien, 1959, 1964).

With the recent development of tertiary care centers within NICUs, the role of monitoring and reporting has expanded. Training programs for pediatric residents, neonatal fellows, and developmental-behavioral pediatric fellows incorporate experiences in neonatal follow-up programs. Most neonatal centers maintain a database and conduct clinical single-center studies or participate in larger multicenter studies to monitor the outcomes of high-risk neonates and to determine the effects of NICU interventions on outcomes. Examples of programs collecting multicenter data include the Cochrane Collaborative, the National Institute of Child Health and Development (NICHD) Research Network, and the Vermont Oxford Database.

Most follow-up programs focus on the assessment of VLBW infants. In part, this is related to the fact that very premature infants most often have a high illness severity, require prolonged hospitalization, and are at greatest risk for adverse health and neurodevelopmental sequelae. Smaller and more immature infants are surviving in increasing numbers. The survival rates of infants weighing less than 800 g have risen markedly, going from 0% (1943 to 1945 birth cohort) to 34% (1987 to 1988 birth cohort) to 70% in 1994 (Bennett, Robinson, & Sells, 1982; Dunham, 1948; Hack & Fanaroff, 1988; Hack et al., 1996; Hack et al., 1991; Hoffman & Bennett, 1990; LaPine, Jackson, & Bennett, 1995; Msall, Buck, et al., 1994). It is important to monitor the outcome of these infants to assess the efficacy of new perinatal and neonatal interventions, to provide critical information on child outcomes to parents and primary care providers, and to advocate for quality family support and early childhood education experiences.

RISK CRITERIA FOR FOLLOW-UP PROGRAMS

The criteria for follow-up must be established at each perinatal center. Center-specific criteria may vary related to the illness severity of the infants cared for in the NICU, interventions available for mothers and infants at the perinatal center, cultural and environmental characteristics in the region, and means of support provided to follow-up programs. A small Level II center may have the resources to follow all infants, whereas a large tertiary care center with more than 1,000 admissions annually may have to restrict its criteria to infants with the highest expected morbidity. For example, a center may only follow VLBW infants with IVH Grades III or IV, periventricular leukomalacia, or CLD, whereas other centers may follow all admissions to the NICU.

The criteria established at a specific center depend on the clinical and research goals of its program. Some sites may provide clinical well-child care for NICU graduates. A clinical goal may be to provide a continuum of care for high-risk infants after discharge. This may consist of medical monitoring and management of CLD and nutritional intake, growth monitoring, and management of children with severe illnesses. Another clinical goal may be to monitor the neurologic, developmental, and behavioral outcomes of a specific group of high-risk infants as a quality control indicator for the NICU. Research goals can be quite varied and may, in fact, overlap with the clinical descriptive data collected.

If a hospital serves as a referral center for ECMO, organ transplants, or early treatment of congenital heart disease, then its program will develop follow-up protocols for these specific subgroups of infants. Finally, some urban areas may have increased risks for neurodevelopmental, medical, or behavioral sequelae based on various maternal characteristics, such as depression, teenage parenting status, non–English speaking status, homelessness, or family history of educational underachievement or developmental disabilities.

Table 15 shows 10 different primary domains of risk that should be considered as criteria for follow-up programs. Within these domains, decisions must be made as to how lenient or conservative the program's enrollment principles will be. Factors

Table 15. Suggested criteria for neonatal follow-up programs

Risk Factor	Definition
LBW	Weighing less than 2,500 g (LBW), 1,500 g (VLBW), 1,000 g (ELBW), or 750 g (micropreemie); SGA
Asphyxia	5-minute Apgar score of less than 4, seizures, hypoxic-ischemic encephalopathy
Infection	Meningitis, sepsis, or positive TORCH titers
Respiratory problems	Supplemental oxygen required at 28 days (for BPD), at 36 weeks (for CLD), or at home
Neurologic findings	IVH, PVL, hydrocephalus, neuromuscular disorders, ventriculomegaly
Congenital and/or chromosomal syndromes	Down syndrome, CHARGE association, arthrogryposis, cranofacial disorders, tracheoesophageal fistula, and congenital heart disease are examples
Vision/hearing impairments	Cataracts, ROP, failed neonatal hearing screening
ECMO	Diaphragmatic hernia, meconium aspiration
Psychosocial issues	Maternal depression, parental substance abuse, teenage parenting status, limited family supports
Technology dependence	Requirements for apnea monitor, pulse oximeter, oxygen, assisted ventilation, nasogastric tube, or gastric feeding tube

to consider are the degree of risk for poor neurodevelopmental outcome, available staff, and program funding. A site must determine that it has both the funds and the staff to support assessments of the infants identified.

Low Birth Weight

Birth weight is inversely related to the rate of neurodevelopmental morbidity. Therefore, the smaller the infant, the greater the risk of morbidity and the need for neurodevelopmental monitoring (see Chapter 7 for birth weight definitions). It is well known that abnormal or suspect neurologic findings observed at term age—including hypertonicity, tremors, and asymmetries of tone or strength—resolve in the first year of life for most infants. This plasticity or ability to recover from adverse biomedical factors is well documented among infants (see Chapter 3). Longitudinal monitoring of ELBW infants and high-risk term infants is important for identifying the 10%–20% of infants with persistent neuromotor impairments.

As noted previously, growth impairment identified in utero with decreased fetal measurements constitutes IUGR, and infants with birth weights that plot below the 10th percentile on standard intrauterine growth curves are SGA. When weight, length, and head circumference measurements all plot below the 10th percentile, the findings are termed *symmetric growth restriction*. The anthropometric findings in symmetric growth restriction suggest that prolonged nutritional deprivation to the fetus results in increased risk for less optimal neurodevelopmental and growth outcomes.

Perinatal Asphyxia

Perinatal asphyxia is often characterized by signs of intrauterine or neonatal distress and by a variety of neurologic abnormalities—including decreased responsiveness, coma, hyperirritability, and seizures—as well as by impacts on major organ systems (heart, lung, kidney, liver). If all four neurologic abnormalities are present, the infant's neurologic status is defined as *hypoxic-ischemic encephalopathy*. If the findings are associated with multiorgan involvement, then impairment is considered severe, recovery is slow, and the infant is at increased risk of a poor neurologic outcome. Developmental input from professionals in neurology or developmental pediatrics, occupational therapy, and physical therapy should begin in the NICU and continue after discharge.

Infections

Infections that develop prior to delivery or during labor and delivery may have significant neurosensory and physical effects on the fetus and newborn. Serious infections of the neonate include bacterial meningitis, an infection that inflames the membranes that surround the brain and the spinal fluid; bacterial sepsis; and toxoplasmosis, rubella, cytomegalovirus, and herpes simplex (TORCH). Infants with a history of meningitis, sepsis, or TORCH infections are at increased risk of mental retardation, cerebral palsy, hearing impairment, and visual impairment.

Bronchopulmonary Dysplasia and Chronic Lung Disease

BPD (oxygen required at 28 days) and CLD (oxygen required at 36 weeks) are serious disorders secondary to severe respiratory distress syndrome of prematurity. The biologic stresses on infants with CLD may include hypoxemia, acidosis, and circulatory derangements, with periods of right-to-left shunting or hypoperfusion. Environmental stresses for infants with CLD include prolonged hospitalization and more invasive care, including intubation with assisted ventilation, indwelling catheters, frequent blood sampling, and the inability to tolerate oral feedings. Seriously ill infants with respiratory distress also have longer separations from their parents and often are placed in noisy surroundings with bright lights. Pulmonary treatments such as suctioning, chest physical therapy, steroids, and surfactant administration are intended to improve pulmonary function but may be stressful when administered. A subgroup of infants with prolonged or chronic disorders of pulmonary function are sent home on cardiorespiratory monitors, supplemental oxygen, and medications such as bronchodilators, respiratory stimulants, and diuretics. Studies have shown that after NICU discharge, infants with chronic lung disease are at increased risk for feeding problems, growth failure, developmental delay, speech and language delays, and motor delays associated with diminished tone (Gregoire, Lefebvre, & Glorieux, 1998).

Neurologic Findings

IVH is a serious neonatal morbidity of premature infants less than 32 weeks of gestation (Volpe, 1989). Papile, Burstein, Burstein, and Koffler (1978) first reported a radiographic grading system for describing the severity of IVH. This development permitted clinicians to place neonates into IVH categories that reflect the severity: Grade I (subependymal hemorrhage), Grade II (IVH without ventricular dilation), Grade III (IVH with ventricular dilation), and Grade IV (IVH with parenchymal hemorrhage) (see also Chapter 6). Although treatment advances—including prenatal steroids, surfactant, and prophylactic indomethacin—have contributed to a decrease in the incidence of IVH, the range from Grade III to IV IVH remains a significant risk factor for neurologic, neurosensory, developmental, behavioral, functional, and educational sequelae (Ahmann, Lazzara, Dykes, Brann, & Schwartz, 1980; Ment et al., 1994; Ment, Westerveld, Makuch, Vohr, & Allen, 1998; Papile et al., 1978; Philip, Allen, Tito, & Wheeler, 1989; Volpe, 1989). Dilated ventricles (ventriculomegaly) occur more frequently in association with moderate hemorrhage and may or may not be related to posthemorrhagic hydrocephalus. Studies suggest that ventriculomegaly at term is associated with an increased incidence of subsequent motor developmental and learning abnormalities (Allan, Holt, Sawyer, Tito, & Meade, 1982; Hill & Volpe, 1981).

PVL is more often identified in premature infants and is related to the vulnerability of oligodendroglia (a special type of cell in the nervous system). The etiology is believed to be secondary to changes in cerebral blood flow (Szymonowicz, Yu, Bajuk, & Astbury, 1986). PVL is generally a symmetric injury of the periventricular white matter, identified by cranial ultrasonography as echolucencies, echodensities, or cystic lesions. Risk factors for PVL include hypotensive, apneic, and hypocarbic ischemic events that are associated with decreased cerebral blood flow, as well as cytokine (type of protein) mediated brain injury triggered by events such as maternal infection, sepsis, NEC, and/or lung injury. The greatest risk for neurodevelopmental sequelae is the combination of IVH and PVL. It is also important to realize that cystic PVL can occur without IVH. Although all forms of motor, visual, and hearing impairments and developmental abnormalities may occur with PVL, the most frequent clinical correlate of PVL is spastic diplegia (O'Shea & Dammann, 2000).

Seizures are another frequent neurologic finding in NICU infants. The most common neonatal seizures in premature infants are subtle (oral-buccal or oculomotor movements) or generalized tonic. The majority of premature infants with neonatal seizures do not develop epilepsy. Yet, infants with neonatal seizures who have had Grade III or Grade IV IVH, a moderately abnormal EEG, or neurologic findings, are at increased risk and require follow-up with a neurologist. An acceptable approach in a stable infant with no abnormal neurologic findings is to allow the infant to "outgrow" the need for anticonvulsants in the first year of life. Infants who continue to have seizures should be monitored for adverse neurodevelopmental sequelae.

Congenital Abnormalities

Infants with major chromosomal abnormalities—including trisomies 13, 18, and 21; neural tube defects; and multiple congenital malformations—may be identified by prenatal diagnosis or in the delivery suite. Congenital disorders may present with infants who are clinically distressed and include congenital cardiac or pulmonary anomalies, Pierre Robin anomaly, myotonic dystrophy, Prader-Willi syndrome, osteogenesis imperfecta, and skeletal dysplasia. Infants with metabolic disorders such as urea cycle, organic acid, and amino acid disorders may also have catastrophic or neurologically severe illnesses in the newborn period. Depending on the abnormality and the risk for neurosensory sequelae, mental retardation, or death, these infants should immediately be referred for early intervention services and monitoring by a child development and metabolic genetic center.

Neurosensory Abnormalities

In addition to referral to early intervention programs, infants identified with significant risk for hearing or visual impairments require monitoring of sensory status and development. The AAP recommends that all neonates be screened for hearing impairment prior to discharge from the hospital (Task Force on Newborn and Infant Hearing, 1999; Vohr, Carty, Moore, & Letourneau, 1998). Special care nurseries have protocols to screen premature infants at risk for ROP based on guidelines from "An International Classification of Retinopathy of Prematurity" (1984). All infants with sensory impairments need to be monitored by the appropriate subspecialists and be referred for appropriate intervention services.

Extracorporeal Membrane Oxygenation Treatment

ECMO (Davis, 1998), a treatment for severe hypoxemia, has been recognized as a risk factor for sequelae. Near-term infants who have severe hypoxemia despite conventional medical therapy may benefit from the use of ECMO. Primary diagnoses that use ECMO include meconium aspiration syndrome, congenital diaphragmatic hernia, pneumonia, respiratory distress syndrome, and persistent pulmonary hypertension. Infants requiring ECMO are among the sickest in the NICU and are at increased risk of pulmonary, neurologic, and sensory sequelae (i.e., major hearing impairment). It is difficult if not impossible to determine whether neurodevelopmental sequelae are secondary to the preexisting serious disease process or the intervention with ECMO.

Psychosocial Problems

Psychosocial problems of the family are often included in the follow-up criteria because of their known contribution to adverse outcomes. Poverty, the top issue, is followed closely by other parental characteristics that may be highly correlated with one another. One or more psychosocial criteria are often included as program indicators of risk: African American or Hispanic ethnicity, teenage pregnancy, single parenting status, receipt of public assistance, lack of insurance, non–English speaking status, maternal psychiatric disorders, parental education status (i.e., less than a high school education), maternal developmental disabilities, absent prenatal care, parental substance abuse, and social isolation. Studies have begun to collect a larger spectrum of sociodemographic, psychosocial, and family variables to assess their impact on child outcomes. Given the double vulnerability of children with these factors and neonatal biologic risk, coordinated efforts of home visiting, parent education, Early Head Start, and comprehensive family support services are recommended.

Technology Dependence

The increased survival rates of ELBW and critically ill full-term infants, as well as shortened hospital stays, have resulted in more infants being discharged with specialized needs for treatment. ELBW infants are at increased risk of apnea. Apnea, a common cause of technology dependence among premature infants, is usually defined as a cessation of breathing which may be short (6–10 seconds) and self-limited or prolonged (longer than 20 seconds) and associated with bradycardia. A variety of respiratory abnormalities associated with apnea can be found in premature infants. Potentially life-threatening events are called *pathologic apnea* (refer to Chapter 6). Apnea of prematurity becomes problematic when events are associated with bradycardia (fewer than 100 heart beats per minute) and/or oxygen desaturation (below 90%) and/or the requirement of stimulation for recovery. Home cardiorespiratory monitoring for apnea of prematurity is the most common technology used in the home.

Additional examples of technology used at home are intravenous infusions of antibiotics, hyperalimentation, renal dialysis, oxygen, mechanical ventilation, and gastrostomy tube feeding. Infants who depend on technology are at increased risk of neurodevelopmental and behavioral sequelae related to illness severity, illness chronicity, and family factors that arise from providing comprehensive care at home.

ASSESSMENT SCHEDULES

Each follow-up program must identify assessment schedules that achieve the program's objectives and are financially sound. Sites may charge for clinical services provided to infants but not for assessments that are performed solely for a research protocol. In programs that include postdischarge medical management, infants are usually seen on schedules that optimize clinical management of the medical condition. For instance, infants with feeding problems, with severe BPD requiring supplemental oxygen, or with parents who have limited coping skills may be seen within 1–4 weeks of discharge. If the visits are scheduled only to facilitate the transition home, then infants may be seen one or two times or until they are stable. Then, they are referred to appropriate resources for long-term monitoring or intervention. If the program objectives are to assess the neurodevelopmental status of a cohort of high-risk infants, then a schedule of assessment times must be established. Many follow-up clinics have a schedule of assessment at 6, 12, 18, 24, and 36 months. If staff or resources are limited, then one or two key ages for assessment, identification, and referral may be identified.

VLBW infants usually are evaluated at corrected age rather than chronological age for the first 1–2 years. Chronological age is based on the number of weeks or months since the date of delivery. Corrected age is the age calculated from the expected date of delivery. It may also be calculated by subtracting the number of weeks of prematurity from the chronological age. For example, the chronological age 6-month-old infant with a gestational age of 28 weeks (3 months premature) has a corrected age of 3 months. It is important to recognize that evidence-based literature justifying correction after 1 year is not robust or unanimous (Blasco, 1989).

Assessment of Health, Neurodevelopmental, and Functional Outcomes in High-Risk Neonates

Important areas of assessment include health status, neurosensory status, developmental competencies, functional outcomes in daily living activities, and school-age outcomes. Effective assessment in these areas requires a conceptual framework as well as an understanding of the strengths and limitations of assessment measures over time.

Models of Disablement and Enablement

In 1980, the World Health Organization proposed the ICIDH model, an international classification of impairment (disturbance of body structures or organ performance), disability (functional limitations in essential activities), and handicap (difficulty with social role performance). In 1993, the U.S. National Institutes of Health expanded this framework as the National Center for Medical Rehabilitation Research (NCMRR) model (National Advisory Board on Medical Rehabilitation, 1993). The NCMRR model employed five dimensions: 1) pathophysiology, 2) impairment (disturbance of body structures or organ performance), 3) functional limitations of personal activities (self-care, mobility, communication, learning, social interactions), 4) disability in social role performance (play, school, work), and 5) societal limitations (legal, attitudinal, architectural barriers).

Despite explicit warnings, the ICIDH and NCMRR models were misinterpreted to suggest that disease causes impairment that may result in disability or functional limitations and, ultimately, in handicaps. To remedy concerns about this disablement framework and to use person-first language, an enablement model was developed called the ICF model (World Health Organization, 2001). The ICF model explicitly measures functional strengths and functional limitations, social role performance activities, community participation, social role difficulties, and community restrictions, as well as environmental facilitators and environmental barriers. Table 16 illustrates the use of this framework for a 3-year-old boy with asthma and language delays after having CLD, a 5-year-old girl with developmental challenges who is entering kindergarten, and a 4-year-old boy with many functional strengths and participatory experiences despite having the neuromotor impairments of spastic diplegic cerebral palsy.

The ICF model emphasizes three complex categories: 1) body structure and function, 2) activity, and 3) participation. Most experts envision that the ICF model will enhance the focus of intervention and developmental follow-up by changing emphasis from dysfunction and disability to functional strengths, the impact of assistive technology, and social and community participation.

Several assumptions are critical to understanding a functional and strengths-based conceptual framework. First, measures of health status (e.g., growth delays, respiratory tract infections) do not uniformly predict global delays in motor or developmental skills. Second, measures of neurologic integrity (e.g., tone, reflexes, primitive reflexes, postural control) are measures of impairment and do not describe whether a child crawls or walks, feeds or dresses him- or herself, speaks in sentences, maintains continency, or is able to learn in small groups. Understanding the ICF framework allows multidisciplinary professionals to choose appropriate instruments at key ages to understand the complexity of health and developmental tasks and pathways of risk and resiliency.

Purpose of Assessment

In using developmental assessment batteries for motor, developmental, communicative, adaptive, educational, and behavioral skills, evaluators must understand the purpose of the measures (Kirshner & Guyatt, 1985). Discriminative instruments are designed to compare an individual child's performance with his or her peers who do not have disabilities. Examples of discriminative instruments include the Bayley Scales of Infant Development–Second Edition (BSID-II) (Bayley, 1993); the Child Behavior Checklist (Achenbach, 1991); the Peabody Developmental Motor Scales, Second Edition (PDMS-2) (Folio & Fewell, 2000); the Preschool Language Scale, Fourth Edition (PLS-4) (Zimmerman, Steiner, & Pond, 2002); and the Vineland Adaptive Behavior Scales (VABS) (Sparrow, Balla, & Cicchetti, 1984). Although a Bayley Mental Developmental Index (MDI) score of less than 68 at age 18 months indicates that a child has significant developmental delays compared with typically developing 18-month-olds, the score does not indicate the child's basic skills with using his or her hands, prelinguistic communication skills, and potential to go beyond basic sensory-motor processes.

Table 16. Three illustrations of the dimensions of disablement and enablement within the International Classification of Functioning, Disability and Health (ICF) framework (World Health Organization, 2001)

Dimension	Definition of dimension	As illustrated by a 3-year-old boy	As illustrated by a 5-year-old girl	As illustrated by a 4-year-old boy
Pathophysiology	Molecular or biochemical mechanisms interfering with cellular function	Developmental lung injury in an infant who was born at 25 weeks of gestation and weighed 700 g	Infant who was born at 27 weeks of gestation, weighing 900 g with Grade I IVH	An infant who weighed 800 g when born at 26 weeks of gestation
Impairment	Loss of organ structure or physiologic performance	Growth delays, recurrent respiratory tract infections and CLD during the first year of life with asthma sequelae	Myopia, behavioral immaturity	ROP requiring laser surgery, cystic PVL with spastic diplegic cerebral palsy, myopia, hyperactivity
Functional strengths	Performance of daily activities	Climbing, running, drinking with a straw	Learning songs, playing with peers indoors	Ambulatory, using lightweight braces in all community environments, being continent, talking in complete sentences
Functional limitations	Restriction of ability to perform essential activities (e.g., feeding, dressing, bathing, crawling, walking, talking in sentences)	Postural control, feeding inefficiencies, developmental delays in communicative skills	Speech articulation and perceptual delays, attentional control difficulties	Difficulty with eye-hand coordination, difficulty seeing details in material presented from right visual field
Participation	Engagement in activities valued by family/society	Playing on the outdoor playground	Playing dolls with peers	Fully participating in Montessori pre-school
Disability	Difficulty performing roles typical for peers	Requires special home nursing; respiratory, nutrition, and medication supports; early intervention services for language and peer activities	Requires special education supports and structure in her kindergarten class, speech-language and occupational therapy services, and ear-tubes; stimulant medication for attentional difficulties is helping	Unable to ride bike with peers
Contextual factors (facilitators)	Characteristics of the child's environment that support participation	Good hand-washing policies at preschool (to prevent spreading germs that can cause respiratory problems), asthma care plan that optimizes preschool attendance	Kindergarten class structure and tolerance for understanding her strengths	Adapted clothing that allows for independence during the transition to outdoor activities; large print books
Societal limitations (barriers)	Attitudinal, legal, policy, and architectural barriers	Access to quality skilled pediatric community nursing, access to quality respite or quality home child care, access to pediatric speech-language therapy	Access to a creative holistic developmental curriculum	Access to swimming

An evaluative instrument specifies criterion-related tasks (e.g., Gross Motor Function Measure [GMFM], Russell, Rosenbaum, Avery, & Lane, 2002; Functional Independence Measure for Children [WeeFIM], Uniform Data System for Medical Rehabilitation [UDSMR], 1998; Pediatric Evaluation of Disability Inventory [PEDI], Haley, Coster, Ludlow, Haltiwanger, & Andrellos, 1992) and describes current levels of performance in key dimensions that are sensitive to change over time (Guyatt, Walter, & Norman, 1987). For example, the GMFM specifies an individual's performance in the motor tasks of lying and rolling, sitting, crawling and kneeling, and standing and in the upright mobility skills of walking, running, and jumping (Rosenbaum et al., 1990). A predictive measure is designed to assess key skills related to a future state. For example, Bleck (1987) specified components of primitive reflexes that predicted the inability to walk in children with cerebral palsy in middle childhood, whereas Capute and Shapiro (1985) used the Gross Motor Quotient to predict who would be diagnosed with cerebral palsy in the preschool years based on the rate of early motor milestone attainment.

Assessment Methods and Instruments

Although many follow-up studies report specific areas of outcome, such as language or visual-perceptual status, the more recent approach is to report comprehensive neurologic, developmental, functional, and health status outcomes. This approach permits a total view of the child within the context of his or her family, peers, school, and health care system. Key areas in health status include somatic growth measures, head circumference, immunization status, neurologic status, the presence of chronic illness, lead exposure, health care utilization, and parental perception of the child's health status. Table 17 provides a summary of the assessments most frequently used in follow-up studies of VLBW and ELBW infants. Assessments have been divided into 10 major categories: 1) health/growth, 2) neurologic/neurosensory, 3) vision, 4) hearing, 5) developmental/cognitive/educational, 6) behavior, 7) speech/language/vocabulary, 8) motor, 9) functional/adaptive status, and 10) kindergarten readiness.

Health/Growth Assessment

Health

The Health Utilities Index (HUI) is a set of multiattribute health status classification systems, of which there are three editions (HUI:1, HUI:2, and HUI:3) (Feeny, Furlong, Boyle, & Torrance, 1995; Patrick & Erickson, 1993; Torrance, Furlong, Feeny, & Boyle, 1995). There are two core components of each HUI measurement system: 1) a generic multiattribute health status (MAHS) classification system, and 2) a preference-based scoring function (i.e., formula). An original goal of the HUI:2 system was to serve as a generic, preference-based measure of health status and health-related quality of life for assessing the outcomes of treatments for childhood cancer (Feeny et al., 1992). It has since been applied in many other pediatric settings (Feeny, Torrance, Godsmith, Furlong, & Boyle, 1993). The HUI:3 system was developed for applicability to a broader age range (i.e., 6 years of age and older) and has been extended to include preschool populations (Saigal, Feeny, et al., 1994). A 15-item self-administered questionnaire was designed to ask the minimum number of questions required to classify an individual's health status.

Table 17. Assessments most frequently used in follow-up studies of VLBW and ELBW infants

Categories and assessment tools	Age range
Health/growth	
Health Utilities Index (Feeny et al., 1995)	3 years–16 years
Child Health Questionnaire (Landgraf, Abetz, & Ware, 1996)	3 years–16 years
Height, weight, head circumference; health services, including medical, home, and subspecialty access	All ages
Neurologic/neurosensory, standard neurologic examination categorizing child as	
Normal/suspect/abnormal	All ages
Expanded classification of CP specifying hemiplegia, diplegia, triplegia, and quadriplegia	2 years–7 years
Gross Motor Functional Classification System (GMFCS) (Wood & Rosenbaum, 2000)	2 years–16 years
Vision	
Vision/ophthalmologic examination: Teller Acuity Cards (Teller, McDonald, Preston, Sebris, & Dobson, 1986)	All ages
HOTV chart	All ages
Snellen chart	All ages
Hearing	
Otoacoustic emissions: auditory brainstem test	All ages
Tympanometry: vision reinforcement audiometry	Older than 6 months
Developmental/cognitive/educational	
Capute Scales (CAT/CLAMS) (Accardo et al., in press; Capute, 1996)	2 months–36 months
Child Development Inventory (CDI) (Ireton, 1992)	15 months–6 years
Ages & Stages Questionnaires (ASQ), Second Edition (Bricker & Squires, 1999)	Birth–5 years
Bayley Scales of Infant Development–Second Edition (BSID-II) (Bayley, 1993)	1 month–42 months
Stanford-Binet Intelligence Scale (4th ed.) (SB-4) (Thorndike, Hagen, & Sattler, 1986)	2 years–18 years
Wechsler Preschool and Primary Scale of Intelligence–Revised (WPPSI-R) (Wechsler, 1989a)	3 years–7 years, 3 months
Woodcock-Johnson Psychoeducational Battery (Woodcock & Johnson, 1989)	3 years–adult
Differential Ability Scales (Elliott, 1990)	2.5 years–8.5 years
McCarthy Scales (McCarthy, 1972)	2.5 years–18 years
Kaufman Assessment Battery for Children (K-ABC) (Kaufman & Kaufman, 1983)	2.5 years–12.5 years
Behavior	
Child Behavior Checklist (Achenbach, 1991; Achenbach & Rescorla, 2000, 2001)	1.5 years–18 years
Conners' Teacher Rating Scale (Conners, 1997)	3 years–17 years
Conners' Parent Rating Scale (Conners, 1997)	3 years–17 years

Categories and assessment tools	Age range
Speech/language/vocabulary	
Preschool Language Scale, Fourth Edition (PLS-4) (Zimmerman et al., 2002)	Birth–6 years
Peabody Picture Vocabulary Test–III (PPVT-III) (Dunn & Dunn, 1997)	2.5 years–adult
The Expressive One-Word Picture Vocabulary Test–2000 Edition (EOWPVT) (Brownell, 2000)	2 years–11 years, 11 months
Early Language Milestone Scale, Second Edition (ELMS-2) (Coplan, 1993)	Birth–36 months
Sequenced Inventory of Communicative Development–Revised (SICD-R) (Hedrick, Prather, & Tobin, 1984)	4 months–4 years
Clinical Linguistic Auditory Milestone Scale (CLAMS) (Accardo et al., in press; Capute, 1996)	2 months–36 months
Gross and fine motor (including visual perceptual skills)	
Peabody Developmental Motor Scales, Second Edition (PDMS-2) (Folio & Fewell, 2000)	2 years–11 years
Bruininks-Oseretsky Test of Motor Proficiency (Bruininks, 1978)	4.5 years–14.5 years
Early Screening Profiles (ESP) (Harrison et al., 1990)	4.5 years–14.5 years
Alberta Infant Motor Scales (AIMS) (Piper & Darrah, 1995)	Birth–walking age
Gross Motor Function Measure (GMFM) (Russell et al., 1989)	Birth–5 years
Gross Motor Performance Measure (GMPM) (Russell et al., 2002)	Birth–5 years
Beery-Buktenica Developmental Test of Visual-Motor Integration (VMI) (4th ed.) (Beery & Buktenica, 1997)	Short form: 3 years–8 years; long form: 3 years–18 years
Functional/adaptive status	
Pediatric Functional Independence Measure (WeeFIM) (UDSMR, 1998)	6 months–7 years
Vineland Adaptive Behavior Scales (VABS) (Sparrow et al., 1984)	Birth–18 years, 11 months
Battelle Developmental Inventory (BDI) (Newborg, Stock, Wnek, Guidubaldi, & Svinick, 1984)	Birth–8 years
Pediatric Evaluation of Disability Inventory (PEDI)	6 months–7.5 years
Kindergarten readiness	
Miller Assessment for Preschoolers (MAP) (Miller, 1988)	4 years–6 years
Learning Accomplishment Profile (LAP-D) (Nehring, Nehring, Bruni, & Randolph, 1992)	30 months–70 months
Child Development Inventory (CDI) (Ireton, 1992)	15 months–6 years
Mullen Scales of Early Learning (MSEL) (Mullen, 1995)	Birth–68 months
Kindergarten Readiness Test (KRT) (Larson & Vitali, 1988)	4 years–6 years
Kaufman Survey of Early Academic and Language Skills (K-SEALS) (Kaufman & Kaufman, 1993)	3 years–7 years

The MAHS classification system describes both the type and severity of functional limitations of individuals according to seven attributes: 1) sensation, 2) mobility, 3) emotion, 4) cognition, 5) self-care, 6) pain, and 7) fertility in adolescents and adults. The MAHS is based on the concept that health consists of a number of attributes that should be considered collectively. Each attribute has three to five defined functional levels of severity, ranging from normal function to severe dysfunction. The levels for each attribute are meant to be interpreted as developmentally appropriate for the age of the subject. The comprehensive health status of an individual at a particular time may be described by a seven-element vector. This classification system can potentially describe 24,000 unique health states (the product of the number of levels within each of the seven attributes). Saigal and colleagues (1996) had adolescents evaluate their own health status at ages 12–16 years. The adolescents rated their status as a fate "similar to" or "worse than" a range of choices, from 0 (*dead*) to 1 (*perfect health*). The researchers found that 71% of ELBW teens and 73% of peers gave themselves a utility rating greater than 0.95 for health status. Thus, these measures are an important component of long-term assessments and indicate that although there are higher rates of neurodevelopmental impairments in ELBW infants, severe disability with perceived very low quality of life is rare.

The Child Health Questionnaire (CHQ) (Landgraf et al., 1996) measures physical functioning, role/social limitations, general health perception, bodily pain, self-esteem, parental impact on time and emotions, mental health, general behavior, family activities, family cohesion, and change in health. There are three parent-completed versions of the CHQ, each with varying numbers (28, 50, and 98) of questions. The child-completed version consists of 87 questions and is for use with children 10 years of age and older. Administration time varies depending on the version utilized.

The CHQ has been used to evaluate children with cerebral palsy (Liptak et al., 2001). A multisite assessment team evaluated 199 children, ages 2–18 years, with moderate to severe impairments according to the Gross Motor Functional Classification System (GMFCS) (Wood & Rosenbaum, 2000). Caregivers were administered the CHQ and a questionnaire designed to assess demographics, health, and functional status. The mean z score on the CHQ physical summary score was −0.76 (mean = 0). In addition, the children's general health index was significantly associated with the GMFCS. The authors concluded that these children with cerebral palsy overall had poorer health status compared with children without disabilities, and they required more health-related treatments and resources than their peers without disabilities (Liptak et al., 2001). This type of study emphasizes the need to conduct multidimensional assessments of children with special health care needs and the consequences of these needs on health and rehabilitation resources.

The use of health services in a high-risk population is an important assessment question. A checklist of information related to primary care visits, chronic conditions, pediatric subspecialty visits, emergency visits, hospitalizations, and surgeries is important in understanding ongoing health service use. Physical therapy, occupational therapy, speech-language therapy, and behavioral interventions are costly. Insurance companies often only pay for a specified number of visits for such services, but early intervention and school programs provide the services for longer periods of time. When assessing the frequency of these interventions, the time should be evaluated in the number of 15-minute increments utilized per week and the current expected functional goals of the interventions specified.

Growth

Using z scores for growth is a helpful method for comparing height, weight, and head circumference with those of a typically developing population. This allows the identification of children with delayed growth. The EpiInfo software package of international reference curves of the World Health Organization (1978) is available. Rogers et al. (1998) developed a software package to calculate head circumference-for-age z scores using a similar curve to the World Health Organization's international reference for somatic growth. These curves were based on head circumference-for-age data obtained from 1) the National Center for Health Statistics (NCHS) for children from birth to 3 years of age and 2) the Fels Longitudinal Study for children 3 years to 18 years of age (Hammill et al., 1979; Roche, Mukherjee, Guo, & Moore, 1987). The normalized head circumference-for-age references were developed using the same methods as those for creating normalized NCHS length-for-age, weight-for-age, and weight-for-length references.

Neurologic/Neurosensory Assessment

The most severe disabilities are reported in the neurologic/neurosensory category. The incidence of visual impairments, hearing impairments, and cerebral palsy are important health indicators and are significant morbidities for a child and his or her family. The diagnosis of severe neurosensory morbidities is more specific than other areas of cognitive development. A diagnosis of cerebral palsy is obtained by performing a systematic neurologic assessment of a young child. Although severe impairments can be diagnosed within the first year of life, cerebral palsy's varying degrees of severity is more routinely diagnosed by 18 months of age. Diagnosing cerebral palsy in VLBW and ELBW children less than a year of age is a challenge because of the general prevalence of hypertonicity and transient dystonia among these infants. The classification of cerebral palsy is further compromised by lack of uniform protocols for specifying topography between 18 months to 5 years of age (Evans, Johnson, Mitch, & Alberman, 1989). The topographical classification allows for criteria that clearly distinguish hemiplegia, diplegia, triplegia, and quadriplegia based on easily observed postural and hand skills at key ages. This is illustrated in Figure 53. See Msall and Tremont (2000) for further applications of this topography and linking it to the GMFCS.

Vision Assessment

The standard of care within tertiary care centers determines that VLBW infants have ophthalmologic examinations for ROP prior to discharge, with appropriate follow-up and intervention when appropriate (see Chapter 6). This has facilitated the identification of both severe and milder degrees of vision impairment. In addition, ongoing monitoring for the detection of strabismus and myopia are important for VLBW and

   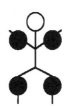

Figure 53.   Topographical classification of cerebral palsy by postural and hand skills.

ELBW infants. One assessment tool, the Teller Acuity Cards, has been used to estimate recognition vision in infants and toddlers (Teller et al., 1986).

Hearing Assessment

Based on recommendations by the Joint Committee on Infant Hearing Screening (1994), the majority of U.S. tertiary care centers have in place or are in the process of developing hearing screening programs using either transient otoacoustic emissions (OAE), automated auditory brainstem response (AABR), or standard ABR. In addition, tympanometry is an important screening tool for middle ear dysfunction. This has resulted in earlier administration of audiology diagnostic tests and earlier identification of significant hearing loss by using diagnostic ABR, tympanometry, and vision reinforcement audiometry.

Developmental/Cognitive/Educational Assessment

The assessment category of developmental/cognitive/educational tests includes the instruments most commonly reported in the literature. Although all of these tests have limitations, they provide important information about a preschooler's level of competence, provided certain precautions are taken. The results, however, must be interpreted relative to the presence of a motor or sensory disability, behavior during the test situation, the language spoken at home, and cultural differences. In addition, the assessor must be experienced with a variety of children who have developmental disabilities and must be skilled at establishing rapport with infants, toddlers, and preschoolers. For an individual child, early test results, especially in the first 6 months, have limited predictive validity. However, children who repeatedly test more than three standard deviations below the mean in language or problem solving in the first 3 years will have complex developmental and academic challenges. Tests administered at younger ages also may not tap into the same psychological capacities as those present in older children. In addition, children reside within a dynamic environment with a spectrum of positive and negative influences on development and test-taking ability. Therefore, the older the child, the greater the predictive validity of these types of assessments.

   The Clinical Adaptive Test (CAT) and the Clinical Linguistic and Auditory Milestone Scale (CLAMS) comprise the Capute Scales, which have established reliability and validity (Accardo et al., in press; Capute, 1996; Capute & Accardo, 1978; Capute, Shapiro, & Palmer, 1987). The CAT and the CLAMS are widely used measures of visual-motor, problem-solving, and auditory functioning in children ages 1–36 months. These assessment instruments are designed to quantify delays in language and problem solving and can be administered in 15–20 minutes. The Capute Scales give the examiner Age Equivalents and Chronological Age scores for visual-motor abilities, problem-solving skills, and language, as well as a composite score of cognitive functioning. Along with a normative population (Capute et al., 1986a), the Capute Scales have been validated for children with motor delays (Capute et al., 1986b; Capute & Shapiro, 1985), children referred for developmental delays (Hoon, Pulsifer, Gopalan, Palmer, & Capute, 1993; Wachtel, Shapiro, Palmer, Allen, & Capute, 1994), children in early intervention programs (Macias et al., 1998; Rossman et al., 1994), and children with chronic illness (Wachtel, Tepper, Houck, McGrath, & Thompson, 1994).

Two developmental screening instruments available to primary health care professionals help rule out serious developmental concerns. The Child Development Inventory (CDI) (Ireton, 1992) is designed for children ages 15 months–6 years of age. The inventory consists of 270 items in 9 scales: social, self-help, gross motor, fine motor, expressive language, language comprehension, letters, numbers, and general development. The CDI was normed in Minnesota with 568 children from ages 1 year to 6 years, 3 months. Adequate reliability and validity data are reported. The second screening device available to primary care professionals, the Ages & Stages Questionnaires (ASQ), Second Edition (Bricker & Squires, 1999), is a parent-completed screening instrument designed for use with children from 4 months to 60 months of age. The areas assessed are communication, gross motor, fine motor, problem solving, and personal-social. It is scored on a three-level scale where the parents answer "yes," "sometimes," or "not yet" for each developmental skill. Completion time ranges from 10 to 30 minutes. The ASQ's reliability and validity are good to excellent. If resources are scarce, the CDI and the ASQ, in conjunction with developmental observations from primary care and educational professionals in early childhood, can help reassure neonatal follow-up professionals. For example, if a 4-year-old speaks clearly in six-word sentences, runs quickly, knows all of the primary colors, and can draw a person with facial and extremity details, the need to obtain IQ testing to rule out developmental disability (standard score of less than 70) is not indicated.

The BSID-II (Bayley, 1993) is the most commonly used test for preschoolers ages 4–42 months and provides information in both the cognitive (mental developmental index, or MDI) and motor (psychomotor developmental index, or PDI) domains. The Differential Ability Scales (Elliott, 1990), the McCarthy Scales of Children's Abilities (McCarthy, 1972), the Stanford-Binet Intelligence Scale (4th ed.) (Thorndike, Hagen, & Sattler, 1986), the Wechsler Preschool and Primary Scale of Intelligence–Revised (Wechsler, 1989a), and the Woodcock-Johnson Psychoeducational Battery–Revised (Woodcock & Johnson, 1989) are tests of cognitive/developmental ability that provide an IQ score as well as subtests providing a preliminary assessment of strengths and weaknesses in specific areas of learning. Caution should be used in interpreting IQ test results for individual children, particularly for children who are slow learners (IQ score of 70–85) or who have mild mental retardation (IQ score of 55–70) in the context of chronic illness and social disadvantages. For studying populations of children, the data will provide information for comparing groups with one another (intervention versus control) or with normative data. Because of the limitations of IQ scores, it is becoming more acceptable to evaluate a child's performance using a battery of tests, which include those for visual-perceptual skills (Beery & Buktenica, 1997; Colarusso & Hamel, 1972), speech and language skills (Coplan, 1993; Dunn & Dunn, 1997; Hedrick, Prather, & Tobin, 1984; Zimmerman et al., 2002), cognition (Elliott, 1990; McCarthy, 1972; Thorndike et al., 1986; Wechsler, 1989b; Woodcock & Johnson, 1989), fine and gross motor function (Bruininks, 1978; Folio & Fewell, 2000; Harrison et al., 1990; Palisano & Haley, 1993), and kindergarten readiness (Kauffman & Kauffman, 1993; Larson & Vitali, 1988; Miller, 1988; Nehring et al., 1992).

The Kaufman Assessment Battery for Children (K-ABC) (Kaufman & Kaufman, 1983) measures cognition and achievement using 16 subtests that distinguish sequential and simultaneous processing. Examples of the sequential tasks include hand movements, number recall, and word order. Simultaneous tasks include face recognition, gestalt closure, and matrix analogies. The Achievement scale possesses excellent prediction of future achievement and internal consistency for preschoolers. The Mental

Processing scales yield stability coefficients in the 0.80s. The K-ABC has been validated against the Slosson Intelligence Test (Lampley & Rust, 1986) and was used to assess the long-term stability with preschoolers who are at risk (Bing & Bing, 1985; Lyon & Smith, 1986; Ricciardi & Boelker, 1987).

Behavioral Assessment

The Child Behavior Checklist (Achenbach, 1991) is a comprehensive measure of children's behaviors. It is designed to assess in a standardized format the social competencies and behavioral problems of children ages 2–3 years (CBCL/2-3) and 4–18 years (CBCL/4-18) as reported by their parents or others who know the child well. Norms are based on 368 children. Internalizing/externalizing and total problem scores are computed. Psychometric properties are excellent (Achenbach, 1991). A revised edition of the Achenbach System of Empirically Based Assessment (Achenbach & Rescorla, 2000) has a preschool profile for ages $1^1/_2$–5 years, a Language Development Survey, and a Caregiver–Teacher Report Form.

The Conners' Rating Scales–Revised (Conners, 1997) evaluate challenging behaviors, as identified by a parent (the Conners' Parent Rating Scales–Revised, CPRS-R) or a teacher (the Conners' Teacher Rating Scales–Revised, CTRS-R), in preschoolers, school-age children, and adolescents. The Conners' Teacher Rating Scale–Revised includes a 59-item form (CTRS-R: L) and a 28-item short form (CTRS-R: S). Testing requires approximately 15 minutes and 5–10 minutes, respectively. The Conners' Parent Rating Scale can be administered with parents of children ages 3–17 years and includes a long (80-item; 15–20 minutes) version (CPRS-R: L) and a short (27-item; 5–10 minutes) version (CPRS-R: S). The Conners' Rating Scales also contain subscales for the assessment of conduct problems, cognitive problems, family problems, emotional problems, anger control problems, hyperactivity, impulsivity, inattention, and anxiety problems. The Conners' Rating Scales were normed with more than 8,000 children of various ethnicities in North America. Internal consistency ranges from 0.75 to 0.90 and test-retest reliability ranges from 0.60 to 0.90. This instrument was validated against previous editions of itself as well as against the Children's Depression Inventory (Kovacs, 1985) and Conners' Continuous Performance Test (1994).

Speech/Language/Vocabulary Assessment

Six tests of speech/language/vocabulary abilities are shown in Table 17. The PLS-4 (Zimmerman et al., 2002), is a standardized assessment that includes two subscales—auditory comprehension and expressive communication—to assess attention, vocal development, social communication, semantics, language structure, and integrative thinking skills. The Peabody Picture Vocabulary Test–Third Edition (PPVT-III) (Dunn & Dunn, 1997) is a nonverbal, multiple-choice test that measures receptive vocabulary. The Expressive One-Word Picture Vocabulary Test–2000 Edition (EOWPVT) (Brownell, 2000) measures expressive vocabulary. The Early Language Milestone Scale, Second Edition (ELMS-2), (Coplan, 1993) assesses speech and language development according to three areas: Auditory Expressive, Auditory Receptive, and Visual. The Sequenced Inventory of Communication Development–Revised Edition (SICD-R) (Hedrick et al., 1984) is a diagnostic test that evaluates the communication abilities of children who are functioning between 4 months and 4 years of age. It has been used successfully with children who have sensory impairments and with children who have varying degrees of mental retardation. The Clinical Linguistic Auditory Milestone Scale (CLAMS) (Accardo et al., in press; Capute et al., 1987) is used to measure children's developing strengths and limitations in relation to prelinguistic, linguistic expressive, and receptive language milestones.

Gross and Fine Motor Function Assessment

The Peabody Developmental Motor Scales, Second Edition (PDMS-2) (Folio & Fewell, 2000), is a test of gross and fine motor skills for children birth through 83 months of age. Grasping, use of hands, eye-hand coordination, and manual dexterity are assessed. Scores range from 0 (*cannot or will attempt*) to 2 (*child accomplishes the task*) and administration time is 45–60 minutes. Test-retest reliability is 0.99 for the Total Score, 0.95 for the Gross Motor Scale, and 0.8 for the Fine Motor Scale (Folio & Fewell, 2000). The authors claim good construct validity with other instruments and good discriminate validity. The PDMS activity cards form an additional component that can be used to provide an instructional curriculum that strengthens emerging skills and sets objectives for skills not attained. Palisano and Haley (1993) used these activity cards to evaluate interventions for children with cerebral palsy and other developmental disabilities.

The Bruininks-Oseretsky Test of Motor Proficiency (Bruininks, 1978) was developed to assess gross and fine motor skills and thereby determine therapeutic and educational placement. It is designed for use in children ages $4^1/_2$–$14^1/_2$ years. The normative sample consisted of 765 children who were stratified by sex, age, community size, and geographic location. Fine motor subtests include coordination of upper limbs, speed of response, visual-motor control, and speed and dexterity of the upper limbs. The gross motor subtests assess speed and agility while running, turning, balance, bilateral coordination, and strength. Administration time is 45–60 minutes. The test's reliability and validity are reported as good, and it is a useful measure for determining limitations in children with no obvious disabilities. A 14-item short form was developed from the standardization program. The short form is designed to yield an estimate of general motor development.

The Early Screening Profiles (ESP) (Harrison et al., 1990) tool measures motor, cognitive/language, and developmental skills in children. The ESP consists of three profiles: motor, cognitive/language, and self-help/social. Four surveys complement the profiles by adding important information from additional sources. These surveys measure health, home environment, articulation, and behavior and can be used in any combination.

The Alberta Infant Motor Scale (AIMS) (Piper & Darrah, 1995) measures gross motor maturation of infants from birth to the time of independent ambulation. Postural control is rated in terms of supine, prone, sitting, and standing positions. The norming sample consisted of 2,200 infants who were stratified by age and sex. Reliability and validity sampling was established on 506 infants using the AIMS, the Bayley Scales, and the Peabody. Concurrent validity scores with the Bayley and Peabody scales were 0.98 and 0.97, respectively (Piper, Pinnell, Darrah, Maguire, & Byrne, 1992).

The GMFM (Russell et al., 2002), a test for children with cerebral palsy, is specifically designed and validated for measuring change over time in gross motor function. This test contains 88 items of gross motor function, which are distributed across five dimensions to measure how much children can do, not the quality with which they do it. These categories include lying and rolling; sitting; crawling and kneeling; standing; and walking, running, and jumping. All of these skills are achievable by 5-year-old children with typical motor function. Reliability and validity studies show good responsiveness to change and interrater reliability.

The authors of the original GMFM (Russell et al., 1989) also developed the Gross Motor Performance Measure (GMPM) (Boyce et al., 1991; Boyce et al., 1995; Gowland et al., 1995). This test was specifically designed to evaluate the quality of movement in children with cerebral palsy. The test measures alignment, stability, coordination, weight shift, and dissociation. Scores range from 1 (*severely abnormal*) to 5 (*consistently normal*). Correlations between the GMFM and GMPM were not consistent across age groups and diagnoses. The researchers confirm that more studies are needed to support the reliability and validity of the GMPM.

The Beery-Buktenica Developmental Test of Visual-Motor Integration (VMI) (4th ed.) (Beery & Buktenica, 1997) assesses the degree to which visual perception and motor behavior are integrated. It can help identify visual-motor problems before they develop into more serious difficulties. The VMI consists of geometric figures arranged in order of increasing difficulty. The child uses a pencil and paper to copy the figures as accurately as possible. The Motor-Free Visual perceptual test measures visual perception and visual memory without requiring a motor response (Colarusso & Hamel, 1972).

Functional/Adaptive Status Assessment

The ninth area of assessment includes functional assessment of daily living skills (often called *adaptive skills*) to understand children's functional strengths and limitations. Key areas include essential activities of self-care, mobility, communication, and social learning (Msall et al., 1994; Newborg et al., 1984; Sparrow et al., 1984). Functional assessment determines as accurately as possible an individual's ability to perform the tasks of daily living and to fulfill the social roles expected of a typically developing peer from the same culture (Granger, Seltzer, & Fishbein, 1987). The key tasks include feeding, dressing, bathing, maintaining continency, mobility, communication, play, and social interaction (Msall, 1996). The social roles expected include involvement with peers and attending school.

Until the 1980s, the functional status of VLBW or ELBW survivors had received relatively little empirical study despite general recognition that survivors were at greater risk than full-term children for major neurodevelopmental impairments (e.g., cerebral palsy, mental retardation, visual and hearing impairments), minor neurodevelopmental impairments (e.g., communicative, perceptual, coordination, learning, and attentional disorders), and educational achievement difficulties (e.g., reading, math, and written language disorders) (Allen, 1993; Bregman & Kimberlin, 1993; Flynn, 1995; Hack & Fanaroff, 1988; Hack et al., 1994; Herrgard, Karjalainen, Martikainen, & Heinonen, 1995; Lipkin, 1996; McCormick, 1989; Msall, Buck, Rogers, & Catanzaro, 1992; Msall, DiGaudio, & Duffy, 1993; Victorian Infant Collaborative Study Group, 1991). Part of the difficulty in measuring functional status was the lack of an appropriate model for defining functional limitations and relating their impact on performance status at home, at school, and in the community (Msall et al., 1993).

As noted in Table 17, four functional outcome measures are available to pediatric professionals. The PEDI (Haley et al., 1992) assesses developmental skills in self-care, mobility, and social function; caregiver assistance; and modification of environment for children from ages 6 months to $7^{1}/_{2}$ years. Social function includes communication, problem resolution, play, peer and adult interaction, memory, household chores, self-protection, and community safety. It has been used for children with traumatic brain injury and children with cerebral palsy after rhizotomy (DiScala, Grant, Brooke, & Gans, 1992; McLaughlin et al., 1994). Rasch analysis has been used to clarify item difficulties and help prioritize rehabilitation goals (Haley, Ludlow, & Coster, 1993). The caregiver assistance areas overlap with the WeeFIM, and the tool has the advantages of multiregional norms and Spanish version availability.

The WeeFIM (UDSMR, 1998) consists of 18 items in six domains: self-care, sphincter control, transfers, locomotion, communication, and social cognition. The child is given a rating for all 18 items based on his or her level of independence. The WeeFIM has been normed on a Western New York population of more than 500 children ages 1–7 years without disabilities; it has been used extensively in children with neurodevelopmental disabilities ($n = 700$) to monitor functional status (Msall, 1996). Pilot validation studies included extreme prematurity, spina bifida, cerebral palsy, Down syndrome, congenital limb disorders, traumatic brain injuries, and ROP (Msall et al., 2000). The WeeFIM proves to have excellent test–retest reliability as well as concurrent validity with psychological and educational measures of adaptive functioning (Ottenbacher et al., 1997, 1999). An additional feature of the WeeFIM is excellent equivalence reliability of face-to-face or telephone interviews (Ottenbacher et al., 1996). Parents, educators, and allied health professionals have reported that the WeeFIM provides useful information about functional strengths and challenges for both typically developing children and children with developmental delays.

The Vineland Adaptive Behavior Scales (VABS) measures communication, daily living, socialization, and motor skills in children from birth to 18 years (Sparrow et al., 1984). The VABS has been used with children with motor, cognitive, and sensory disabilities. Rosenbaum, Saigal, Szatmari, and Hoult (1995) advocated its use for describing degrees of disability in children who were born with very low birth weights. In older children, the communication domain includes reading and written language; the daily living skills include domestic skills and extended activities of daily living such as shopping, accessing transportation, and meal preparation. The socialization domain includes play and leisure skills as well as coping skills. The VABS consists of 301 items and takes 45–60 minutes to administer. Internal consistency, test-retest reliability, and the interrater reliability range from good to excellent. High concurrent validity has been reported between the communication domain of the VABS and other cognitive and achievement tests.

The Battelle Developmental Inventory (BDI) is a developmental educational assessment battery for children from birth to 8 years with or without developmental delays (Newborg et al., 1984). The BDI consists of five domains: personal-social, adaptive, motor, communicative, and cognitive. It is widely used in early intervention programs and preschools, and it can be used in educational settings to determine kindergarten readiness and the need for special education services. The number of items in the early age range is quite limited, restricting its utility for young infants.

Kindergarten Readiness Assessment

The following components are embedded in the concept of kindergarten readiness: cognitive skills, language skills, perceptual skills, motor coordination, attention abilities, and social maturity. When applying readiness batteries to at-risk populations, investigators must obtain essential information to document developmental competencies but should not subject children to extensive neuropsychological evaluations unless complex motor, cognitive, communicative, perceptual, or attentional impairments are of concern to parents or teachers.

Several approaches have been used to measure kindergarten readiness. One approach used in European and Australian studies define some children as slow learners—that is, children with IQ scores more than one standard deviation below the mean (IQ score of less than 85) are not ready for kindergarten. A second approach to establish readiness is the discrepancy model—that is, children with a 10- to 15-point (or more) discrepancy between dimensions of the test (e.g., verbal IQ score = 80, performance IQ score = 95) are not ready for kindergarten. Neither the slow learner model nor the discrepancy model accurately predicts learning. The third approach is to use a standardized global developmental screening instrument, such as the Denver II (Frankenburg, Dodds, Archer, Shapiro, & Bresnick, 1990), Florida Kindergarten Screening Battery (1982), or the Revised Gesell Scales (Knobloch, Stevens, & Malone, 1980), These global screening tools, however, do not have adequate sensitivity and specificity to predict academic performance when applied to large populations of children. The fourth strategy is to use formal educationally specific instruments, including the CDI (Ireton, 1992), the Kaufman Survey of Early Academic and Language Skills (K-SEALS) (Kaufman & Kaufman, 1993), the Kindergarten Readiness Test (KRT) (Larson & Vitali, 1988), the Learning Accomplishment

Table 18. Kindergarten readiness scales

	Miller Assessment for Preschool (MAP) (Miller, 1988)	Learning Accomplishment Profile (LAP-D) (Nehring et al., 1992)	Child Development Inventory (CDI) (Ireton, 1992)	Mullen Scales of Early Learning (MSEL): AGS Edition (Mullen, 1995)
Purpose	Discriminate measure of Sensory and Motor, Cognitive, and Combined Skills for children ages 2 years, 9 months–5 years, 8 months	Norm-referenced tool to assess Fine Motor, Cognitive, Language, and Gross Motor skills for children ages 30–72 months	Norm-referenced tool to assess Social, Self-Help, Gross Motor, Fine Motor, Expression, Comprehension, Letters, Numbers, and General Development for children ages 15 months–6 years	Tool that measures Cognitive and Motor function for preschool children birth through age 68 months
Standardization	Normative sample of 1,204 children without disabilities stratified by age, sex, race, community size, and socioeconomic status	Sample of 792 children stratified by sex, race, community size, and receipt of public or private child care	Convenience sample of 568 children, including 14 with disabilities 95% of children in the sample were Caucasian	1,849 children without disabilities standardized on a national sample of children from English-speaking homes
Reliability	Interrater: 0.84–0.99 Test–Retest: 72%–94% Internal consistency: 0.82	Internal Consistency: 0.74 to 0.92	Scale by age: 0.33–0.96	Internal Consistency: 0.75–0.91 Test–Retest: 0.71–0.96 Interrater: 0.91–0.99

Profile (LAP-D) (Nehring et al., 1992), the Miller Assessment for Preschoolers (MAP) (Miller, 1988), and the Mullen Scales of Early Learning (MSEL) (Mullen, 1995). These instruments are described in Table 18. A fifth strategy is to use the criteria of school districts combining independent psychoeducational assessments, parents' reports, and teachers' reports of classroom skills. Overall, by having a broad perspective on the transition to kindergarten, investigators and clinicians can understand the interaction among developmental competencies, functional skills, and neurobehavioral maturity. Perspectives on determining kindergarten readiness should also include preschool experiences and community resources available to populations that are ethnically diverse and of low socioeconomic status (Meisels, 1987).

NEONATAL FOLLOW-UP TEAM

Table 19 lists the members of the neonatal follow-up team and their typical responsibilities. A follow-up program functions most efficiently with a closely coordinated team and a director who is responsible for overseeing the program's clinical and administrative components. The clinic coordinator is in charge of scheduling patients, tracking, preparing charts, scheduling clinic visits, distributing reports and letters, and collecting data.

One issue that may arise centers on which professional should perform follow-up assessments. A variety of professionals—physicians, nurse practitioners, and therapists—can administer medical and neuromotor assessments. The key for individuals administering the neuromotor assessments is to establish interrater reliability. The developmental assessments can be administered by a psychologist, a school psychologist, a developmental therapist, or a psychometrist as long as the examiner has had the proper training and has established interrater reliability.

Because the children in the follow-up clinic may be socially at risk in addition to biologically at risk, having a social worker as a resource is important. Another

Table 19. Members of the neonatal follow-up team and their responsibilities

Position	Responsibilities
Clinic coordinator	Coordinates daily clinic activities
Data analyst	Manages the database and completes analyses as needed
Data entry personnel	Enters necessary data for clinic database
Developmental pediatrician	Participates in the weekly clinic to complete medical, sensory, neurologic, functional, developmental, and family assessments
Neonatal fellow	
Neonatologist	
Pediatric nurse practitioner	
Therapist (occupational, physical, or speech-language)	
Medical director	Oversees the clinic's activities
Nutritionist	Provides nutritional assessments and intervention
Psychologist/psychometrist	Conducts psychometric assessments
Secretary	Provides support for director and coordinator as needed
Social worker	Provides consultation as needed
Student volunteer	Obtains histories and anthropometrics as needed

professional who is taking on a greater role in follow-up is the nutritionist. Many of these children have feeding and growth problems requiring intensive support and intervention.

Additional contributors to the program may be medical or undergraduate students who assist for a semester as part of a clinical rotation. Once trained, students can perform a basic history assessment, obtain anthropometric measurements, assist during physical exams, and help entertain siblings in the waiting room. Programs collecting data for quality assurance or for research studies have data forms, which are handled by data entry personnel and data analysts. The clinic's secretary assists in preparing and sending clinic reports and letters to primary care providers, early intervention providers, and school departments.

The goal of any follow-up program must be to achieve a comprehensive, coordinated, culturally sensitive interdisciplinary assessment that minimizes stress for the child and family. Family members take active roles in the assessment process by sharing their concerns, joys, and wishes for their child and family. After the evaluation has been completed and discussed with the family, the team then makes final recommendations to the family.

Service for Families of NICU Graduates

Having an infant as an unexpected resident of the NICU, with its high-technology atmosphere, is stressful for all families. Hospitalization is often described as a roller coaster ride, with ups and downs related to alternating periods of increased medical acuity and recovery. During the hospitalization, certain professionals provide the majority of the day-to-day care. The joyful prospect of taking a baby home is often overshadowed by anxiety about taking over the infant's care. Fears about the child's outcome are very real for most families. Preparing a family for discharge by having the parents gradually assume more responsibility for their infant's care is an important contribution to a successful discharge. Assisting the family in gaining access to community resources begins while the infant is still in the NICU. NICU staff need to provide both the parents and the primary physician with information regarding 1) the infant's medical and developmental conditions; 2) all medications and doses; 3) nutritional needs, the specifics of formula mixing, and a copy of the hospital growth chart; 4) recommendations regarding a home monitor, supplemental oxygen, or other life-support equipment. In addition, the following arrangements should be made: a primary care appointment within 2 weeks of discharge; appointments with the follow-up program staff and other consultants; and schedules for support services, including home care, visiting nurse services, WIC (Special Supplemental Nutrition Program for Women, Infants and Children), Supplemental Security Income (SSI), and early intervention services.

Teaching within the Follow-Up Program

Follow-up programs provide an ideal environment for educating health care professionals (physicians, psychologists, therapists, nurses, social workers and educators) and families. Involved in the longitudinal evaluation of high-risk infants, professionals learn to recognize both the resiliencies and challenges that these children and their families face. Participation in follow-up programs enables health professionals to appreciate the impact of conditions such as CLD, GER, NEC, and apnea on family life and health services. Professionals also realize the strengths and weaknesses of primary care systems and community supports for children. Understanding the complexity of cerebral palsy and other neurologic syndromes is also a key component of longitudinal participation in neonatal follow-up. Learning to observe and describe emerging postural control, hand skills, and prelinguistic milestones contributes to an appreciation of developmental competencies in early childhood. Family stressors resulting from technology dependency (e.g., tracheostomy, gastrostomy, colostomy), sensory impairments (vision and hearing), and severe developmental disabilities can also be appreciated.

Physical and occupational therapists learn that the majority of NICU graduates do not have cerebral palsy or severe developmental disabilities. They may begin to understand that central hypotonia (i.e., low tone without weakness) is not a neuromuscular disorder precluding motor progress and that transient dystonia is not the same as cerebral palsy. Finally, they would begin to appreciate the positive changes that are part of the natural history of children with diplegia and hemiplegia and to celebrate the inherent resiliency of children.

Another educational function of NICU follow-up programs is to provide an environment for better understanding the need for family supports, for facilitating early intervention professionals' recognition of the complexity of children at highest risk, and for the education of policy makers. Although the majority of NICU graduates do not have neurosensory disabilities, high rates of speech, perceptual, attention, educational, and learning difficulties exist. When training health professionals, the importance of functional observation, family support, and an enablement framework can ensure quality home visiting services, comprehensive early intervention services, early childhood education services, and family supports. In this way, children's resiliency can be celebrated, and family supports and quality of life can be optimized among children with complex challenges.

Data Management

Accurate measurement of the quality indicators for a NICU requires a dependable and user-friendly data management program. The data analyst has the important role of coordinating the data entry and then analyzing the data on the baseline descriptive data collected by the program and on all ongoing research protocols. The data analyst's specific responsibilities include implementing and managing a database system, setting up the databases for specific research protocols, maintaining the computer software to accurately collect and analyze data, and analyzing and assisting in the interpretation of data for the clinical and research staff. Inherent in these responsibilities is the preservation and protection of patient rights and confidentiality. Data may be collected and coordinated for the single site, or it may be linked to other databases for multicenter data analyses. The data analyst assists in the preparation of presentations and publications from the site.

Each site must establish its own quality indicators. Possible neonatal benchmarks may include survival, length of stay, the incidence of BPD, and the incidence of IVH. Additional benchmarks might include the number of referrals to the follow-up program, the number of NICU graduates who receive visiting nursing services, and the implementation of early intervention plans. Examples of outcome benchmarks could relate to growth on a standard growth curve (e.g., greater than 10%), normal neurologic status, and developmental status within 2 standard deviations of the norm.

Parental compliance and participation in the follow-up program and the need for community resource referrals should also be considered.

CONCLUSION

Maternal, neonatal and postneonatal, biological, and environmental factors contribute to the outcomes of NICU infants. As increasing numbers of infants at the limits of viability survive, a large number of children with complex neurologic, genetic, and medical disorders face new challenges. Primary care providers and neonatal follow-up programs must remain vigilant in neurodevelopmental and psychosocial surveillance and advocate for quality comprehensive early childhood family supports.

References

Abad, F., Díaz, N.M., Domenech, E., Robayna, M., & Rico, J. (1996). Oral sweet solution reduces pain-related behaviour in preterm infants. *Acta Paediatrica*, *85*, 854–858.

Accardo, P.J., Capute, A.J., Visintainer, P.F., Leppert, M., Rogers, B., Msall, M., Voight, R., & Whitman, B.Y. (in press). *The Capute Scales.* Baltimore: Paul H. Brookes Publishing Co.

Achenbach, T.M. (1991). *Manual for the Child Behavior Checklist 4–18 and 1991 Profile.* Burlington: University of Vermont Department of Psychiatry.

Achenbach, T.M., & Rescorla, L.A. (2000). *Manual for the Achenbach System of Empirically Based Assessment (ASEBA) Preschool Forms and Profiles: Child Behavior Checklists for Ages 1^1/2–5, Language Development Survey, and Caregiver–Teacher Report Form. An integrated system of multi-informant assessment.* Burlington: University of Vermont, Research Center for Children, Youth, and Families.

Achenbach, T.M., & Rescorla, L.A. (2001). *Manual for the Achenbach System of Empirically Based Assessment (ASEBA) School-Age Forms and Profiles: Child Behavior Checklists for Ages 6–18, Teacher's Report Form, and Youth Self-Report.* Burlington: University of Vermont, Research Center for Children, Youth, and Families.

Adams, J.A., Zabaleta, I.A., & Sackner, M.A. (1994). Comparison of supine and prone noninvasive measurements of breathing patterns is fullterm newborns. *Pediatric Pulmonology*, *18*, 8–12.

Affleck, G., & Tennen, H. (1991). The effect of newborn intensive care on parents' psychological well-being. *Child Health Care*, *20*, 6–14.

Affonso, D., Bosque, E., Wahlberg, V., & Brady, J.P. (1993). Reconciliation and healing for mothers through skin-to-skin contact provided in an American tertiary level intensive care nursery. *Neonatal Network*, *12*(3), 25–32.

Ahmann, P.A., Lazzara, A., Dykes, F.D., Brann, A.W., & Schwartz, J.F. (1980). Intraventricular hemorrhage in the high risk preterm infant: Incidence and outcome. *Annals of Neurology*, *7*, 118–124.

Allan, W.C., Holt, P.J., Sawyer, L.R., Tito, A.M., & Meade, S.K. (1982). Ventricular dilatation after neonatal periventricular-intraventricular hemorrhage. *American Journal of Disease of Children*, *136*, 589–593.

Allen, M.C. (1993). The high-risk infant. *Pediatric Clinics of North America*, *40*, 479–490.

Allen, M.C., & Capute, A.J. (1989). Neonatal neurodevelopment examination as a predictor of neuromotor outcome in premature infants. *Pediatrics*, *83*, 498–505.

Allen, M.C., & Capute, A.J. (1990). Tone and reflex development before term. *Pediatrics*, *85*(3, Pt. 2), 393–399.

Als, H. (1982). Toward a synactive theory of development: Promise for the assessment and support of infant individuality. *Infant Mental Health Journal*, *3*, 229–243.

Als, H. (1986). A synactive model of neonatal behavioral organization: Framework for the assessment of neurobehavioral development in the premature infant and for support of infants and parents in the neonatal intensive care environment. *Physical & Occupational Therapy in Pediatrics*, *6*, 3–53.

Als, H. (1995). *Manual for the Naturalistic Observation of Newborn Behavior: Newborn Individualized Developmental Care and Assessment Program (NIDCAP).* Unpublished document, Harvard Medical School, Boston.

Als, H. (1997a). Earliest intervention for preterm infants in the newborn intensive care unit. In M.J. Guralnick (Ed.), *The effectiveness of early intervention* (pp. 47–76). Baltimore: Paul H. Brookes Publishing Co.

Als, H. (1997b). The role of relationship-based developmentally supportive newborn intensive care in strengthening outcome of preterm infants. *Seminars in Perinatology, 21*, 178–189.

Als, H., & Duffy, F.H. (1989). Neurobehavioral assessment in the newborn period: Opportunity for early detection of later learning disabilities and for early intervention. *Birth Defects, 25*, 127–152.

Als, H., & Gibes, R. (1986). *Newborn individualized developmental care and assessment program (NID-CAP): Training guide.* Unpublished document, Department of Psychiatry at Children's Hospital, Boston.

Als, H., Lawhon, G., Brown, E., Gibes, R., Duffy, F.H., & McAnulty, G. (1986). Individualized behavioral and environmental care for the very low birth weight preterm infant at high risk for bronchopulmonary dysplasia: Neonatal intensive care unit and developmental outcome. *Pediatrics, 78*, 1123–1132.

Als, H., Lawhon, G., Duffy, F.H., McAnulty, G.B., Gibes-Grossman, R., & Blickman, J.G. (1994). Individualized developmental care for the very low-birth-weight preterm infant: Medical and neurofunctional effects. *Journal of the American Medical Association, 272*(11), 853–858.

Als, H., Lester, B.M., & Brazelton, T.B. (1979). Dynamics of the behavioral organization of the premature infant: A theoretical perspective. In T.M. Field, A.M. Sostek, S. Goldberg, & H.H. Shuman (Eds.), *Infants born at risk* (pp. 173–193). New York: Spectrum Publications.

Als, H., Lester, B.M., Tronick, E.Z., & Brazelton, T.B. (1982a). Manual for the Assessment of Preterm Infants' Behavior (APIB). In H.E. Fitzgerald, B.M. Lester, & M.W. Yogman (Eds.), *Theory and research in behavioral pediatrics: Vol. 1.* (pp. 65–132). New York: Kluwer Academic/Plenum Publishers.

Als, H., Lester, B.M., Tronick, E.Z., & Brazelton T.B. (1982b). Toward a research instrument for the Assessment of Preterm Infants' Behavior (APIB). In H.E. Fitzgerald, B.M. Lester, & M.W. Yogman (Eds.), *Theory and research in behavioral pediatrics* (pp. 36–63). New York: Kluwer Academic/Plenum Publishers.

Amemiya, F., Vos, J.E., & Prechtl, H.F. (1991). Effects of prone and supine position on heart rate, respiratory rate and motor activity in fullterm newborn infants. *Brain & Development, 13*, 148–154.

American Academy of Pediatrics. (1996). Positioning and sudden infant death syndrome (SIDS) update: American Academy of Pediatrics Task Force on Infant Positioning and SIDS. *Pediatrics, 98*(6, Pt. 1), 1216–1218.

American Academy of Pediatrics Committee on Environmental Health. (1997). Noise: A hazard for the fetus and newborn. *Pediatrics, 100*, 724–727.

American Medical Association. (1974). *American Medical Association Committee on Maternal and Child Care: Action guide for maternal and child care committees.* Chicago: Author.

American Occupational Therapy Association. (1997). *Neonatal therapy services for children and youth under the Individuals with Disabilities Education Act.* Bethesda, MD: Author.

Amiel-Tison, C. (1996). Does neurological assessment still have a place in the NICU? *Acta Paediatrica Supplement, 416*, 31–38.

Amiel-Tison, C., & Grenier, A. (1986). *Neurological assessment during the first year of life.* New York: Oxford University Press.

Anand, K.J. (1998). Clinical importance of pain and stress in preterm neonates. *Biology of the Neonate, 73*, 1–9.

Anand, K.J. (2000). Effects of perinatal pain and stress. *Progress in Brain Research, 122*, 117–129.

Anderson, C.L., & Stewart, J.E. (1997). Retinopathy of prematurity. In J.P. Cloherty & A.R. Stark (Eds.), *Manual of neonatal care* (4th ed., pp. 643–648). Philadelphia: Lippincott, Williams & Wilkins.

Andrews, K.A., & Fitzgerald, M. (1994). The cutaneous withdrawal reflex in human neonates: sensitization, receptive fields, and the effects of contralateral stimulation. *Pain, 56*, 95–101.

Anzalone, M. (1994). Neonatal therapy in neonatology: What is our ethical responsibility? *American Journal of Occupational Therapy, 48*, 563–566.

Appleton, S.M. (1997). Handle with care: An investigation of the handling received by preterm infants in intensive care. *Journal of Neonatal Nursing, 3*(3), 23–27.

Arango, P. (1999). A parent's perspective on family-centered care. *Journal of Developmental and Behavioral Pediatrics, 20*, 123–124.

Ashbaugh, J.B., Leick-Rude, M.K., & Kilbride, H.W. (1999). Developmental care teams in the neonatal intensive care unit: Survey on current status. *Journal of Perinatolgy, 19*, 48–52.

Askie, L.M., & Henderson-Smart, D.J. (2001). Gradual versus abrupt discontinuation of oxygen in preterm or low birth weight infants. *Cochrane Database Systematic Review, 4,* CD001075.

Avery, G.B. (1987). *Neonatolgy: Pathophysiology and management of the newborn.* Philadelphia: Lippincott, Williams & Wilkins.

Ayres, J.A. (1972). *Sensory integration and learning disorders.* Los Angeles: Western Psychological Services.

Bachman, D.H., & Lind, R.F. (1997). Perinatal social work and the family of the newborn intensive care infant. *Social Work in Health Care, 24*(3/4), 21–37.

Bader, D., Tirosh, E., Hodgins, H., Abend, M., & Cohen, A. (1998). Effect of increased environmental temperature on breathing patterns in preterm and term infants. *Journal of Perinatology, 18,* 5–8.

Bailey, D.B., Jr., Bruer, J.T., Symons, F.J., & Lichtman, J.W. (Eds.). (2001). *Critical thinking about critical periods.* Baltimore: Paul H. Brookes Publishing Co.

Baird, D. (1969a). An area maternity service. *The Lancet, 1*(7593), 515–519.

Baird, D. (1969b). Perinatal mortality. *The Lancet, 1*(7593), 511–515.

Baird, T.M., Paton, J.B., & Fisher, D.E. (1992, July/August). Improved oxygenation with prone positioning in neonates: Stability of increased transcutaneous PO_2. *Neonatal Intensive Care,* 43–46.

Ballard, J.L., Khoury, J.C., Wedig, K., Wang, L., Eilers-Walsman, B.L., & Lipp, R. (1991). New Ballard score, expanded to include extremely premature infants. *Journal of Pediatrics, 119,* 417–423.

Barnard, K.E. (1978). NCAST publication CDMRC, Res. 110, WJ-10. Seattle: University of Washington.

Barr, R.G., Chen, S., Hopkins, B., & Westra, T. (1996). Crying patterns in preterm infants. *Developmental Medicine and Child Neurology, 38,* 345–355.

Barr, R.G., Quek, V.S., Cousineau, D., Oberlander, T.F., Brian, J.A., & Young, S.N. (1994). Effects of intra-oral sucrose on crying, mouthing, and hand-to-mouth contact in newborn and six-week-old infants. *Developmental Medicine and Child Neurology, 36,* 608–618.

Barratt, M.S., Roach, M.A., & Leavitt, L.A. (1992). Early channels of mother–infant communication: Preterm and term infants. *Journal of Child Psychology and Psychiatry, 33,* 1193–1204.

Bartlett, D. (1997). Primitive reflexes and early motor development. *Journal of Developmental and Behavioral Pediatrics, 18,* 151–157.

Bass, L.S. (1991). What do parents need when their infant is a patient in the NICU? *Neonatal Network, 10*(4), 25–33.

Bates, J.E. (1987). Temperament in infancy. In J.D. Osofsky (Ed.), *Handbook of infant development* (2nd ed., pp. 1101–1149). New York: John Wiley & Sons.

Bateson, P. (1996). Design for a life. In D. Magnusson (Ed.), *The lifespan development of individuals: Behavioral, neurobiological, and psychosocial perspectives* (pp. 1–20). New York: Cambridge University Press.

Bauer, K., Pyper, A., Sperling, P., Uhrig, C., & Versmold, H. (1998). Effects of gestational and postnatal age on body temperature, oxygen consumption, and activity during early skin-to-skin contact between preterm infants of 25–30 week gestation and their mothers. *Pediatric Research, 44,* 247–251.

Bayley, N. (1969). *Bayley Scales of Infant Development: Birth to two years.* San Antonio, TX: The Psychological Corporation.

Bayley, N. (1993). *Bayley Scales of Infant Development—Second Edition (BSID-II) Manual.* San Antonio, TX: The Psychological Corporation.

Beal, J.A., & Quinn, M. (2002). The nurse practitioner role in the NICU as perceived by parents. *American Journal of Maternal and Child Nursing, 27,* 183–188.

Beauchamp, G.K., Cowart, B.J., Mennella, J.A., & Marsh, R.R. (1994). Infant salt taste: Developmental, methodological, and contextual factors. *Developmental Psychobiology, 27,* 353–365.

Becker, P.T., Grunwald, P.C., Moorman, J., & Stuhr, S. (1991). Outcomes of developmentally supportive nursing care for very low birthweight infants. *Nursing Research, 40,* 150–155.

Becker, P.T., Grunwald, P.C., Moorman, J., & Stuhr, S. (1993). Effects of developmental care on behavioral organization in very-low-birth-weight infants. *Nursing Research, 42,* 214–220.

Beers, M.H., & Berkow, M.H. (Eds.). (1999). *The Merck manual of diagnosis and therapy* (17th ed./ centennial ed.). New York: McGraw-Hill.

Beery, K.E., & Buktenica, N.A. (1997). *The Beery-Buktenica Developmental Test of Visual-Motor Integration* (4th ed.). Parsippany, NJ: Modern Curriculum Press.

Bell, P.L. (1997). Adolescent mothers' perceptions of the neonatal intensive care unit environment. *Journal of Perinatal and Neonatal Nursing, 11,* 77–84.

Bellefeuille-Reid, D., & Jakubek, S. (1989). Adaptive positioning intervention for premature infants: Issues for paediatric occupational therapy practice. *British Journal of Occupational Therapy, 52*(3), 93–96.

Bennett, F.C., Robinson, N.M., & Sells, C.J. (1982). Hyaline membrane disease, birth weight, and gestational age. Effects on development in the first two years. *American Journal of Diseases of Children, 136,* 888–891.

Berger, S.P., Holt-Turner, I., Cupoli, J.M., Mass, M., & Hageman, J.R. (1998). Caring for the graduate from the neonatal intensive care unit. At home, in the office, and in the community. *Pediatric Clinics of North America, 45,* 701–712.

Bier, J.B., Ferguson, A., Anderson, L., Solomon, E., Voltas, C., Oh, W., & Vohr, B.R. (1993). Breast-feeding of very low birth weight infants. *Journal of Pediatrics, 123,* 773–778.

Bier, J.B., Ferguson, A.E., Morales, Y., Liebling, J.A., Archer, D., Oh, W., & Vohr, B.R. (1996). Comparison of skin-to-skin contact with standard contact in low-birthweight infants who are breast-fed. *Archives of Pediatrics & Adolescent Medicine, 150,* 1265–1269.

Bigsby, R. (1994). *Motor behaviors as cues to cardiorespiratory reactivity in full-term and preterm infants at three months corrected age.* Unpublished dissertation, Sargent College of Allied Health Professions, Boston University.

Bigsby, R., Coster, W., Lester, B.M., & Peucker, M.R. (1996). Motor behavioral cues of term and preterm infants at 3 months. *Infant Behavior and Development, 19,* 295–307.

Bing, S.G., & Bing, J.R. (1985). Comparison of the K-ABC and PPVT-R with Head Start children. *Psychology in the Schools, 22,* 245–249.

Biringen, Z., & Robinson, J. (1991). Emotional availability in mother–child interactions: A reconceptualization for research. *American Journal of Orthopsychiatry, 61,* 258–271.

Birren, J.E., Kinney, D.K., Schaie, K.W., & Woodruff, D.S. (Eds.). (1981). *Developmental psychology: A lifetime approach.* Boston: Houghton Mifflin.

Bishop, G.C., & Lobo, M.L. (1994). Case study of a high-risk neonate failing to thrive post-extracorporeal membrane oxygenation and post-necrotizing enterocolitis. *Journal of Pediatric Nursing, 9,* 166–174.

Bjornson, K.F., Deitz, J.C., Blackburn, S., Billingsley, F., Garcia, J., & Hays, R. (1992). The effect of body position on the oxygen saturation of ventilated preterm infants. *Pediatric Physical Therapy, 5,* 109–115.

Blackburn, S.T. (1996). Research utilization: Modifying the NICU light environment. *Neonatal Network, 15*(4), 63–66.

Blackburn, S.T., & Loper, D.L. (1992). *Maternal, fetal and neonatal physiology: A clinical perspective.* Philadelphia: W.B. Saunders.

Blasco, P.A. (1989). Preterm birth: To correct or not to correct. *Developmental Medicine and Child Neurology, 31,* 816–826.

Blass, E.M. (1997). Infant formula quiets crying human newborns. *Journal of Developmental and Behavioral Pediatrics, 18,* 162–165.

Blass, E.M., & Ciaramitaro, V. (1994). A new look at some old mechanisms in human newborns: Taste and tactile determinants of state, affect, and action. *Monographs of the Society for Research in Child Development, 59*(1, I–V), 1–81.

Bleck, E.E. (1987). Orthopedic management of cerebral palsy. *Clinics in Developmental Medicine, 100,* 142–147.

Bloom, B.T. (2001). Invited commentary: "In search of excellence—the Neonatal Intensive Care Quality Improvement Collaborative." *Baylor University Medical Center Proceedings, 14,* 97–98.

Blumenthal, I., & Lealman, G.T. (1982). Effect of posture on gastro-esophageal reflux in the newborn. *Archives of Disease in Childhood, 57,* 555–556.

Bobath, K., & Bobath, B. (1984). Neurodevelopmental treatment. In D. Scrutton (Ed.), *Clinics in developmental medicine: No. 90. Management of the motor disorders of children with cerebral palsy* (pp. 6–18). New York: Cambridge University Press.

Bohnhorst, B., Heyne, T., Peter, C.S., & Poets, C.F. (2001). Skin-to-skin (kangaroo) care, respiratory control, and thermoregulation. *Journal of Pediatrics, 138,* 193–197.

Boyce, W.F., Gowland, C., Hardy, S., Rosenbaum, P.L., Lane, M., Plews, N., Goldsmith, C., & Russell, D.J. (1991). Development of a quality of movement measure for children with cerebral palsy. *Physical Therapy, 71,* 820–828.

Boyce, W.F., Gowland, C., Rosenbaum, P.L., Lane, M., Plews, N., Goldsmith, C.H., Russell, D.J., Wright, V., Potter, S., & Harding, D. (1995). The Gross Motor Performance Measure (GMPM): Validity and responsiveness of a measure of quality of movement. *Physical Therapy, 71,* 603–613.

Bozynski, M.E.A., Naglie, R.A., Nicks, J.J., Burpee, B., & Johnson, R.V. (1988). Lateral positioning of the stable ventilated very-low-birthweight infant: Effect on transcutaneous oxygen and carbon dioxide. *American Journal of Diseases of Children, 142,* 200–202.

Brackbill, Y. (1970). Acoustic variation and arousal level in infants. *Psychophysiology, 6,* 517–526.

Brandon, D.B.H., Holditch-Davis, D., & Beylea, M. (1999). Nursing care and the development of sleeping and waking behaviors in preterm infants. *Research in Nursing & Health, 22,* 217–229.

Braun, M.A., & Palmer, M.M. (1985). A pilot study of oral-motor dysfunction in "at-risk" infants. *Physical & Occupational Therapy in Pediatrics, 5,* 13–25.

Brazelton, T.B. (1973). Neonatal Behavioral Assessment Scale. *Clinics in developmental medicine: No. 50.* Philadelphia: Lippincott, Williams & Wilkins.

Brazelton, T.B. (1984). Neonatal Behavioral Assessment Scale, Second Edition. *Clinics in developmental medicine: No. 88.* Philadelphia: Lippincott, Williams & Wilkins.

Brazelton, T.B. (1998). *Housecall.* Retrieved April 13, 2003 from http://www.babycenter.com/general/toddler/toilettraining/4526.html

Brazelton, T.B., & Nugent, J.K. (1995). *The Neonatal Behavioral Assessment Scale, Second Edition.* London: Mac Keith Press.

Bregman, J., & Kimberlin, L.V.S. (1993). Developmental outcome in extremely premature infants: Impact of surfactant. *Pediatric Clinics of North America, 40,* 937–953.

Bricker, D., & Squires, J. (1999). *Ages & Stages Questionnaires (ASQ): A parent-completed, child-monitoring system* (2nd ed.). Baltimore: Paul H. Brookes Publishing Co.

Browne, J.V. (2000). Considerations for touch and massage in the neonatal intensive care unit. *Neonatal Network, 19,* 61–64.

Brownell, R. (Ed.). (2000). *The Expressive One-Word Picture Vocabulary Test–2000 Edition.* Novato, CA: Academic Therapy Publications.

Bruer, J.T. (2001). A critical and sensitive period primer. In D.B. Bailey, Jr., J.T. Bruer, F.J. Symons, & J.W. Lichtman (Eds.), *Critical thinking about critical periods* (pp. 3–26). Baltimore: Paul H. Brookes Publishing Co.

Bruininks, R.H. (1978). *Bruininks-Oseretsky Test of Motor Proficiency: Examiners' Manual.* Circle Pines, MN: American Guidance Service.

Budin, P. (1907). *The Nursling: The feeding and hygiene of premature and full term infants* (W.J. Maloney, Trans.). London: The Caxton Publishing Co.

Bu'Lock, F., Woolridge, M.W., & Baum, J.D. (1990). Development of co-ordination of sucking, swallowing and breathing: Ultrasound study of term and preterm infants. *Developmental Medicine and Child Neurology, 32,* 669–78.

Burke, J.P. (1998). Play: The Life role of the infant and young child. In J. Case-Smith (Ed.), *Pediatric occupational therapy and early intervention* (2nd ed., pp. 189–206). Burlington, MA: Butterworth-Heinemann.

Campbell, M.K., Ostbye, T., & Irgens, L.M. (1997). Post-term birth: Risk factors and outcomes in a 10-year cohort of Norwegian births. *Obstetrics and Gynecology, 89,* 543–548.

Candilis-Huisman, D., & Bydlowski, M. (1997). Soothing and swaddling infants: Ancient practices, modern implications for consoling. *Ab Initio, 4,* 1.

Capute, A.J. (1996). *The Capute Scales: CAT/CLAMS instruction manual.* Baltimore: Kennedy Fellows Association.

Capute, A.J., & Accardo, P.J. (1978). Linguistic and auditory milestones during the first two years of life. *Clinical Pediatrics, 17,* 847–853.

Capute, A.J., Palmer, F.B., Shapiro, B.K., Wachtel, R.C., Schmidt, S., & Ross, A. (1986a). Clinical Linguistic and Auditory Milestone Scale: Prediction of cognition in infancy. *Developmental Medicine and Child Neurology, 128,* 762–771.

Capute, A.J., Palmer, F.B., Shapiro, B.K., Wachtel, R.C., Schmidt, S., & Ross, A. (1986b). The Clinical Linguistic and Auditory Milestone Scale (CLAMS): Identification of cognitive defects in motor delayed children. *American Journal of Diseases of Children, 140,* 694–698.

Capute, A.J., & Shapiro, B.K. (1985). The motor quotient: A method for the early detection of motor delay. *American Journal of Diseases of Children, 139,* 940–942.

Capute, A.J., Shapiro, B.K., & Palmer, F.B. (1987). Marking the milestones of language development. *Contemporary Pediatrics, 4,* 24–41.

Cartlidge, P.H.T., & Rutter, N. (1988). Reduction of head flattening in preterm infants. *Archives of Disease in Childhood, 63,* 755–757.

Case-Smith, J. (1998). Defining the early intervention process. In J. Case-Smith (Ed.), *Pediatric occupational therapy and early intervention* (2nd ed., pp. 27–48). Burlington, MA: Butterworth-Heinemann.

Case-Smith, J., & Bigsby, R. (2000). *Posture and Fine Motor Assessment of Infants*. San Antonio, TX: The Psychological Corporation.

Cashore, W.J. (1999, March). *Gastroesophageal reflux*. Unpublished lecture, Brown University School of Medicine, Providence, RI.

Chang, Y., Anderson, G.C., Dowling, D., & Lin, C. (2002). Decreased activity and oxygen desaturation in prone ventilated preterm infants during the first postnatal week. *Heart & Lung: Journal of Acute & Critical Care, 31*, 34–42.

Chang, Y., Anderson, G.C., & Lin, C. (2002). Effects of prone and supine positioning on sleep state and stress responses in mechanically ventilated preterm infants during the first postnatal week. *Journal of Advanced Nursing, 40*, 161–169.

Chang, Y.J., Lin, C.H., & Lin, L.H. (2001). Noise and related events in a neonatal intensive care unit. *Acta Paediatrica, 42*, 212–217.

Charpak, N., Ruiz-Pelaez, J.G., & Charpak, Y. (2001). A randomized, controlled trial of kangaroo mother care: Results of follow-up at 1 year corrected age. *Pediatrics, 108*, 1072–1079.

Chatoor, I., Getson, P., Menvielle, E., Brasseaux, C., O'Donnell, R.R., Rivera, Y., & Mrazek, D.A. (1997). A feeding scale for research and clinical practice to assess mother-infant interactions in the first three years of life. *Infant Mental Health, 18*, 76–91.

Chatson, K., Fant, M.E., & Cloherty, J.P. (1997). Temperature control. In J.P. Cloherty & A.R. Stark (Eds.), *Manual of neonatal care* (4th ed., pp. 139–142). Philadelphia: Lippincott, Williams & Wilkins.

Cheour-Luhtanen, M., Alho, K., Sainio, K., Rinne, T., Reinikainen, K., Pohjavuori, M., Renlund, M., Aaltonen, O., Eerola, O., & Naatanen, R. (1996). The ontogenetically earliest discriminative response of the human brain. *Psychophysiology, 33*, 478–481.

Cioni, G., Prechtl, H.F., Ferrari, F., Paolicelli, P.B., Einspieler, C., & Roversi, M.F. (1997). Which better predicts later outcome in full-term infants: quality of general movements or neurological examination? *Early Human Development, 50*, 71–85.

Clarici, A., Travan, L., Accardo, A., DeVonderweid, U., & Bava, A. (2002). Crying of a newborn child: Alarm signal or protocommunication. *Perceptual Motor Skills, 94*, 752–754.

Cloherty, J.P. (1997). Diabetes mellitus. In J.P. Cloherty & A.R. Stark (Eds.), *Manual of neonatal care* (4th ed., pp. 11–20). Philadelphia: Lippincott, Williams & Wilkins.

Cochran, W.D. (1997). Assessment of the newborn. In J.P. Cloherty & A.R. Stark (Eds.), *Manual of neonatal care* (4th ed., pp. 31–37). Philadelphia: Lippincott, Williams & Wilkins.

Coffman, S., Levitt, M.J., & Deets, C. (1991). Personal and professional support for mothers of NICU and healthy newborns. *Journal of Gynecological and Neonatal Nursing, 20*, 406–415.

Cohen, S.E. (1987). Longitudinal studies of preterm infants. In H.W. Tauesch & M.W. Yogman (Eds.), *Follow-up management of the high-risk infant* (pp. 21–28). New York: Little, Brown and Company.

Colarusso, R.P., & Hamel, D.D. (1972). *Motor-Free Visual Perception Test*. San Antonio, TX: The Psychological Corporation.

Colombo, J. (2001). The development of visual attention in infancy. *Annual Reviews in Psychology, 52*, 37–67.

Committee on Fetus and Newborn; Committee on Drugs, Section on Anesthesiology, Section on Surgery; Fetus and Newborn Committee. (2000). Prevention and management of pain and stress in the neonate. *Pediatrics, 105*, 454–461.

Conners, C.K. (1994). *Conners' Continuous Performance Test—Computer program* (Version 3.0). North Tonawanda, NY: Multi-Health Systems.

Conners, C.K. (1997). *Conners' Rating Scales–Revised*. North Tonawanda, NY: Multi-Health Systems.

Consensus Committee to Establish Recommended Standards for Newborn ICU Design. (2002). Recommended Standards for Newborn ICU Design. *Report of the Fifth Consensus Conference on Newborn ICU Design*. Clearwater Beach, FL.

Coplan, J. (1993). *Early Language Milestone, Second Edition (ELMS-2)*. Austin, TX: PRO-ED.

Corwin, M.J., Lester, B.M., Sepkoski, C., Peucker, M., Kayne, H., & Golub, H.L. (1995). Newborn acoustic cry characteristics of infants subsequently dying of sudden infant death syndrome. *Pediatrics, 96*, 73–77.

Coster, W. (1998). Occupation-centered assessment of children. *American Journal of Occupational Therapy, 52*, 337–344.

Coster, W.J. (1996, April). Toward an occupation-based view of children's development. *University of Southern California IX Occupational Science Symposium Proceedings*. Los Angeles: University of Southern California.

Cryotherapy for Retinopathy of Prematurity Cooperative Group. (2001). Multicenter trial of cryotherapy for retinopathy of prematurity: Ophthalmological outcomes at 10 years. *Archives of Ophthalmology, 119,* 1110–1118.

Curley, M.A.Q., & Meyer, E.C. (1996). The impact of the critical care experience on the family. In M.A.Q. Curley, J.B. Smith, & P.A. Moloney-Harmon (Eds.), *Critical care nursing of infants and children* (pp. 47–67). Philadelphia: W.B. Saunders.

Curzi-Dascalova, L., Peirano, P., & Christova, E. (1996). Respiratory characteristics during sleep in healthy small-for-gestation age newborns. *Pediatrics, 97,* 554–559.

Dalton, T.C. (1996, Winter). Reconstructing John Dewey's Unusual Collaboration with Myrtle McGraw in the 1930's. *Newsletter of the Society for Research in Child Development,* 1–3, 8–10.

Daniels, H., Devlieger, H., Minami, T., Eggermont, E., & Casaer, P. (1990). Infant feeding and cardiorespiratory maturation. *Neuropediatrics, 21,* 9–10.

Dann, M., & Levine, S.Z. (1958). New I: The development of prematurely born children with birth weights or minimal postnatal weights of 1000 grams or less. *Pediatrics, 22,* 1037.

D'Argassies, S.S. (1977). *Neurological development in the full-term and premature neonate.* Hillsborough, NJ: Excerpta Medica.

Davis, B.E., Moon, R.Y., Sachs, H.C., & Ottolini, M.C. (1998). Effects of sleep position on infant motor development. *Pediatrics, 102,* 1135–1140.

Davis, D.W. (1998). Long-term outcome of neonatal ECMO: What do we really know? *Pediatric Nursing, 4,* 343–347.

Davis, P.G., Thorpe, K., Roberts, R., Schmidt, B., Doyle, L.W., & Kirpalani, H. (Trial Indomethacin Prophylaxis in Preterm Investigators). (2002). Evaluating "old" definitions for the "new" bronchopulmonary dysplasia. *Journal of Pediatrics, 140*(5), 555–560.

Davis, P.M., Robinson, R., Harris, L., & Cartlidge, P.H.T. (1993). Persistent mild hip deformation in preterm infants. *Archives of Disease in Childhood, 69,* 597–598.

Davison, T.H., Karp, W.B., & Kanto, W.P. (1994). Clinical characteristics and outcomes of infants requiring long-term neonatal intensive care. *Journal of Perinatology, 14,* 461–466.

Dayton, G.O., & Jones, M.H. (1964). Analysis of characteristics of fixation reflex in infants by use of direct current electrooculography. *Neurology, 14,* 1152–1156.

Desor, J.A. (1973). Taste in acceptance of sugars by human infants. *Journal of Comparative Physiology and Psychology, 84,* 496–501.

Desor, J.A. (1975). Ingestive responses of human newborns to salty, sour, and bitter stimuli. *Journal of Comparative Physiology and Psychology, 89,* 966–970.

Dimitriou, G., Greenough, A., Pink, L., McGhee, A., Hickey, A., & Rafferty, G.F. (2002). Effects of posture on oxygenation and respiratory muscle strength in convalescent infants. *Archives of Disease in Childhood, Fetal and Neonatal Edition, 86,* F147–F150.

DiPietro, J.A., Caughy, M.O., Cusson, R., & Fox, N.A. (1994). Cardiorespiratory functioning of preterm infants: Stability and risk associations for measures of heart rate variability and oxygen saturation. *Developmental Psychobiology, 27,* 137–152.

DiScala, C., Grant, C.C., Brooke, M.A., & Gans, G.M. (1992). Functional outcome in children with traumatic brain injury: Agreement between clinical judgment and the functional independence measure. *American Journal of Physical Medicine & Rehabilitation, 71,* 145–148.

Dobbins, N., Bohlig, C., & Sutphen, J. (1994). Partners in growth: Implementing family-centered changes in the neonatal intensive care unit. *Children's Health Care, 23,* 115–126.

Dodd, V. (1996). Gestational age assessment. *Neonatal Network, 15*(1), 27–36.

Doussard-Roosevelt, J., Porges, S.W., & McClenny, B.D. (1996). Behavioral sleep states in very low birth weight preterm neonates: Relation to neonatal health and vagal maturation. *Journal of Pediatric Psychology, 21,* 785–802.

Downs, J.A., Edwards, A.D., McCormick, D.C., Roth, S.C., & Stewart, A.L. (1991). Effect of intervention on development of hip posture in very preterm infants. *Archives of Disease in Childhood, 66,* 797–801.

Drillien, C.M. (1959). Physical and mental handicaps in the prematurely born. *Journal of Obstetrics & Gynaecology of the British Commonwealth, 66,* 721.

Drillien, C.M. (1964). *The growth and development of the prematurely born infant.* Edinburgh, Scotland: E & S Livingston Ltd.

Dubowitz, L., & Dubowitz, V. (1981). The neurological assessment of the preterm and full-term infant. *Clinics in developmental medicine: No.79.* Philadelphia: Lippincott, Williams & Wilkins.

Dubowitz, L.M.S., Dubowitz, V., & Goldberg, C. (1970). Clinical assessment of gestational age in the newborn infant. *Journal of Pediatrics, 77,* 1–10.

Dunham, E.C. (1948). *Premature infants* (Children's Bureau Publication Nos. 325, 4243). Washington, DC: U.S. Government Printing Office.

Dunn, L.M., & Dunn, L.M. (1997). *Peabody Picture Vocabulary Test–Third Edition (PPVT–III)*. Circle Pines, MN: American Guidance Service.

Dunst, C.J., Trivette, C.M., & Deal, A.G. (1988). *Enabling and empowering families: Principles and guidelines for practice*. Newton-Upper Falls, MA: Brookline Books.

Ecklund-Flores, L., & Turkewitz, G. (1996). Asymmetric headturning to speech and nonspeech in human newborns. *Developmental Psychobiology, 29*, 205–217.

Education of the Handicapped Act Amendments of 1986, PL 99-457, 20 U.S.C. §§ 1400 *et seq.*

Eichenwald, E.C. (1997). Mechanical ventilation. In J.P. Cloherty & A.R. Stark (Eds.), *Manual of neonatal care* (4th ed., pp. 336–348). Philadelphia: Lippincott, Williams & Wilkins.

Elliott, C.D. (1990). *Differential Ability Scales. Introductory and technical handbook*. San Antonio, TX: The Psychological Corporation.

Emery, J.R., & Peabody, J.L. (1983). Head position affects intracranial pressure in newborn infants. *Journal of Pediatrics, 103*, 950–953.

Engler, A.J., Ludington-Hoe, S.M., Cusson, R.M., Adams, R., Bahnsen, M., Brumbaugh, E., Coates, P., Grieb, J., McHargue, L., Ryan, D.L., Settle, M., & Williams, D. (2002). Kangaroo care: National survey of practice, knowledge, barriers, and perceptions. *MCN American Journal of Maternal and Child Nursing, 27*, 146–1153.

Epstein, M.F. (1987). Major causes of neonatal mortality and morbidity. In H.W. Tauesch & M.W. Yogman (Eds.), *Follow-up management of the high-risk infant* (pp. 15–20). New York: Little, Brown and Company.

Evanochko, C., Janes-Kelley, S., Boyle, R., Fox, M., Molesky, M., & Byrne, P. (1996). Facilitating early discharge from the NICU: The development of a home gavage program and neonatal outpatient clinic. *Neonatal Network, 15*(8), 44.

Evans, P.M., Johnson, A., Mitch, L., & Alberman, A. (1989). A standard form for recording clinical findings in children with motor deficit of central origin. *Developmental Medicine and Child Neurology, 31*, 119–127.

Fanaroff, A.A., & Merkatz, I.R. (1993). Antenatal and intrapartum care of the high-risk infant. In M.H. Klaus & A.A. Fanaroff (Eds.), *Care of the high-risk neonate* (pp. 1–37). Philadelphia: W.B. Saunders.

Fantz, R.L. (1973). The origin of form perception. In R.L. Fantz (Ed.), *The nature and nurture of behavior, developmental psychobiology* (p. 36). New York: W.H. Freeman and Co.

Fantz, R.L., & Miranda, S.B. (1975). Newborn infant attention to form of contour. *Child Development, 46*, 224–228.

Fay, M.J. (1988, April). The positive effects of positioning. *Neonatal Network*, 23–28.

Feeny, D., Furlong, W., Barr, R.D., Torrance, G.W., Rosenbaum, P., & Weitzman, S.A. (1992). Comprehensive multiattribute system for classifying the health status of survivors of childhood cancer. *Journal of Clinical Oncology, 10*, 923–928.

Feeny, D., Furlong, W., Boyle, M., & Torrance, G.W. (1995). Multi-attribute health status classification systems: Health Utilities Index. *Pharmacoeconomics, 7*, 490–502.

Feeny, D.H., Torrance, G.W., Godsmith, C.H., Furlong, W., & Boyle, M. (1993). A multi-attribute approach to population health status. In *Proceedings of the Social Statistics Section: American Statistical Association* (pp. 161–166). Alexandria, VA: American Statistical Association.

Feinberg, B.B., & Repke, J.T. (1997). Preeclampsia and related conditions. In J.P. Cloherty & A.R. Stark (Eds.), *Manual of neonatal care* (4th ed., pp. 26–29). Philadelphia: Lippincott, Williams & Wilkins.

Feldman, R., Weller, A., Sirota, L., & Eidelman, A. (2002). Skin-to-skin contact (kangaroo care) promotes self-regulation in premature infants: Sleep-wake cyclicity, arousal modulation, and sustained exploration. *Developmental Psychology, 38*, 194–207.

Fenton, T.R., Geggie, J.H., Warners, J.N., & Tough, S.C. (2000). Nutrition services in Canadian neonatal intensive care: the role of the dietitian. *Canadian Journal of Dietetic Practice and Research, 61*, 172–175.

Ferrari, F., Prechtl, H.F., Cioni, G., Roversi, M.F., Einspieler, C., Gallo, C., Paolicelli, P.B., & Cavazzuti, G.B. (1997). Posture, spontaneous movements, and behavioural state organisation in infants affected by brain malformations. *Early Human Development, 50*, 87–113.

Field, T. (1980). Supplemental stimulation of preterm neonates. *Early Human Development, 4*, 301–314.

Field, T.M., Dempsey, J.R., Hatch, J., Ting, G., & Clifton, R.K. (1979). Cardiac and behavioral responses to repeated tactile and auditory stimulation by preterm and term neonates. *Developmental Psychology, 15,* 406–416.

Fiorentino, M. (1965). *Reflex testing methods for evaluating CNS development* (2nd ed.). Springfield, IL: Charles C Thomas.

Florida Kindergarten Screening Battery. (1982). Lutz, FL: Psychological Assessment Resources.

Flynn, J.T. (1995). Retinopathy of prematurity: Perspective for the nineties. *Acta Opthalmologica Scandinavica, 73,* 12–14.

Folio, M.R., & Fewell, R.R. (1983). *Peabody Developmental Motor Scales and Activity Cards.* Allen, TX: Developmental Learning Materials Teaching Resources.

Folio, M.R., & Fewell, R.R. (2000). *The Peabody Developmental Motor Scales, Second Edition (PDMS-2).* Austin, TX: PRO-ED.

Fox, H. (1997). Aging of the placenta. *Archives of Disease in Childhood, Fetal and Neonatal Edition, 77*(3), 171F–175F.

Fox, M., & Molesky, M. (1990). The effects of prone and supine positioning on arterial oxygen pressure. *Neonatal Network, 8*(4), 25–29.

Fox, R.E., Viscardi, R.M., Taciak, V.L., Niknafs, H., & Cinoman, M.I. (1993). Effect of position on pulmonary mechanics in healthy preterm newborn infants. *Journal of Perinatology, 8*(3), 205–211.

Franco, P., Pardou, A., Hassid, S., Lurquin, P., Groswasser, J., & Kahn, A. (1998). Auditory arousal thresholds are higher when infants sleep in the prone position. *Journal of Pediatrics, 132,* 240–243.

Frank, D.I., Paredes, S.D., & Curtin, J. (1997). Perceptions of parent and nurse relationships and attitudes of parental participation in caring for infants in the NICU. *Florida Nurse, 45*(5), 9–10.

Frank, J.E., Mullanery, D.M., Darnall, R.A., & Stashwick, C.A. (2000). Teaching residents in the neonatal intensive care unit: A non-traditional approach. *Journal of Perinatology, 20,* 111–113.

Frankenburg, W.K., Dodds, J., Archer, P., Shapiro, H., & Bresnick, B. (1990). *Denver II.* Denver, CO: Denver Developmental Materials.

Furdon, S.A., Pfeil, V.C., & Snow, K. (1998). Operationalizing Donna Wong's principle of atraumatic care: Pain management protocol in the NICU. *Pediatric Nursing, 24,* 336–342.

Furman, L. (1995, June/July). Nursing the premature infant. *Zero to Three,* 24–29.

Furman, L., Minich, N.M., & Hack, M. (1998). Breastfeeding of very low birthweight infants. *Journal of Human Lactation, 14,* 29–34.

Gaining and Growing: Assuring Nutritional Care of Preterm Infants. (2000). *A discussion of growth of preterm infants.* Retrieved February 27, 2003, from http://staff.washington.edu/growing/Assess/Grdis.htm

Gale, G., & VandenBerg, K.A. (1998). Kangaroo care. *Neonatal Network, 17*(5), 69.

Galland, B.C., Bolton, D.P.G., Taylor, B.J., Sayers, R.M., & Williams, S.M. (2000). Ventilatory sensitivity to mild asphyxia: Prone versus supine sleep position. *Archives of Disease in Childhood, 83,* 423–428.

Galland, B.C., Taylor, B.J., & Bolton, D.P.G. (2002). Prone versus supine sleep position: A review of the physiological studies in SIDS research. *Journal of Pediatrics & Child Health, 38,* 332–338.

Gamblian, V., Hess, D.J., & Kenner, C. (1998). Early discharge from the NICU. *Journal of Pediatric Nursing, 13,* 296–301.

Gannon, B.A. (2000). Theophylline or caffeine: Which is best for apnea of prematurity? *Neonatal Network, 19*(8), 33–36.

Garbarino, J. (1990). The human ecology of early risk. In S.J. Meisels & J.P. Shonkoff (Eds.), *Handbook of early childhood intervention* (pp. 78–96). New York: Cambridge University Press.

Gardner, J.M., Karmel, B.Z., & Freedland, R.L. (2001). Determining functional integrity in neonates: A Rapid Neurobehavioral Assessment Tool. In L. Singer & P.S. Zeskind (Eds.), *Biobehavioral assessment of the infant* (pp. 398–422). New York: The Guilford Press.

Gardner, M.F. (1990). *Expressive One-Word Picture Vocabulary Test–Revised.* Novato, CA: Academic Therapy Publications.

Gerard, C.M., Harris, K.A., & Thach, B.T. (2002). Physiologic studies on swaddling: An ancient child care practice, which may promote supine position for infant sleep. *Journal of Pediatrics, 141,* 398–404.

Gesell, A. (1928). *Infancy and human growth.* New York: Macmillan.

Gibson, J.J. (1979). *The ecological approach to visual perception.* Boston: Houghton Mifflin.

Gilfoyle, E., Grady, A., & Moore, J. (1981). *Children adapt.* Thorofare, NJ: Slack.

Glass, L.S., & Wolff, R.P. (1998). Feeding and Oral-Motor Skills. In J. Case-Smith (Ed.), *Pediatric occupational therapy and early intervention* (2nd ed., pp. 127–166). Burlington, MA: Butterworth-Heinemann.

Goldberg, R.N., Joshi, A., Moscoso, P., & Castillo, T. (1983). The effect of head position on intracranial pressure in the neonate. *Critical Care Medicine, 11,* 428–430.

Gomella, T.L. (Ed.). (1999). *Neonatology: Management, procedures, on-call problems, diseases, and drugs* (4th ed.). Stamford, CT: Appleton & Lange.

Gorga, D., Anzalone, M., Holloway, E., Bigsby, R., Holloway, E., Hunter, J., Strzyzewski, S., & Vergara, E.R. (2000). Specialized knowledge and skills for neonatal therapy practice in the neonatal intensive care unit. *American Journal of Neonatal Therapy, 54,* 641–648.

Gorski, P., Davison, M.F., & Brazelton, T.B. (1979). Stages of behavioral organization in the high-risk neonate: Theoretical and clinical considerations. *Seminars in Perinatology, 3,* 61–72.

Gorski, P.A., Hole, W.T., Leonard, C.H., & Martin, J.A. (1983). Direct computer scoring of premature infants and nursery care: Distress following two interventions. *Pediatrics, 72,* 198–202.

Goto, K., Mirmiran, M., Adams, M.M., Longford, R.V., Baldwin, R.B., Boeddiker, M.A., & Ariagno, R.L. (1999). More awakenings and heart rate variability during supine sleep in preterm infants. *Pediatrics, 103,* 603–609.

Gottfried, A.W. (1990). Touch as an organizer of development and learning. In K. Barnard & T.B. Brazelton (Eds.), *Touch: the foundation of experience* (pp. 349–361). Madison, CT: International Universities Press.

Gottfried, A.W., Wallace-Lande, P., Sherman-Brown, S., King, J., & Coen, C. (1981). Physical and social environment of newborn infants in special care units. *Science, 214,* 673–675.

Gowland, C., Boyce, W.F., Wright, V., Russell, D.J., Goldsmith, C.H., & Rosenbaum P.L. (1995). Reliability of the Gross Motor Performance Measure. *Physical Therapy, 75,* 597–602.

Graillon, A., Barr, R.G., Young, S.N., Wright, J.H., & Hendricks, L.A. (1997). Differential response to intraoral sucrose, quinine and corn oil in crying human newborns. *Physiology and Behavior, 62,* 317–325.

Granger, C.V., Seltzer, G.B., & Fishbein, C.F. (1987). *Primary care of the functionally disabled: Assessment and management* (p. 15). Philadelphia: Lippincott, Williams & Wilkins.

Graven, S.N. (1997). Clinical research data illuminating the relationship between the physical environment & patent medical outcomes. *Journal of Healthcare, 9,* 115–19.

Graven, S.N. (2000). Sound and the developing infant in the NICU: Conclusions and recommendations for care. *Journal of Perinatology, 20*(8, Pt. 2), S88–S93.

Graves, J.K., & Ware, M.E. (1990). Parents' and health professionals' perceptions concerning parental stress during a child's hospitalization. *Children's Health Care, 19,* 37–42.

Green, M. (Ed.). (1994). *Bright Futures: Guidelines for health supervision of infants, children, and adolescents.* Washington, DC: National Center for Education in Maternal and Child Health.

Gregoire, M.C., Lefebvre, F., & Glorieux, J. (1998). Health and developmental outcomes at 18 months in very preterm infants with bronchopulmonary dysplasia. *Pediatrics, 101*(5), 856–860.

Grenier, I.R., Bigsby, R., Vergara, E.R., & Lester, B.M. (2003). Comparison of motor self-regulatory and stress behaviors of preterm infants across body positions. *American Journal of Occupational Therapy, 57,* 289–297.

Griffin, T., Wishba, C., & Kavanaugh, K. (1998). Nursing interventions to reduce stress in parents of hospitalized preterm infants. *Journal of Pediatric Nursing, 13,* 290–295.

Groome, L.J., Swiber, M.J., Atterbury, J.L., Bentz, L.S., & Holland, S.B. (1997). Similarities and differences in behavioral state organization during sleep periods in the perinatal infant before and after birth. *Child Development, 68,* 1–11.

Guyatt, G., Walter, S., & Norman, G. (1987). Measuring change over time: Assessing the usefulness of evaluative instruments. *Journal of Chronic Diseases, 40,* 171–178.

Hack, M., & Fanaroff, A.A. (1988). How small is too small? Considerations in evaluating the outcome of the tiny infants. *Clinics in Perinatology, 15,* 773–788.

Hack, M., & Fanaroff, A.A. (1989). Outcomes of extremely low-birth weight infants between 1982 and 1988. *The New England Journal of Medicine, 321,* 1642–1647.

Hack, M., Fanaroff, A.A., & Merkatz, I.R. (1979). The low birth-weight infant. Evolution of a changing outlook. *The New England Journal of Medicine, 301,* 1162–1165.

Hack, M., Flannery, D.J., Schluchter, M., Cartar, L., Borawski, E., & Klein, N. (2002). Outcomes in young adulthood for very-low-birth-weight infants. *The New England Journal of Medicine, 346,* 149–157.

Hack, M., Friedman, H., & Fanaroff, A.A. (1996). Outcomes of extremely low-birth weight infants. *Pediatrics, 98,* 931–937.

Hack, M., Horbar, J.D., Malloy, M.H., Tyson, J.E., Wright, E., & Wright, L. (1991). Very low birth weight outcomes of the National Institute of Child Health and Human Development Neonatal Network. *Pediatrics, 87,* 587–597.

Hack, M., Taylor, H.G., Klein, N., Eiben, R., Schatschneider, C., & Mercuri-Minich, N. (1994). School-age outcomes in children with birth weights under 750 g. *The New England Journal of Medicine, 331*(12), 753–759.

Hadders-Algra, M., & Prechtl, H.F. (1992). Developmental course of general movements in early infancy. I. Descriptive analysis of change in form. *Early Human Development, 28,* 201–213.

Hadjistavropoulos, H.D., Craig, K.D., Grunau, R.E., & Whitfield, M.F. (1997). Judging pain in infants: behavioral, contextual, and developmental determinants. *Pain, 73,* 319–324.

Hagedorn, M.I., Gardner, S.L., & Abman, S.H. (1989). Respiratory diseases. In G.B. Merenstein & S.L. Gardner (Eds.), *Handbook of neonatal intensive care* (pp. 365–426). St. Louis: Mosby.

Hainline, L., & Lemerise, E. (1982). Infants' scanning of geometric forms varying in size. *Journal of Experimental Child Psychology, 33,* 235–256.

Haley, S.M., Coster, W.J., Ludlow, L.H., Haltiwanger, J.T., & Andrellos, P.J. (1992). *Pediatric Evaluation of Disability Inventory (PEDI), Version 1: Development, standardization and administration manual.* Boston: New England Medical Center, PEDI Research Group.

Haley, S.M., Ludlow, L.H., & Coster, W.J. (1993). Pediatric evaluation: Clinical interpretation of summary scores using Rasch scaling methodology. *Physical Medicine and Rehabilitation Clinics of North America, 4,* 529–540.

Hallsworth, M. (1995). Positioning the preterm infant. *Paediatric Nursing, 7,* 18–20.

Hamill, P.V., Drizd, T.A., Johnson, C.L., Reed, R.B., Roche, A.F., & Moore, W.M. (1979). Physical growth: National center for health statistics percentiles. *American Journal of Clinical Nutrition, 32,* 607–629.

Hamrick, W.B., & Riley, L. (1992). A comparison of infection rates in a newborn intensive care unit before and after adoption of open visitation. *Neonatal Network, 11*(1), 15–18.

Han, T.R., Bang, M.S., Lim, J.Y., Yoon, B.H., & Kim, I.W. (2002). Risk factors of cerebral palsy in preterm infants. *American Journal of Physical Medicine and Rehabilitation, 81*(4), 297–303.

Hanft, B. (1988). The changing environment of early intervention services: Implications for practice. *American Journal of Occupational Therapy, 42,* 724–731.

Hanzlik, J.R. (1998). Parent–child relations: Interaction and intervention. In J. Case-Smith (Ed.), *Pediatric occupational therapy and early intervention* (2nd ed., pp. 207–222). Burlington, NJ: Butterworth-Heinemann.

Harlow, H.F. (1958). The nature of love. *American Psychologist, 13,* 673–685.

Harper, R.M. (1996). The cerebral regulation of cardiovascular and respiratory functions. *Seminars in Perinatology, 3,* 13–22.

Harrison, H. (1983). *The premature baby book: A parent's guide to coping and caring in the first years.* New York: St. Martin's Press.

Harrison, H., & Kositsky, A. (1987). *The premature baby book: A parent's guide to coping and caring in the first years* (2nd ed.). New York: St. Martin's Press.

Harrison, L. (1997). Research utilization: Handling preterm infants in the NICU. *Neonatal Network, 16*(3), 65–69.

Harrison, P., Kaufman, A.S., Kaufman, N.L., Bruininks, R.H., Rynders, J., Ilmer, S., Sparrow, S., & Cicchetti, D.V. (1990). *Early Screening Profiles (ESP).* Circle Pines, MN: American Guidance Service.

Hashimoto, T., Hiura, K., Endo, S., Fukuda, K., Mori, A., Tayama, M., & Miyao, M. (1983). Postural effects on behavioral states of newborn infants: A sleep polygraphic study. *Brain and Development, 5,* 286–291.

Heller, R., & McKlindon, D. (1996). Families as "faculty": Parents educating caregivers about family-centered care. *Pediatric Nursing, 22,* 428–431.

Hemingway, M.M., & Oliver, S.K. (1991). Water bed therapy and cranial molding of the sick preterm infant. *Neonatal Network, 10*(3), 53–56.

Henrick, D.L., Prather, M., & Tobin, A.R. (1984). *Sequenced Inventory of Communication Development–Revised Edition (SICDR-R).* Austin, TX: PRO-ED.

Heriza, C.B., & Sweeney, J.K. (1990). Effects of NICU intervention of preterm infants: Part 1. Implications for neonatal practice. *Infants and Young Children, 2*(3), 31–47.

Herrgard, E., Karjalainen, S., Martikainen, A., & Heinonen, K. (1995). Hearing loss at the age of 5 years of children born preterm: A matter of definition. *Acta Paediatrica, 84,* 1160–1164.

Hess, J.H. (1953). Experiences gained in a thirty year study of prematurely born infants. *Pediatrics, 11*, 425–434.

Heyman, M.A., Teitel, D.F., & Liebman, J. (1993). The heart. In M.H. Klaus & A.A. Fanaroff (Eds.), *Care of the high-risk neonate* (4th ed., pp. 345–373). Philadelphia: W.B. Saunders.

Hill, A., & Volpe, J. (1981). Normal pressure hydrocephalus in the newborn. *Pediatrics, 68*, 623–629.

Hoffman, E.L., & Bennett, F.C. (1990). Birth weight less than 800 grams: Changing outcomes and influences of gender and gestation number. *Pediatrics, 86*, 27–34.

Hohlagschwandtner, M., Husslein, P., Klebermass, K., Weninger, M., Nardi, A., & Langer, M. (2001). Perinatal mortality and morbidity. Comparison between maternal transport, neonatal transport and inpatient antenatal treatment. *Archives of Gynecology & Obstetrics, 265*, 113–118.

Holloway, E. (1990). Adaptation of neonatal intensive care units as an occupational therapy intervention. In S.C. Merrill (Ed.), *Environment: Implications for occupational therapy practice* (pp. 45–64). Bethesda, MD: American Occupational Therapy Association.

Holloway, E. (1994). Parent and occupational therapist collaboration in the neonatal intensive care unit. *American Journal of Occupational Therapy, 48*, 535–538.

Holloway, E. (1998). Relationship-based occupational therapy in the neonatal intensive care unit. In J. Case-Smith (Ed.), *Pediatric occupational therapy and early intervention* (2nd ed., pp. 111–126). Burlington, NJ: Butterworth-Heinemann.

Hoon, A.H., Pulsifer, M.B., Gopalan, R., Palmer, F.B., & Capute, A.J. (1993). Clinical Adaptive Test/Clinical Linguistic Auditory Milestone Scale in early cognitive assessment. *Journal of Pediatrics, 123*(1), S1–S8.

Horton, J.C. (2001). Critical periods in the development of the visual system. In D.B. Bailey, Jr., J.T. Bruer, F.J. Symons, & J.W. Lichtman (Eds.), *Critical thinking about critical periods* (pp. 45–65). Baltimore: Paul H. Brookes Publishing Co.

Hubin-Gayte, M. (1997). Research in brief: Newborn consolability and maternal soothing behavior. *Ab Initio, 4*, 1.

Hughes, M., McCollum, J., Scheffel, D., & Sanchez, G. (1994). How parents cope with the experience of neonatal intensive care. *Children's Health Care, 23*, 1–14.

Humphry, R. (2002). Young children's occupations: Explicating the dynamics of developmental processes. *American Journal of Occupational Therapy, 56*, 171–179.

Hunter, J., Mullen, J., & Dallas, D.V. (1994). Medical considerations and practice guidelines for the neonatal occupational therapist. *American Journal of Occupational Therapy, 48*, 546–560.

Hunter, J.G. (1996). The neonatal intensive care unit. In J. Case-Smith (Ed.), *Occupational therapy for children* (3rd ed., pp. 583–647). St. Louis: Mosby.

Hutchinson, A.A. (1989, February). *Perinatal respiration.* Workshop presented at the University of Florida, Gainesville.

Individuals with Disabilities Education Act Amendments of 1997, PL 105-17, 20 U.S.C. §§ 1400 *et seq.*

An international classification of retinopathy of prematurity. (1984). *Pediatrics, 74*, 127–133.

Ireton, H. (1992). *Child Development Inventory (CDI) Manual.* Minneapolis, MN: Behavior Science Systems.

Jahnukainen, T., van Ravenswaaij-Arts, C., Jalonen, J., & Valimaki, I. (1993). Dynamics of vasomotor thermoregulation of the skin in term and preterm neonates. *Early Human Development, 33*, 133–143.

Jantz, J.W., Blosser, C.D., & Fruechting, L.A. (1997). A motor milestone change noted with a change in sleep position. *Archives of Pediatrics & Adolescent Medicine, 151*, 565–568.

Jarrett, M.H. (1996a). Parent Partners: A parent-to-parent support program in the NICU: Part I. Program development. *Pediatric Nursing, 22*, 60–63.

Jarrett, M.H. (1996b). Parent Partners: A parent-to-parent support program in the NICU: Part II. Program implementation. *Pediatric Nursing, 22*, 142–144.

Jenni, O.G., von Siebenthal, K., Wolf, M., Keel, M., Duc, G., & Bucher, H.U. (1997). Effect of nursing in head elevated tilt position (15 degrees) on the incidence of bradycardic and hypoxemic episodes in preterm infants. *Pediatrics, 100*, 622–625.

Johnston, C.C., Sherrard, A., Stevens, B., Franck, L., Stremler, R., & Jack, A. (1999). Do cry features reflect pain intensity in preterm neonates? A preliminary study. *Biology of the Neonate, 76*(2), 120–124.

Johnston, C.C., Stremler, R., Horton, L., & Friedman, A. (1999). Effect of repeated doses of sucrose during heel stick procedure in preterm neonates. *Biology of the Neonate*, 75(3), 160–166.

Johnston, C.C., Stremler, R.L., Stevens, B.J., & Horton, L. (1997). Effectiveness of oral sucrose and simulated rocking on pain response in preterm neonates. *Pain*, 72, 193–199.

Joint Committee on Infant Hearing Screening. (1994). Position statement. *ASHA*, 36, 38–41.

Jones, H.E., & Kassity, N. (2001). Varieties of alternative experience: Complementary care in the neonatal intensive care unit. *Clinical Obstetrics and Gynecology*, 44, 750–768.

Jones, M.W., McMurray, J.L., & Englestad, D. (2002). The "geriatric" NICU patient. *Neonatal Network*, 21(6), 49–58.

Jones, R., Wincott, E., Elbourne, D., & Grant, A. (1995). Controlled trial of dexamethasone in neonatal chronic lung disease: A 3-year follow-up. *Pediatrics*, 96, 897–906.

Kajiura, H., Cowart, B.J., & Beauchamp, G.K. (1992). Early developmental change in bitter taste responses in human infants. *Developmental Psychobiology*, 25, 375–386.

Karlowicz, M.G., & McMurray, J.L. (2000). Comparison of neonatal nurse practicioners' and pediatric residents' care of extremely low-birth-weight infants. *Archives of Pediatrics & Adolescent Medicine*, 154, 1123–1126.

Kasper, J., & Nyamathi, A. (1988). Parents of children in the pediatric intensive care unit: What are their needs? *Heart & Lung: Journal of Acute & Critical Care*, 17, 574–581.

Kaufman, A.S., & Kaufman, N.L. (1983). *Interpretive manual for the Kaufman Assessment Battery for Children*. Circle Pines, MN: American Guidance Service.

Kaufman, A.S., & Kaufman, N.L. (1993). *Kaufman Survey of Early Academic and Language Skills (K-SEALS)*. Circle Pines, MN: American Guidance Service.

Keating, R.F., Spence, C.A., & Lynch, D. (2002). The brain and nervous system: Normal and abnormal development. In M.L. Batshaw (Ed.), *Children with disabilities* (5th ed., pp. 243–262). Baltimore: Paul H. Brookes Publishing Co.

Kemp, J.S., & Thach, B.T. (1991). Sudden death in infants sleeping on polystyrene-filled cushions. *The New England Journal of Medicine*, 324, 1858–1864.

Kessel, J., & Ward, R.M. (1998). Congenital malformations presenting during the neonatal period. *Clinics in Perinatology*, 25, 351–369.

King, L.J. (1978). Toward a science of adaptive responses. In American Occupational Therapy Association (Ed.), *A professional legacy: The Eleanor Clark Slagle Lectures in Occupational Therapy, 1955–1984* (pp. 311–328). Bethesda, MD: American Occupational Therapy Association.

Kinneer, M.D., & Beachy, P. (1994). Nipple feeding premature infants in the neonatal intensive-care unit: Factors and decisions. *Journal of Gynecologic and Neonatal Nursing*, 23, 107–112.

Kirschbaum, M.S. (1990). Needs of parents of critically ill children. *Dimensions of Critical Care Nursing*, 9, 344–352.

Kirshner, B., & Guyatt, G. (1985). A methodological framework for assessing health indices. *Journal of Chronic Diseases*, 38, 27–36.

Kliegman, R.M., Walker, W.A., & Yolken, R.H. (1994). Research agenda for a disease of unknown etiology & pathogenesis. In B.J. Stoll & R.B.M. Kliegman (Eds.), Necrotizing enterocolitis. *Clinics in Perinatology*, 21(2), 437–456.

Kliethermes, P.A., Cross, M.L., Lanese, M.G., Johnson, K.M., & Simon, S.D. (1999). Transitioning preterm infants with nasogastric tube supplementation: Increased likelihood of breastfeeding. *Journal of Obstetric Gynecological and Neonatal Nursing*, 28, 264–73.

Knobloch, H., Stevens, F., & Malone, A.F. (1980). *Manual of developmental diagnosis: The administration and interpretation of the Revised Gesell Developmental and Neurological Examination*. New York: Harper & Row.

Konishi, Y., Takaya, R., Kimura, K., Konishi, K., Fulii, Y., Saito, M., & Sudo, M. (1994). Development of posture in prone and supine positions during the prenatal period in low risk preterm infants. *Archives of Disease in Childhood, Fetal and Neonatal Edition*, 70(1), F188–F191.

Korner, A.F., & Constantinou, J. (2001). The neurobehavioral assessment of the preterm infant: Reliability and developmental and clinical validity. In L. Singer & P.S. Zeskind (Eds.), *Biobehavioral assessment of the infant* (pp. 381–397). New York: The Guilford Press.

Korner, A.F., Constantinou, J., Dimiceli, S., & Brown, B.W. (1991). Establishing the reliability and developmental validity of neurobehavioral assessment for preterm infants: A methodological process. *Child Development*, 62, 1200–1208.

Korner, A.F., & Thom, V.A. (1990). *Neurobehavioral Assessment of the Preterm Infant.* San Antonio, TX: The Psychological Corporation.

Kotagal, U.R., Perlstein, P.H., Gamblian, V., Donovan, E.F., & Atherton, H.D. (1995). Description and evaluation of a program for the early discharge of infants from a neonatal intensive care unit. *Journal of Pediatrics, 127,* 285–290.

Kovacs, M. (1985).The Children's Depression Inventory (CDI). *Psychopharmacological Bulletin, 21,* 995–998.

Kuban, K.C.K., & Filiano, J. (1997). Neonatal seizures. In J.P. Cloherty & A.R. Stark (Eds.), *Manual of neonatal care* (4th ed., pp. 493–505). Philadelphia: Lippincott, Williams & Wilkins.

Kurlak, L.O., Ruggins, N.R., & Stephenson, T.J. (1994). Effect of nursing position on incidence, type, and duration of clinically significant apnoea in preterm infants. *Archives of Disease in Childhood, Fetal and Neonatal Edition, 71*(1), F16–F19.

Lampley, D.A., & Rust, J.O. (1986). Validation of the Kaufman Assessment Battery for Children with a sample of preschool children. *Psychology in the Schools, 23,* 131–137.

Landgraf, J.M., Abetz, L., & Ware, J.E. (1996). *Child Health Questionnaire (CHQ): A user's manual.* Boston: The Health Institute, New England Medical Center.

Landry, R.J., Scheidt, P.C., & Hammond, R.W. (1985). Ambient light and phototherapy conditions of eight neonatal care units: A summary report. *Pediatrics, 75,* 434–441.

Laneau, S., Evangelista, J.K., Pizzi, A.M., Mobassaleh, M., Fulton, D.R., & Berul, C.I. (1998). Proarrhythmia associated with cisapride in children. *Pediatrics, 101*(6), 1053–1056.

LaPine, T.R., Jackson, C., & Bennett, F.C. (1995). Outcome of infants weighing less than 800 grams at birth: 15 years experience. *Pediatrics, 96,* 479–483.

Largo, R.H., & Duc, G. (1978). Head growth changes in head configuration in healthy preterm and term infants during the first six months of life. *Helvetica Paediatrica Acta, 32,* 431–442.

Larson, S.L., & Vitali, G.J. (1988). *Kindergarten Readiness Test (KRT).* East Aurora, NY: Slosson Educational Publications.

Lasky, R. (1995). Sound in the NICU and its effect on the newborn. *10th Canadian Ross Conference in Pediatrics: Optimizing the Neonatal Intensive Care Environment, September 8–11, 1994* (pp. 26–41). Montreal, Quebec, Canada: Abott Laboratories.

Lawhon, G. (2002). Facilitation of parenting the premature infant within the newborn intensive care unit. *Journal of Perinatal and Neonatal Nursing, 16,* 71–82.

Lawhon, G., & Melzan, A. (1988). Developmental care of the very low birth weight infant. *Perinatal and Neonatal Nursing, 2,* 56–65.

Lawson, M.E. (1997). Transient tachypnea of the newborn. In J.P. Cloherty & A.R. Stark (Eds.), *Manual of neonatal care* (4th ed., pp. 369–371). Philadelphia: Lippincott, Williams & Wilkins.

Lee, S. (1999). Retinopathy of prematurity in the 1990s. *Neonatal Network, 18*(2), 31–38.

Lee, S.K., McMillan, D.D., Ohlsson, A., Pendray, M., Synnes, A., Whyte, R., Chien, L.Y., & Sale, Y. (2000). Variations in practice and outcomes in the Canadian NICU network: 1996–1997. *Pediatrics, 106*(5), 1070–1079.

Lester, B., Bigsby, R., High, P., & Wu, S. (1995). Principles of intervention for preterm infants in the NICU. In *Optimizing the Neonatal Intensive Care Environment: Proceedings of the Tenth Conference in Pediatrics* (pp. 59–72). Canadian Paediatric Society. Montreal, Quebec, Canada: Abbott Laboratories.

Lester, B.M., Boukydis, C.F., & LaGasse, L. (1996). Cardiorespiratory reactivity during the Brazelton Scale in term and preterm infants. *Journal of Pediatric Psychology, 21,* 771–783.

Lester, B.M., McGrath, M.M., Garcia-Coll, C.T., Brem, F.S., Sullivan, M.C., & Mattis, S.B. (1994). Relationship between risk and protective factors, developmental outcome, and the home environment at 4-years-of-age in term and preterm infants. In H. Fitzgerald, B.M. Lester, & B. Zuckerman (Eds.), *Children in poverty: Research, health care, and policy issues* (pp. 197–227). New York: Garland.

Lester, B.M., & Tronick, E. (2001). Behavioral assessment scales: The NICU Network Neurobehavioral Scale, the Neonatal Behavioral Assessment Scale, and the Assessment of Premature Infant Behavior. In L.T. Singer & P.S. Zeskind (Eds.), *Biobehavioral assessment of the infant* (pp. 363–380). New York: The Guilford Press.

Lester, B.M., & Tronick, E. (in press). *The NICU Network Neurobehavioral Scale.* Baltimore: Paul H. Brookes Publishing Co.

Levy, M., & Fackler, J. (1997). Extracorporeal membrane oxygenation. In J.P. Cloherty & A.R. Stark (Eds.), *Manual of neonatal care* (4th ed., pp. 348–353). Philadelphia: Lippincott, Williams & Wilkins.

Lichtman, J.W. (2001). Developmental neurobiology overview: Synapses, circuits, and plasticity. In D.B. Bailey, Jr., J.T. Bruer, F.J. Symons, & J.W. Lichtman (Eds.), *Critical thinking about critical periods* (pp. 27–42). Baltimore: Paul H. Brookes Publishing Co.

Liley, H.G., & Stark, A.R. (1997). Respiratory distress syndrome/hyaline membrane disease. In J.P. Cloherty & A.R. Stark (Eds.), *Manual of neonatal care* (4th ed., pp. 329–336). Philadelphia: Lippincott, Williams & Wilkins.

Lindeke, L.L., Stanley, J.R., Else, B.S., & Mills, M.M. (2002). Neonatal predictors of school-based services used by NICU graduates at school age. *American Journal of Maternal & Child Nursing, 27*, 41–46.

Lindh, V., Wiklund, U., Sandman, P.O., & Hakansson, S. (1997). Assessment of acute pain in preterm infants by evaluation of facial expression and frequency domain analysis of heart rate variability. *Early Human Development, 48*, 131–142.

Linn, P.L., Horowitz, F.D., & Fox, H.A. (1985). Stimulation in the NICU: Is more necessarily better? *Clinics in Perinatology, 12*, 407–422.

Lipkin, P.H. (1996). Epidemiology of the developmental disabilities. In A.J. Capute & P.J. Accardo (Eds.), *Developmental disabilities in infancy and childhood, Second Edition: Vol. 1. Neurodevelopmental diagnosis and treatment* (pp. 137–156). Baltimore: Paul H. Brookes Publishing Co.

Liptak, G.S. (2002). Neural tube defects. In M.L. Batshaw (Ed.), *Children with disabilities* (5th ed., pp. 467–492). Baltimore: Paul H. Brookes Publishing Co.

Liptak, G.S., O'Donnell, M., Conaway, M., Chumlea, W., Worley, G., Henderson, R.C., Fung, E., Stallings, V., Samson-Fang, L., Calvert, R., Rosenbaum, P., & Stevenson, R.D. (2001). Health status of children with moderate to severe cerebral palsy. *Developmental Medicine and Child Neurology, 43*, 364–370.

Littlefield, T.R., Kelly, K.M., Pomatto, J.K., & Beals, S.P. (1999). Multiple-birth infants at higher risk for development of deformational plagiocephaly. *Pediatrics, 103*, 565–569.

Littlefield, T.R., Kelly, K.M., Pomatto, J.K., & Beals, S.P. (2002). Multiple-birth infants at higher risk for development of deformational plagiocephaly: II. Is one twin at greater risk? *Pediatrics, 109*, 19–25.

Llorens, L.A. (1969). Facilitation growth and development: The promise of occupational therapy. In American Occupational Therapy Association (Ed.), *A professional legacy: The Eleanor Clark Slagle Lectures in Occupational Therapy, 1955–1984* (pp. 311–328). Bethesda, MD: American Occupational Therapy Association.

Lloyd-Thomas, A.R., & Fitzgerald, M. (1996). Reflex responses do not necessarily signify pain. *British Medical Journal, 313*(7060), 797–798.

Lubchenco, L.O. (1976). *The high risk infant.* Philadelphia: W.B. Saunders.

Lubchenco, L.O., Bard, H., Goldman, A.L., Coyer, W.E., McIntyre, C., & Smith, D.M. (1974). Newborn intensive care and long term prognosis. *Developmental Medicine and Child Neurology, 16*, 421–423.

Lubchenco, L.O, Delivoria-Papadopoulos, M., Butterfield, L.J., Metcalf, D., Hix, I.E., Danick, J., Dodds, J., Downs, M., & Freeland, E. (1972). Long term follow-up studies of prematurely born infants: I. Relationship of handicaps to nursery routines. *Journal of Pediatrics, 80*, 501–508.

Lubchenco, L.O., Delivoria-Papadopoulos, M., & Searls, D. (1972). Long term follow-up studies of prematurely born infants: II. Influence of birth weight and gestational age on sequelae. *Journal of Pediatrics, 80*, 509–512.

Lubchenco, L.O., Horner, F.A., Reed, L.H., Hix. I.E., Metcalf, D., Cohig, R., Elliott, H.C., & Bourg, M. (1963). Sequelae of premature birth. *American Journal of Diseases of Children, 106*, 101–155.

Ludington-Hoe, S.M., Cong, X., & Hashemi, F. (2002). Infant crying: Nature, physiologic consequences, and select interventions. *Neonatal Network, 21*(2), 29–36.

Ludington-Hoe, S.M., & Swinth, J.Y. (1996). Developmental aspects of kangaroo care. *Journal of Obstetric, Gynecologic, & Neonatal Nursing, 25*, 691–703.

Lynch, A.Y. (1997, July). Prone to good positioning? The nursing cost of bad positioning of neonates. *Journal of Neonatal Nursing*, 16–20.

Lyon, M.A., & Smith, D.K. (1986). A comparison of at-risk preschool children's performance on the K-ABC, McCarthy Scales, and Stanford-Binet. *Journal of Psychoeducational Assessment, 4,* 35–43.

MacFarlane, A. (1975). Olfaction in the development of social preferences in the human neonate. In *Ciba Foundation Symposium 33: Parent Interaction* (pp. 103–113). New York: Elsevier.

Macias, M.M., Saylor, C.F., Greer, M.K., Charles, J.M., Bell, N., & Katikanen, L.D. (1998). Infant screening: The usefulness of the Bayley Infant Neurodevelopmental Screener and the Clinical Adaptive Test/Clinical Linguistic Auditory Milestone Scale. *Journal of Developmental and Behavioral Pediatrics, 19,* 155–161.

Madden, S.L. (2000). *The preemie parents' companion.* Boston: Harvard Common Press.

Maekawa, K., & Ochiai, Y. (1975). Electromyographic studies on flexor hypertonia of the extremities of newborn infants. *Developmental Medicine and Child Neurology, 17,* 440–446.

Maone, T.R., Mattes, R.D., & Beauchamp, G.K. (1992). Cocaine-exposed newborns show an exaggerated sucking response to sucrose. *Physiological Behavior, 51,* 487–491.

Maone, T.R., Mattes, R.D., Bernbaum, J.C., & Beauchamp, G.K. (1990). A new method for delivering a taste without fluids to preterm and term infants. *Developmental Psychobiology, 23,* 179–191.

Marlier, L., Schaal, B., & Soussignan, R. (1997). Orientation responses to biological odours in the human newborn. Initial pattern and postnatal plasticity. *Comptes Rendus de L'Académie des Sciences, Série III, 320,* 999–1005.

Martin, J.H. (1991). Coding and processing of sensory information. In E.R. Kandel, J.H. Schwartz, & T.M. Jessell (Eds.), *Principles of neural science* (pp. 329–340). New York: Elsevier.

Martin, R.J., DiFiore, J.M., Korenke, C.B., Randal, H., Miller, M.J., & Brooks, L.J. (1995). Vulnerability of respiratory control in healthy preterm infants placed supine. *Journal of Pediatrics, 127,* 609–614.

Martin, R.J., Herrell, N., Rubin, D., & Fanaroff, A. (1979). Effect of supine and prone positioning on arterial oxygen tension in the preterm infant. *Pediatrics, 63,* 528–531.

Masterson, J., Zucker, C., & Schulze, K. (1987). Prone and supine positioning effects on energy expenditure and behavior of low birth weight neonates. *Pediatrics, 80,* 689–692.

McAlmon, K.R. (1997). Necrotizing enterocolitis. In J.P. Cloherty & A.R. Stark (Eds.), *Manual of neonatal care* (4th ed., pp. 609–615). Philadelphia: Lippincott, Williams & Wilkins.

McCanless, L.L. (1994). Work redesign in the neonatal intensive care unit: Role development and training from an educational perspective. *Journal of Perinatology and Neonatal Nursing, 8,* 69–82.

McCarthy, D.A. (1972). *Manual for the McCarthy Scales of Children's Abilities.* San Antonio, TX: The Psychological Corporation.

McCormick, M.C. (1989). Long-term follow-up of infants discharged from neonatal intensive care units. *Journal of the American Medical Association, 261,* 1767–1772.

McCubbin, H.I., McCubbin, M.A., Thompson, A.I., Han, S., & Allen, C.T. (1997, June). Families under stress: What makes them resilient. *1997 American Association of Family and Consumer Sciences Commemorative Lecture.* Retrieved February 5, 2003, from http://www.cyfernet.org/research/resilient.html

McCubbin, M.A., & McCubbin, H.I. (1996). Resilience in families: A conceptual model of family adjustment and adaptation in response to stress and crises. In H.I. McCubbin, A.I. Thompson, & M.A. McCubbin (Eds.), *Family assessment: Resiliency, coping, and adaptation: Inventories for research and practice* (pp. 1–64). Madison: University of Wisconsin.

McEvoy, C., Mendoza, M.E., Bowling, S., Hewlett, V., Sardesai, S., & Durand, M. (1997). Prone positioning decreases episodes of hypoxemia in extremely low birthweight infants (1000 grams or less) with chronic lung disease. *Journal of Pediatrics, 130,* 305–309.

McGrath, J.M., & Conliffe-Torres, S. (1996). Integrating family centered developmental assessment and intervention into routine care in the neonatal intensive care unit. *Nursing Clinics of North America, 31,* 367–368.

McGrath, M.M., & Meyer, E.C. (1992). Maternal self-esteem: From theory to clinical practice in a special care nursery. *Children's Health Care, 21,* 199–205.

McLaughlin, J.F., Bjornson, K.F., Astley, S.J., Hays, R.M., Hoffinger, S.A., Armantrout, E.A., & Roberts, T.S. (1994). The role of selective dorsal rhizotomy in cerebral palsy: Critical evaluation of a prospective clinical series. *Developmental Medicine and Child Neurology, 36,* 755–769.

McNamara, F., Wulbrand, H., & Thach, B.T. (1998). Characteristics of the infant arousal response. *Journal of Applied Physiology, 85,* 2314–2321.

McVey, C. (1998). Pain in the very preterm baby: "Suffer little children?" *Pediatric Rehabilitation, 2,* 47–55.

Meisels, S.J. (1987). Uses and abuses of developmental screening and school readiness testing. *Young Children, 42*, 4–9.

Meisels, S.J., & Shonkoff, J.P. (2000). Early intervention: A continuing evaluation. In J.P. Shonkoff & S.J. Meisels (Eds.), *Handbook of early childhood education* (2nd ed., pp. 3–31). New York: Cambridge University Press.

Mendoza, J., Roberts, J., & Cook, L. (1991). Postural effects on pulmonary function and heart rate of preterm infants with lung disease. *Journal of Pediatrics, 118*, 445–448.

Menon, G., Anand, K.J., & McIntosh, N. (1998). Practical approach to analgesia and sedation in the neonatal intensive care unit. *Seminars in Perinatology, 22*, 417–424.

Ment, L.R., Oh, W., Ehrenkranz, R.A., Philip, A.G., Vohr, B., Allan, W., Duncan, C.C., Scott, D.T., Taylor, K.J., & Katz, K.H. (1994). Low dose indomethacin and preventional intraventricular hemorrhage: A multicenter randomized trial. *Pediatrics, 93*, 543–550.

Ment, L.R., Westerveld, M., Makuch, R., Vohr, B., & Allen, W.C. (1998). Cognitive outcome at $4^{1}/2$ years of very low birth weight infants enrolled in a multicenter indomethacin prevention trial. *Pediatrics, 102*, 159–160.

Merchant, J.R., Worwa, C., Porter, S., Coleman, J.M., & deRegnier, R.O. (2001). Respiratory instability of term and near-term healthy newborn infants in car safety seats. *Pediatrics, 108*, 647–652.

Merenstein, G.B. (1994). Teamwork: The key to quality neonatal care. *Neonatal Network, 13*(6), 53–55.

Merritt, T.A., & Raddish, M. (1998). A review of guidelines for the discharge of premature infants: Opportunities for improving cost effectiveness. *Journal of Perinatology, 18*, S27–S37.

Meyer, E.C., Garcia Coll, C.T., Lester, B.M., Boukydis, Z., McDonough, S.M., & Oh, W. (1994). Family-based intervention improves maternal psychological well-being and feeding interaction of preterm infants. *Pediatrics, 93*, 241–246.

Meyer, E.C., Kennally, K.F., Zika-Beres, E., Cashore, W.J., & Oh, W. (1996). Attitudes about sibling visitation in the neonatal intensive care unit. *Archives of Pediatrics & Adolescent Medicine, 150*, 1021–1026.

Meyer, E.C., Lester, B.M., Boukydis, C.F.Z., & Bigsby, R. (1998). Family-based intervention with high-risk infants and their families. *Journal of Clinical Psychology in Medical Settings, 5*, 49–69.

Meyer, E.C., Snelling, L.K., & Myren-Manbeck, L.K. (1998). Pediatric intensive care: The parents' experience. *AACN Clinical Issues, 19*, 64–74.

Miles, M.S., Funk, S.G., & Carlson, J. (1993). Parental stressor scale: Neonatal intensive care unit. *Nursing Research, 42*, 148–152.

Miles, M.S., Funk, S.G., & Kasper, M.A. (1992). The stress response of mothers and fathers of preterm infants. *Research in Nursing and Health, 15*, 261–269.

Miller, C.L., Landry, S.H., Smith, K.E., Wildin, S.R., Anderson, A.E., & Swank, P.R. (1995). Developmental change in the neuropsychological functioning of very low birth weight infants. *Child Neuropsychology, 1*, 224–236.

Miller, L.J. (1988). *Miller Assessment for Preschoolers (MAP)*. San Antonio, TX: The Psychological Corporation.

Mirmiran, M., & Ariagno, R.L. (2000). Influence of light in the NICU on the development of circadian rhythms in preterm infants. *Seminars in Perinatology, 24*, 247–257.

Molteno, C.D., Thompson, M.C., Buccimazza, S.S., Magasiner, V., & Hann, F.M. (1999). Evaluation of the infant at risk for neurodevelopmental disability. *South African Medical Journal, 89*, 1084–1087.

Monfort, K., & Case-Smith, J. (1997). The effects of a neonatal positioner on scapular rotation. *American Journal of Occupational Therapy, 51*, 378–384.

Monterosso, L., Coenen, A., Percival, P., & Evans, S. (1995). Effect of a postural support nappy on "flattened posture" of the lower extremities in very preterm infants. *Journal of Pediatrics & Child Health, 31*, 350–354.

Monterosso, L., Kristianson, L., & Cole, J. (2002). Neuromotor development and the physiologic effects of positioning in very low birth weight infants. *Journal of Obstetric, Gynecologic, and Neonatal Nursing, 31*, 138–146.

Moore, K.L., & Persaud, T.V.N. (1993). *Before we are born: Essentials of embryology and birth defects* (4th ed.). Philadelphia: W.B. Saunders.

Moore, K.L., & Persaud, T.V.N. (1998). *The developing human: Clinically oriented embryology*. Philadelphia: W.B. Saunders.

Moran, M., Radzyminski, S.G., Higgins, K.R., Dowling, D.A., Miller, M.J., & Anderson, G.C. (1999). Maternal kangaroo (skin-to-skin) care in the NICU beginning 4 hours postbirth. *Materal Child Nursing, 24*, 74–79.

Morante, A., Dubowitz, L.M., Leverne, M., & Dubowitz, V. (1982). The development of visual function in normal and neurologically abnormal preterm and fullterm infants. *Developmental Medicine and Child Neurology, 24*, 771–784.

Morison, S.J., Grunau, R.E., Oberlander, T.R., & Whitfield, M.F. (2001). Relations between behavioral and cardiac autonomic reactivity to acute pain in preterm neonates. *Clinical Journal of Pain, 17*, 350–358.

Morris, B.H., Philbin, M.K., & Bose, C. (2000). Physiological effects of sound on the newborn. *Journal of Perinatology, 20*(8, Pt. 2), S55–S60.

Morris, K.M., & Burns, Y.R. (1994). Reduction of craniofacial and palatal narrowing in very low birthweight infants. *Journal of Paediatric Child Health, 30*, 518–522.

Msall, M.E. (1996). Functional assessment in neurodevelopmental disability. In A.J. Capute & P.J. Accardo (Eds.), *Developmental disabilities in infancy and children, Second Edition: Vol. I. Neurodevelopmental diagnosis and treatment* (pp. 371–392). Baltimore: Paul H. Brookes Publishing Co.

Msall, M.E., Buck, G.M., Rogers, B.T., & Catanzaro, N.L. (1992). Kindergarten readiness after extreme prematurity. *American Journal of Diseases of Children, 146*, 1371–1375.

Msall, M.E., Buck, G.M., Rogers, B.T., Merke, D.P., Wan, C.C., Catanzaro, N.L., & Zorn, W.A. (1994). Multivariate risks among extremely premature infants. *Journal of Perinatology, 4*, 41–47.

Msall, M.E., DiGaudio, K.M., & Duffy, L.C. (1993). Use of functional assessment in children with developmental disabilities. *Physical Medicine and Rehabilitation Clinics of North America, 4*, 517–527.

Msall, M.E., DiGaudio, K., Duffy, L.C., La Forest, S., Braun, S., & Granger, C.V. (1994). WeeFIM: Normative sample of an instrument for tracking functional independence in children. *Clinical Pediatrics, 33*, 431–438.

Msall, M.E., Phelps, D.L., DiGaudio, K.M., Dobson, V., Tung, B., McClead, R.E., Quinn, G.E., Reynolds, J.D., Hardy, R.J., & Palmer, E.A. (2000). Severity of neonatal retinopathy of prematurity (ROP) is predictive of neurodevelopmental functional outcome at age 5.5 years. *Pediatrics, 106*, 998–1005.

Msall, M.E., & Tremont, M.R. (2000). Functional outcomes of self-care, mobility, communication and learning in extremely low birth weight infants. *Clinics in Perinatology, 27*, 381–401.

Muir, D.W., Humphrey, D.E., & Humphrey, G.K. (1994). Pattern and space perception in young infants. *Spatial Vision, 8*, 141–165.

Mullen, E. (1995). *Mullen Scales of Early Learning: AGS Edition.* Circle Pines, MN: American Guidance Service.

Murray, B., & Campbell, D. (1971). Sleep states in the newborn: Influence of sound. *Neuropediatrie, 2*, 335–342.

Murray, L., Fiori-Cowley, A., Hooper, R., & Cooper, P. (1996). The impact of postnatal depression and associated adversity on early mother–infant interactions and later infant outcome. *Child Development, 67*, 2512–2526.

Myers, M.M., Fifer, W.P., Schaeffer, L., Sahni, R., Ohira-Kist, K., Stark, R.I., & Schulze, K.F. (1998). Effects of sleeping position and time after feeding on the organization of sleep/wake states in prematurely born infants. *Sleep, 21*, 343–349.

National Advisory Board on Medical Rehabilitation Research. (1993). *Research plan for the National Center for Medical Rehabilitation Research* (NIH Publication 93-3509). Bethesda MD: National Institutes of Health.

National Center for Health Statistics. (1998a). *1998 Fact sheet: New study identifies infants at greatest health risk.* Retrieved April 14, 2003, from http://www.cdc.gov/nchs/releases/98facts/linkedbd.htm

National Center for Health Statistics. (1998b). *1998 News release: Latest birth statistics for the nation released.* Retrieved April 14, 2003, from http://www.cdc.gov/nchs/releases/98news/natal96.htm

National Center for Health Statistics. (1999). Birthweight and gestation. *Birth and deaths: United States, July 1996–June 1997.* Retrieved April 14, 2003, from http://www.cdc.gov/nchs/fastats/birthwt.htm

National Health Planning and Resources Development Act of 1974, PL 93-641, 42 U.S.C. §§ 217a *et seq.*

Nehring, A.D., Nehring, E.F., Bruni, J.R., & Randolph, P.L. (1992). *Learning Accomplishment Profile–Diagnostic Standardized Assessment.* Lewisville, NC: Kaplan Press.

Newborg, J., Stock, J.R., Wnek, L., Guidubaldi, J., & Svinicki, J. (1984). *Battelle Developmental Inventory with recalibrated technical data and norms: Examiner's manual.* Allen, TX: Developmental Learning Materials Teaching Resources.

Nugent, J.K. (1985). *Using the NBAS with infants and their families.* White Plains, NY: March of Dimes Birth Defects Foundation.

Nyqvist, K.H., & Lutes, L.M. (1998). Co-bedding twins: A developmentally supportive care strategy. *Journal of Obstetric, Gynecologic, and Neonatal Nursing, 27*, 450–456.

Oates, P.R., & Oates, R.K. (1996). Stress and work relationships in the neonatal intensive care unit: Are they worse than in the wards? *Journal of Pediatric Child Health, 32*, 57–59.

Occupational Safety and Health Act of 1970, PL 91-596, 29 U.S.C. §§ 651 *et seq.*

Olson, J.A., & Baltman, K. (1994). Infant mental health in occupational therapy practice in the neonatal intensive care unit. *American Journal of Occupational Therapy, 48*, 499–505.

Omari, T., Snel, A., Barnett, C., Davidson, G., Haslam, R., & Dent, J. (1999). Measurement of upper esophageal sphincter tone and relaxation during swallowing in premature infants. *Journal of Applied Physiology Online: Gastrointestinal and Liver Physiology, 277*(4), G862–G866.

Onozawa, K., Glover, V., Adams, D., Modi, N., & Kumar, R.C. (2001). Infant massage improves mother–infant interaction for mothers with postnatal depression. *Journal of Affective Disorders, 63*, 201–207.

O'Rahilly, R., & Muller, F. (Eds.). (1987). *Developmental stages in human embryos* (Publication 637). Washington, DC: Carnegie Institution of Washington.

Orenstein, S.R., & Whitington, P.F. (1983). Positioning for prevention of infant gastroesophageal reflux. *Journal of Pediatrics, 103*, 534–357.

O'Shea, T.M. (2002). Cerebral palsy in very preterm infants: New epidemiological insights. *Mental Retardation Development Disability Research Reviews, 8*, 135–146.

O'Shea, T.M., & Dammann, O. (2000). Antecedents of cerebral palsy in very low birth weight infants. *Clinical Perinatology, 27*(2), 285–302.

Ottenbacher, K.J., Msall, M.E., Lyon, N., Duffy, L.C., Granger, C.V., & Braun, S. (1997). Interrater agreement and stability of the Functional Independence Measure for Children (Wee-FIM): Use in children with developmental disabilities. *Archives of Physical Medicine & Rehabilitation, 78*, 1309–1315.

Ottenbacher, K.J., Msall, M.E., Lyon, N., Duffy, L.C., Granger, C.V., & Braun, S. (1999). Measuring developmental and functional status in children with disabilities. *Developmental Medicine and Child Neurology, 41*, 186–194.

Ottenbacher, K.J., Muller, L., Brandt, D., Heintzelman, A., Hojem, P., & Sharpe, P. (1987). The effectiveness of tactile stimulation as a form of early intervention: A quantitative evaluation. *Developmental and Behavioral Pediatrics, 8*, 68–76.

Ottenbacher, K.J., Taylor, E.T., Msall, M.E., Braun, S., Lane, S.J., Granger, C.V., Lyons, N., & Duffy, L.C. (1996). The stability and equivalence reliability of the Functional Independence Measure for Children (WeeFIM). *Developmental Medicine and Child Neurology, 38*, 907–916.

Ounsted, M., Moar, V.A., & Scott, A. (1988). Neurological development of small-for-gestational age babies during the first year of life. *Early Human Development, 16*, 163–172.

Page, J., & Lunyk-Child, O. (1995). Parental perceptions of infant transfer from an NICU to a community nursery: Implications for research and practice. *Neonatal Network, 14*(8), 69–71.

Palisano, R.J., & Haley, S.M. (1993). Validity of Goal Attainment Scaling in infants with motor delays. *Physical Therapy, 73*, 651–660.

Palmer, M., & Heyman, M.B. (1993). Assessment and treatment of sensory- versus motor-based feeding problems in very young children. *Infants and Young Children, 6*, 67–73.

Palmer, M.M., Crawley, K., & Blanco, I. (1993). The Neonatal Oral-Motor Assessment Scale: A reliability study. *Journal of Perinatology, 13*, 28–35.

Paneth, N., Keily, J.L., Wallenstein, S., & Suser, M. (1987). The choice of place of delivery: Effect of hospital level on mortality in all singleton births in New York City. *American Journal of the Disabled Child, 141*, 60–64.

Papile, L.A., Burstein, J., Burstein, R., & Koffler, H. (1978). Incidence and evolution of subependymal and intraventricular hemorrhage: A study of infants with birth weights less than 1500 grams. *Journal of Pediatrics, 92*, 529–534.

Parad, R.B., & Berger, T.M. (1997). Chronic lung disease. In J.P. Cloherty & A.R. Stark (Eds.), *Manual of neonatal care* (4th ed., pp. 378–388). Philadelphia: Lippincott, Williams & Wilkins.

Patrick, D.L., & Erickson, P. (1993). *Health status and health policy: Quality of life in health care evaluation and resource allocation.* New York: Oxford University Press.

Peiper, A. (1924). Beitrage Zur Sinnesphysiologie der Fruhgeburt. *J Kinderheilkd, 104*, 195.

Peiper, A. (1931). Die Atemstorungen der Fruhgeburten Ergeb. *Inn Med Kinderheilkd 401*, 1931.

Peitsch, W.K., Keefer, C.H., LaBrie, R.A., & Mulliken, J.B. (2002). Incidence of cranial asymmetry in healthy newborns. *Pediatrics, 110*(6), 72.

Pettett, G., Bonnabel, C., & Bird, C. (1989). Regionalization and transport in perinatal care. In G.B. Merenstein & S.L. Gardner (Eds.), *Handbook of neonatal intensive care* (pp. 3–30). St. Louis: Mosby.

Phelps, D.L. (1992). Retinopathy of prematurity. In A.A. Fanaroff & R.J. Martin (Eds.), *Neonatal-perinatal medicine: Vol. 2. Diseases of the fetus and infant* (5th ed., p. 1393). St. Louis: Mosby-Year Book.

Philip, A.G.S., Allan, W.C., Tito, A.M., & Wheeler, L.R. (1989). Intraventricular hemorrhage in preterm infants: Declining incidence in the 1980's. *Pediatrics, 84*, 797–801.

Piaget, J. (1952). *The origins of intelligence in children.* Madison, CT: International Universities Press.

Piaget, J. (1976). *The psychology of intelligence.* Totowa, NJ: Littlefield, Adams & Co.

Pickler, R.H., Higgins, K.E., & Crummette, B.D. (1993). The effect of nonnutritive sucking on bottle-feeding stress in preterm infants. *Journal of Obstetric, Gynecologic, and Neonatal Nursing, 22*, 230–234.

Pickler, R.H., Mauck, A.G., & Geldmaker, B. (1997). Bottle-feeding histories of preterm infants. *Journal of Obstetrical, Gynecological and Neonatal Nursing, 26*, 414–420.

Piontelli, A., Bocconi, L., Kustermann, A., Tassis, B., Zoppini, C., & Nicolini, U. (1997). Patterns of evoked behaviour in twin pregnancies during the first 22 weeks of gestation. *Early Human Development, 50*, 39–45.

Piper, M.C., & Darrah, J. (1995). *Alberta Infant Motor Scale (AIMS).* Philadelphia: W.B. Saunders.

Piper, M.C., Pinnell, L.E., Darrah, J., Maguire, T., & Byrne, P.J. (1992). Construction and validation of the Alberta Infant Motor Scale (AIMS). *Canadian Journal of Public Health, 83*(Suppl. 2), S46–S50.

Plaas, K.M. (1994). The evolution of parental roles in the NICU. *Neonatal Network, 13*(6), 31–33.

Pollack, H.A., & Frohna, J.G. (2001). A competing risk model of sudden infant death syndrome incidence in two US birth cohorts. *Journal of Pediatrics, 138*, 661–667.

Pollin, I. (1995). *Medical crisis counseling: Short-term therapy for long-term illness.* New York: W.W. Norton & Company.

Powers, W.F. (1997). Multiple births. In J.P. Cloherty & A.R. Stark (Eds.), *Manual of neonatal care* (4th ed., pp. 77–85). Philadelphia: Lippincott, Williams & Wilkins.

Prechtl, H.F.R., & Beintema, J. (1968). The neurological examination of the full-term newborn infant. *Clinics in Developmental Medicine: No. 28.* London: SIMP with Heinemann Medical.

Prechtl, H.F.R., Fargel, J.W., Weinmann, H.M., & Bakker, H.H. (1979). Postures, motility, and respiration of low-risk pre-term infants. *Developmental Medicine and Child Neurology, 21*, 3–27.

Primeau, L.A. (1998). Orchestration of work and play within families. *American Journal of Occupational Therapy, 52*, 188–195.

Prudhoe, C.M., & Peters, D.L. (1995). Social support of parents and grandparents in the neonatal intensive care unit. *Pediatric Nursing, 21*, 1140–1146.

Pursley, D.M., & Cloherty, J.P. (1997). Identifying the high-risk newborn and evaluating gestational age, prematurity, postmaturity, large-for-gestational-age, and small-for-gestational-age infants. In J.P. Cloherty & A.R. Stark (Eds.), *Manual of neonatal care* (4th ed., pp. 37–51). Philadelphia: Lippincott, Williams & Wilkins.

Raddish, M., & Merritt, T.A. (1998). Early discharge of premature infants. A critical analysis. *Clinics in Perinatology, 25*, 499–520.

Raeside, L. (1997). Perceptions of environmental stressors in the neonatal unit. *British Journal of Nursing, 6*, 914–923.

Raines, D.A. (1996). Parents' values: A missing link in the neonatal intensive care equation. *Neonatal Network, 15*(3), 7–12.

Rakic, P. (1991). Plasticity of cortical development. In S.E. Brauth, S.S. Hall, & R.J. Dooling (Eds.), *Plasticity of development* (pp. 127–161). Cambridge, MA: The MIT Press.

Ratliff-Schaub, K., Hunt, C.E., Crowell, D., Golub, H., Smok-Pearsall, S., Palmer, P., Schafer, S., Bak, S., Cantey-Kiser, J., & O'Bell, R. (CHIME Study Group). (2001). Relationship between infant sleep position and motor development in preterm infants. *Journal of Developmental and Behavioral Pediatrics, 22*, 293–299.

Read, P.A., Horne, R.S., Cranage, S.M., Walker, A.M., Walker, D.M., & Adamson, T.M. (1998). Dynamic changes in arousal threshold during sleep in the human infant. *Pediatric Research, 43*, 697–703.

Reddick, B.H., Catlin, E., & Jellinek, M. (2001). Crisis within crisis: Recommendations for defining, preventing, and coping with stressors in the NICU. *Journal of Clinical Ethics, 12*, 264–265.

Redshaw, M.E., & Harris, A. (1995). Maternal perceptions of neonatal care. *Acta Paediatrica, 84*, 593–598.

Rehan, V.K., Nakashima, J.M., Gutman, A., Rubin, L., & McCool, F.D. (2000). Effects of the supine and prone position on diaphragm thickness in healthy term infants. *Archives of Disease in Childhood, 83*, 234–238.

Reiterer, F., Abbasi, S., & Bhutani, V.K. (1994). Influence of head-neck posture on airflow and pulmonary mechanics in preterm neonates. *Pediatric Pulmonology, 17,* 149–154.

Rezaie, P., & Dean, A. (2002). Periventricular leukomalacia, inflammation and white matter lesions within the developing nervous system. *Neuropathology, 22*(3), 106–103.

Ricciardi, P.W.R., & Boelker, S.L. (1987). *Measuring cognitive skills of language impaired preschoolers.* Paper presented at the meeting of the American Psychological Association, New York.

Richardson, D.K. (1997). Tests of pulmonary surfactant. In J.P. Cloherty & A.R. Stark (Eds.), *Manual of neonatal care* (4th ed., pp. 7–9). Philadelphia: Lippincott, Williams & Wilkins.

Ritchie, S.K. (2002). Primary care of the premature infant discharged from the neonatal intensive care unit. *American Journal of Maternal and Child Nursing, 27,* 76–85.

Robb, M.P., & Goberman, A.M. (1997). Application of an acoustic cry template to evaluate at-risk newborns: Preliminary findings. *Biology of the Neonate, 71,* 131–136.

Roberts, K.E. (1999). Ventilatory strategies for the critically ill infant and child. *Critical Care Nursing Clinics of North America, 11,*(4), 501–509.

Robison, M., Pirak, C., & Morrell, C. (2000). Multidisciplinary discharge assessment of the medically and socially high-risk infant. *Journal of Perinatology and Neonatal Nursing, 13,* 67–86.

Roche, A.F., Mukherjee, D., Guo, S., & Moore, W.M. (1987). Head circumference reference data: Birth to 18 years. *Pediatrics, 79,* 706–712.

Rogers, B., Andrus, J., Msall, M.E., Arvedson, J., Sim, J., Rossi, T., Martin, D., & Hudak, M. (1998). Growth of preterm infants with cystic periventricular leukomalacia. *Developmental Medicine and Child Neurology, 40,* 580–586.

Rogoff, B. (1990). *Apprenticeship in thinking.* New York: Oxford.

Roman, L.A., Lindsay, J.K., Boger, R.P., deWys, M., Beaumont, E.J., Jones, A.S., & Haas, B. (1995). Parent-to-parent support initiated in the neonatal intensive care unit. *Research in Nursing Health, 18,* 385–394.

Ronca, A.E., Abel, R.A., & Alberts, J.R. (1996, Oct.). Perinatal stimulation and adaptation of the neonate. *Acta Paediatrica, 416*(Suppl.), 8–15.

Rosenbaum, P., Saigal, S., Szatmari, P., & Hoult, L. (1995). Vineland Adaptive Behavior Scales as a summary of functional outcome of extremely low birth weight children. *Developmental Medicine and Child Neurology, 37,* 577–586.

Rosenbaum, P.L., Russell, D.J., Cadman, E.T., Gowan, C., Jarvis, S., & Hardy, S. (1990). Issues in measuring changes in motor function in children with cerebral palsy. *Physical Therapy, 70,* 125–131.

Rosenthal, S.L., Schmid, K.D., & Black, M.M. (1989). Stress and coping in a NICU. *Research in Nursing and Health, 12,* 257–265.

Rossman, M.J., Hyman, S.L., Rorabaugh, M.L., Berlin, L.E., Allen, M., & Modlen, J.F. (1994). The CAT/CLAMS assessment for early intervention services. *Clinical Pediatrics, 33,* 404–409.

Rothbart, M.K., Derryberry, D., & Posner, M.I. (1994). A psychobiological approach to the development of temperament. In J.E. Bates & T.D. Wachs (Eds.), *Temperament: Individual differences at the interface of biology and behavior* (pp. 83–116). Washington, DC: American Psychological Association.

Rushforth, J.A., & Levene, M.I. (1994). Behavioural response to pain in healthy neonates. *Archives of Disease in Childhood, Fetal and Neonatal Edition, 70,* F174–F176.

Rushton, C.H. (1990). Family-centered care in the critical care setting: Myth or reality? *Children's Health Care, 19,* 68–77.

Russell, D.J., Rosenbaum, P.L., Avery, L.M., & Lane, M. (2002). *Gross Motor Function Measure (GMFM-66 and GMFM-88) user's manual.* London: Mac Keith Press.

Russell, D.J., Rosenbaum, P.L., Cadman, D.T., Gowland, C., Hardy, S., & Jarvis, S. (1989). The Gross Motor Function Measure: A means to evaluate the effects of physical therapy. *Developmental Medicine and Child Neurology, 31,* 341–352.

Rutter, N., Hinchliffe, W., & Cartlidge, P.H.T. (1993). Do preterm infants always have flattened heads? *Archives of Disease in Childhood, 68,* 606–607.

Sadeh, A., Dark, I., & Vohr, B.R. (1996). Newborns' sleep-wake patterns: The role of maternal, delivery, and infant factors. *Early Human Development, 44,* 113–126.

Sahni, R., Schulze, K.F., Kashyap, S., Ohira-Kist, K., Myers, M.M., & Fifer, W.P. (2002). Quality of diet, body position, and time after feeding influence behavioral states in low birth weight infants. *Pediatric Research, 52,* 399–404.

Saigal, S., Feeny, D., Furlong, W., Rosenbaum, P., Burrows, E., & Torrance, G. (1994). Comparison of the health-related quality of life of extremely low birth weight children and a reference group of children at age eight years. *Journal of Pediatrics, 125,* 418–425.

Saigal, S., Feeny, D., Rosenbaum, P., Furlong, W., Burrows, E., & Stoskopf, B. (1996). Self-perceived health status and health-related quality of life of extremely low-birth-weight infants at adolescence. *Journal of the American Medical Association, 14,* 453–459.

Saigal, S., Rosenbaum, P., Stoskopf, B., Hoult, L., Furlong, W., Feeny, D., Burrows, E., & Torrance, G. (1994). Comprehensive assessment of the health status of extremely low birth weight children at eight years of age: Comparison with a reference group. *Journal of Pediatrics, 125,* 411–417.

Saigal, S., Stoskopf, B.L., Rosenbaum, P.L., Hould, L.A., Furlong, W.J., & Feeny, D.H. (1998). Development of a multiattribute pre-school health status classification system. *Pediatric Research,* Abstract No. 1333.

Sameroff, A.J., & Chandler, M.J. (1975). Reproductive risk and the continuum of caretaking casualty. In F.D. Horowitz, M. Hetherington, S. Scarr-Salapatek, & G. Siegel (Eds.), *Review of child development research: Vol. 4* (pp. 187–244). Chicago: University of Chicago Press.

Sammon, M.P., & Darnall, R.A. (1994). Entrainment of respiration to rocking in premature infants: Coherence analysis. *Journal of Applied Physiology, 77,* 1548–1554.

Sarnat, H.B., & Sarnat, M.S. (1976). Neonatal encephalopathy following fetal distress: A clinical and electroencephalographic study. *Archives of Neurology, 33,* 696–705.

Saunders, A.N. (1995). Incubator noise: A method to decrease decibels. *Pediatric Nursing, 21,* 265–268.

Sawyer, G., Kemp, T., Shaw, R., Patchett, K., Siebers, R., Lewis, S., Beasley, R., Crane, J., & Fitzharris, P. (1998). Biologic pollution in infant bedding in New Zealand: High allergen exposure during a vulnerable period. *Journal of Allergy and Clinical Immunology, 102,* 765–770.

Scafidi, F.A., Field, T., & Schanberg, S.M. (1993). Factors that predict which preterm infants benefit most from massage therapy. *Developmental and Behavioral Pediatrics, 14,* 176–180.

Schaal, B., Marlier, L., & Soussignan, R. (1998). Olfactory function in the human fetus: Evidence from selective neonatal responsiveness to the odor of amniotic fluid. *Behavioral Neuroscience, 112,* 1438–1449.

Schanler, R.J., Hurst, N.M., & Lau, C. (1999). The use of human milk and breastfeeding in premature infants. *Clinics in Perinatology, 26,* 379–397.

Scher, M.S. (1998). Understanding sleep ontogeny to assess brain dysfunction in neonates and infants. *Journal of Child Neurology, 13,* 467–474.

Schmidt, K., Rose, S.A., & Bridger, W.H. (1980). Effect of heartbeat sound on the cardiac and behavioral responsiveness to tactual stimulation in sleeping preterm infants. *Developmental Psychology, 16,* 175–184.

Schraeder, B.D. (1993). Assessment of measures to detect preschool academic risks in very low birth weight children. *Nursing Research, 42,* 17–21.

Schwab, F., Tolbert, B., Bagnato, S., & Maisels, M.J. (1983). Sibling visiting in a neonatal intensive care unit. *Pediatrics, 71,* 835–838.

Sconyers, S.M., Ogden, B.E., & Goldberg, H.S. (1987). The effect of body position on the respiratory rate of infants with tachypnea. *Journal of Perinatology, 7,* 118–121.

Seideman, R.Y., Watson, M.A., Corff, K.E., Odle, P., Haase, J., & Bowerman, J.L. (1997). Parent stress and coping in NICU and PICU. *Journal of Pediatric Nursing, 12,* 169–177.

Shaker, C.S. (1999). Nipple feeding preterm infants: An individualized, developmentally supportive approach. *Neonatal Network, 18*(3), 15–22.

Shannon, J.D., & Gorski, P.A. (1994). Health care professionals' attitudes toward the current level and need for developmental services in neonatal intensive care units. *Journal of Perinotology, 14,* 467–472.

Shelton, T.L., Jeppson, E.S., & Johnson, B.H. (1987). *Family-centered care for children with special health care needs.* Wahington, DC: Association for the Care of Children's Health.

Shen, X.M., Zhoa, W., Huang, D.S., Lin, F.G., & Wu, S.M. (1996). Effect of positioning on pulmonary function of newborns: Comparison of supine and prone position. *Pediatric Pulmonology, 21,* 167–170.

Shiao, S.Y. (1997). Comparison of continuous versus intermittent sucking in very-low-birthweight infants. *Journal of Obstetrical, Gynecological and Neonatal Nursing, 26,* 313–319.

Shields-Poe, D., & Pinelli, J. (1997). Variables associated with parental stress in neonatal intensive care units. *Neonatal Network, 16*(1), 29–37.

Shogan, M.G., & Schumann, L.L. (1993). The effect of environmental lighting on the oxygen saturation of preterm infants in the NICU. *Neonatal Network, 12*(5), 7–13.

Short, M.A., Brooks-Brunn, J.A., Reeves, D.S., Yeager, J., & Thorpe, J.A. (1996). The effects of swaddling versus standard positioning on neuromuscular development in very low birth weight infants. *Neonatal Network, 15*(4), 25–31.

Siegel, D.J. (1999). *The developing mind.* New York: The Guilford Press.

Silverman, G.A. (1997). Air leak: Pneumothorax, pulmonary interstitial emphysema, pneumonmediastinum, pneumopericardium. In J.P. Cloherty & A.R. Stark (Eds.), *Manual of neonatal care* (4th ed., pp. 358–364). Philadelphia: Lippincott, Williams & Wilkins.

Simeonsson, R.J., & Bailey, D.B., Jr. (1990). Family dimensions in early intervention. In S.J. Meisels & J.P. Shonkoff (Eds.), *Handbook of early childhood intervention* (pp. 428–444). New York: Cambridge University Press.

Skeels, H.M., Updegraff, R., Wellman, B.L., & Williams, H.L. (1938). A study of environmental stimulation: An orphanage preschool project. *University of Iowa Studies in Child Welfare, 15*(4), 7–191.

Skoczenski, A.M., & Norcia, A.M. (1998). Neural noise limitations on infant visual sensitivity. *Nature, 391*(6668), 697–700.

Slater, A., & Kirby, R. (1998). Innate and learned perceptual abilities in the newborn infant. *Experimental Brain Research, 123,* 90–94.

Slevin, M., Farrington, N., Duffy, G., Daly, L., & Murphy, J.F. (2000). Altering the NICU and measuring infants' responses. *Acta Paediatrica, 89,* 501–502.

Snyder, E.Y., & Cloherty, J.P. (1997). Perinatal asphyxia. In J.P. Cloherty & A.R. Stark (Eds.), *Manual of neonatal care* (4th ed., pp. 515–533). Philadelphia: Lippincott, Williams & Wilkins.

Sparrow, S., Balla, D.A., & Cicchetti, D.V. (1984). *Vineland Adaptive Behavior Scales (VABS).* Circle Pines, MN: American Guidance Service.

Spear, M. (2002). Family reactions during infants' hospitalization in the neonatal intensive care unit. *American Journal of Perinatology, 19,* 205–213.

Spieker, M.R., & Brannen, S.J. (1996). Supine infant sleep: What do family physicians recommend? *Journal of the American Board of Family Practice, 9,* 319–323.

Sporns, O., & Edelman, G.M. (1993). Solving Bernstein's problem: A proposal for the development of coordinated movement by selection. *Child Development, 64,* 960–981.

St. John, D., Mulliken, J.B., Kaban, L.B., & Padwa, B.L. (2002). Anthropometric analysis of mandibular asymmetry in infants with deformational posterior plagiocephaly. *Journal of Oral Maxillofacial Surgery, 60,* 873–877.

Stallings-Sahler, S. (1998). Sensory integration: Assessment and intervention with infants and young children. In J. Case-Smith (Ed.), *Pediatric occupational therapy and early intervention* (2nd ed., pp. 223–254). Burlington, NJ: Butterworth-Heinemann.

Stark, A. (1997). Apnea. In J.P. Cloherty & A.R. Stark (Eds.), *Manual of neonatal care* (4th ed., pp. 374–378). Philadelphia: Lippincott, Williams & Wilkins.

Stevens, B., Taddio, A., Ohlsson, A., & Einarson, T. (1997). The efficacy of sucrose for relieving procedural pain in neonates: A systematic review and meta-analysis. *Acta Paediatrica, 86,* 837–842.

Stevens, B.J., Johnston, C.C., & Horton, L. (1994). Factors that influence the behavioral pain responses of premature infants. *Pain, 59,* 101–109.

Sun, Y., Awnetwant, E.L., Collier, S.B., Gallagher, L.M., Olsen, I.E., & Stewart, J.E. (1997). Nutrition. In J.P. Cloherty & A.R. Stark (Eds.), *Manual of neonatal care* (4th ed., pp. 101–135). Philadelphia: Lippincott, Williams & Wilkins.

Swanson, S.C., & Naber, M.M. (1997). Neonatal integrated home care: Nursing without walls. *Neonatal Network, 16*(7), 33–38.

Sweeney, J.K., Heriza, C.B., Reilly, M.A., Smith, C., & VanSant, A.F. (1999). Practice guidelines for the physical therapist in the neonatal intensive care unit (NICU). *Pediatric Physical Therapy, 11,* 119–132.

Sweeney, J.K., & Swanson, M.W. (1990). At-risk neonates and infants NICU management and follow-up. In D.A. Umphred (Ed.), *Neurological rehabilitation* (pp. 183–238). St. Louis: Mosby.

Sweeney, M.M. (1997). The value of a family-centered approach in the NICU and PICU: One family's perspective. *Pediatric Nursing, 23,* 64–66.

Symington, A., & Pinelli, J. (2001). Developmental care for promoting development and preventing morbidity in preterm infants. *Cochrane Database Systematic Review, 4,* CD001814. Retrieved February 5, 2003, from http://www.nichd.nih.gov/cochrane/symington/symington.htm

Symon, A. (1995). Handling premature neonates: A study using time-lapse video. *Nursing Times, 91*(17), 35–37.

Szymonowicz, W., Yu, V.Y., Bajuk, B., & Astbury, J. (1986). Neurodevelopmental outcome of periventricular hemorrhage and leukomalacia in infants 1250 g or less at birth. *Early Human Development, 14*, 1–7.

Task Force on Newborn and Infant Hearing. (1999). Detection and intervention. *Pediatrics, 103*, 527–530.

Teller, D.Y., McDonald, M.A., Preston, K., Sebris, S.L., & Dobson, V. (1986). Assessment of visual acuity in infants and children: The acuity card procedure. *Developmental Medicine and Child Neurology, 28*, 779–789.

Ten Hof, J., Nijhuis, I.J.M., Mulder, E.J.H., Nijhuis, J.G., Narayan, H., Taylor, D.J., Westers, P., & Visser, G.H.A. (2002). Longitudinal study of fetal body movements: Nomograms, intrafetal consistency, and relationship with episodes of heart rate patterns A and B. *Pediatric Research, 52*, 568–575.

Thach, B.T., & Lijowska, A. (1996). Arousals in infants. *Sleep, 19*(Suppl. 10), S271–S273.

Thelen, E. (1995). Motor development: A new synthesis. *American Psychologist, 50*, 79–95.

Thelen, E., & Fogel, A. (1989). Toward an action-based theory of infant development. In J.J. Lockman & N.Y. Hazen (Eds.), *Action in social context: Perspectives on early development* (pp. 23–63). New York: Kluwer Academic/Plenum Publishers.

Thomas, A., & Chess, S. (1989). Issues in the clinical application of temperament. In G.A. Kohnstamm, J.E. Bates, & M.K. Rothbart (Eds.), *Temperament in childhood* (pp. 377–386). New York: John Wiley & Sons.

Thomas, K.A. (1989). How the NICU environment sounds to a preterm infant. *Maternal and Child Nursing, 14*, 249–251.

Thorndike, R.L., Hagen, E.P., & Sattler, J.M. (1986). *Stanford-Binet Intelligence Scale* (4th ed.). Itasca, IL: The Riverside Publishing Co.

Thoyre, S.M. (2000). Mothers' ideas about their role in feeding their high-risk infants. *Journal of Obstetrical, Gynecological and Neonatal Nursing, 29*, 613–624.

Thurman, S.K. (1991). Parameters for establishing family-centered neonatal intensive-care services. *Children's Health Care, 26*, 34–39.

Torrance, G.W., Furlong, W., Feeny, D., & Boyle, M. (1995). Multi-attribute preference functions Health Utilities Index. *Pharmacoeconomics, 7*, 503–520.

Touch, S.M., Epstein, M.L., Pohl, C.A., & Greenspan, J.S. (2002). The impact of cobedding on sleep patterns. *Clinical Pediatrics, 41*, 425–431.

Trevarthen, C. (1982). Basic patterns of psychogenetic change in infancy. In T.G. Bever (Ed.), *Regressions in mental development: Basic phenomena and theories* (pp. 7–46). Mahwah, NJ: Lawrence Erlbaum Associates.

Trombly, C.A. (1995). Occupation: Purposefulness and meaningfulness as therapeutic mechanisms. *American Journal of Occupational Therapy, 49*, 960–972.

Tronick, E.Z., & Lester B.M. (1996). The NICU Network Neurobehavioral Scale: A comprehensive instrument to assess substance-exposed and high-risk infants. *NIDA Research Monographs, 166*, 198–294.

Twinstuff. (2002). *What type of twins are there?* Retrieved February 5, 2003, from http://www.twinstuff.com/twinfopg.htm

Uniform Data System for Medical Rehabilitation. (1998). *WeeFIM manual (Version 2)*. Buffalo, NY: Author.

Updike, C., Schmidt, R.E., Macke, C., Cahoon, J., & Miller, M. (1986). Positional support for premature infants. *The American Journal of Occupational Therapy, 40*, 712–715.

Urlesberger, B., Muller, W., Ritschl, E., & Reiterer, F. (1991). The influence of head position on the intracranial pressure in preterm infants with posthemorrhagic hydrocephalus. *Child's Nervous System, 7*(2), 85–87.

U.S. Department of Health and Human Services, Public Health Service, Centers for Disease Control and Prevention. (1999). Decrease in infant mortality and sudden infant death syndrome among Northwest American Indians and Alaskan natives: Pacific Northwest, 1985–1996 [Electronic version]. *Morbidity and Mortality Weekly Report, 48*(9), 181–184. Retrieved April 14, 2003, from http://www.cdc.gov/mmwr/PDF/wk/mm4809.pdf

Valenza, E., Simion, F., Cassia, V.M., & Umilta, C. (1996). Face preference at birth. *Journal of Experimental Psychology: Human Perception and Performance, 22*, 892–903.

Van Marter, L.J. (1997). Persistent pulmonary hypertension of the newborn. In J.P. Cloherty & A.R. Stark (Eds.), *Manual of neonatal care* (4th ed., pp. 364–369). Philadelphia: Lippincott, Williams & Wilkins.

Van Reempts, P.J., Wouters, A., De Cock, W., & Van Acker, K.J. (1996). Stress responses in preterm neonates after normal and at-risk pregnancies. *Journal of Pediatrics and Child Health, 32*, 450–456.

Van Riper, M. (2001). Family-provider relationships and well-being in families with preterm infants in the NICU. *Heart & Lung: Journal of Acute & Critical Care, 30*, 74–84.

VandenBerg, K.A. (1990). Nippling management of the sick neonate in the NICU: The disorganized feeder. *Neonatal Network, 9*(1), 9–16.

VandenBerg, K.A. (1993). Basic competencies to begin developmental care in the intensive care nursery. *Infants and Young Children, 6*, 52–59.

VandenBerg, K.A. (1996). Developmental competencies for staff in the NICU. *Neonatal Network, 15*(5), 65–68.

VandenBerg, K.A. (1997). Basic principles of developmental caregiving. *Neonatal Network, 16*(2), 69–71.

Vandenplas, Y., Belli, D.C., Dupont, C., Kneepkens, C.M., & Heymans, H.S. (1997). The relation between gastro-oesophageal reflux, sleeping position and sudden infant death and its impact on positional therapy. *European Journal of Pediatrics, 156*, 104–106.

Vaucher, Y.E., Merritt, T.A., Hallman, M., Jarvenpaa, A.L., Telsey, A.M., & Jones, B.L. (1988). Neurodevelopmental and respiratory outcome in early childhood after human surfactant treatment. *American Journal of Diseases of Children, 142*, 927–930.

Vecchi, C.J., Vasquez, L., Radin, T., & Johnson, P. (1996). Neonatal individualized predictive pathway (NIPP): A discharge planning tool for parents. *Neonatal Network, 15*(4), 7–13.

Vergara, E.R. (Ed.). (1993). *Foundations for practice in the neonatal intensive care unit and early intervention: A self-guided practice manual.* Bethesda, MD: American Occupational Therapy Association.

Vickers, A., Ohlsson, A., Lacy, J.B., & Horsley, A. (2002). Massage for promoting growth and development of preterm and/or low birth-weight infants (Cochrane Review). In *The Cochrane Library* (Issue 3). Oxford, England: Update Software.

Victorian Infant Collaborative Study Group. (1991). Eight year outcome in infants with birth weight of 500–999 grams: Continuing regional study of 1979 and 1980 births. *Journal of Pediatrics, 118*, 761–767.

Vohr, B.R., Carty, L.M., Moore, P.E., & Letourneau, K. (1998). The Rhode Island Hearing Assessment Program: Experience with statewide hearing screening (1993–1996). *Journal of Pediatrics, 336*, 353–357.

Vohr, B.R., Cashore, W.J., & Bigsby, R. (1999). Stresses and interventions in the neonatal intensive care unit. In M.D. Levine, W.B. Carey, & A.C. Crocker (Eds.), *Developmental-behavioral pediatrics* (pp. 263–275). Philadelphia: W.B. Saunders.

Vohr, B.R., Wright, L.L., Dusick, A.M., Mele, L., Verter, J., Steichen, J.J., Simon, N.P., Wilson, D.C., Brooyles, S., Bauer, C.R., Delaney-Black, V., Yolton, K.A., Fleisher, B.E., Papile, L., & Kaplan, M.D. (2000). Neurodevelopmental and functional outcomes of extremely low birth weight infants in the National Institute of Child Health and Human Development Neonatal Research Network, 1993–1994. *Pediatrics, 105*(6), 1216–1225.

Volpe, J.J. (1989). Intraventricular hemorrhage in the premature infant: Current concepts, Part 1. *Annals of Neurology, 25*, 3–11.

Volpe, J.J. (2001). *Neurology of the newborn* (4th ed.). Philadelphia: W.B. Saunders.

Wachs, T.D. (1992). *The nature of nurture.* Thousand Oaks, CA: Sage Publications.

Wachtel, R.C., Shapiro, B.K., Palmer, F.B., Allen, M.C., & Capute, A.J. (1994). CAT/CLAMS: A tool for the pediatric evaluation of infants and young children with developmental delay. *Clinical Pediatrics, 33*, 410–415.

Wachtel, R.C., Tepper, V.J., Houck, D., McGrath, C.J., & Thompson, C. (1994). Neurodevelopment in pediatrics HIV infection: The use of CAT/CLAMS. *Clinical Pediatrics, 33*, 416–420.

Ward, K.G. (1999). A TEAM approach to NICU care. *RN, 62*, 47–49.

Ward, R.M., Lemons, J.A., & Molteni, R.A. (1999). Cisapride: A survey of the frequency of use and adverse events in premature newborns. *Pediatrics, 103*(2), 469–472.

Wechsler, D. (1989a). *Manual for the Wechsler Preschool and Primary Scale of Intelligence–Revised.* San Antonio, TX: The Psychological Corporation.

Wechsler, D. (1989b). *Wechsler Intelligence Scale for Children: 3rd ed. manual.* San Antonio, TX: The Psychological Corporation.

Wechsler, S.B., & Wernovsky, G. (1997). Cardiac disorders. In J.P. Cloherty & A.R. Stark (Eds.), *Manual of neonatal care* (4th ed., pp. 393–453). Philadelphia: Lippincott, Williams & Wilkins.

Weinberg, M.L., & Tronick, E.Z. (1998). The impact of maternal illness on infant development. *Journal of Child Psychiatry, 59*(Suppl. 2), 53–61.

Weingerger, B., Laskin, D.L., Heck, D.E., & Laskin, J.D. (2002). Oxygen toxicity in premature infants. *Toxicology and Applied Pharmacology, 181*(1), 60–67.

Werner, E.E. (1990). Protective factors and individual resilience. In S.J. Meisels & J.P. Shonkoff (Eds.), *Handbook of early childhood intervention* (pp. 97–116). New York: Cambridge University Press.

Werner, E.E. (2000). Protective factors and individual resilience. In J.P. Shonkoff & S.J. Meisels (Eds.), *Handbook of early childhood intervention* (2nd ed., pp. 115–132). New York: Cambridge University Press.

Werner, L.A. (1996). The development of auditory behavior (or what the anatomists and physiologists have to explain). *Ear and Hearing, 17,* 438–446.

White, C. (2002). Using evidence to educate birthing center nursing staff about infant states, cues, and behaviors. *American Journal of Maternal and Child Nursing, 27,* 294–298.

White-Traut, R.C., & Nelson, M.N. (1988). Premature infant massage: Is it safe? *Pediatric Nursing, 14,* 285–289.

White-Traut, R.C., Nelson, M.N., Burns, K., & Cunningham, N. (1994). Environmental influences on the developing premature infant: Theoretical issues and applications to practice. *Journal of Obstetric, Gynecologic, and Neonatal Nursing, 23,* 393–401.

Wilkins-Haug, L., & Heffner, L.J. (1997). Fetal assessment and prenatal diagnosis. In J.P. Cloherty & A.R. Stark (Eds.), *Manual of neonatal care* (4th ed., pp. 1–7). Philadelphia: Lippincott, Williams & Wilkins.

Willinger, M., Hoffman, H.J., Wu, K.T., Hou, J.R., Kessler, R.C., Ward, S.L., Keens, T.G., & Corwin, M.J. (1998). Factors associated with the transition to nonprone sleep positions of infants in the United States: The National Infant Sleep Position Study. *Journal of the American Medical Association, 280,* 329–335.

Wolf, L.S., & Glass, R.P. (1992). *Feeding and swallowing disorders in infancy: Assessment and management.* San Antonio, TX: Therapy Skill Builders.

Wolfson, M.R., Greenspan, J.S., Deoras, K.S., Allen, J.L., & Shaffer, T.H. (1992). Effect of positioning on the mechanical interaction between the rib cage and abdomen in preterm infants. *Journal of Applied Physiology, 72,* 1032–1038.

Wolkoff, L.I., & Narula, P. (2000). Issues in neonatal and pediatric oxygen therapy. *Respiratory Care Clinics of North America, 6*(4), 675–692.

Wood, E.P., & Rosenbaum, P.L. (2000). The Gross Motor Function Classification System for cerebral palsy. *Developmental Medicine and Child Neurology, 42,* 292–296.

Woodcock, R.W., & Johnson, M.B. (1989). *Woodcock-Johnson Psychoeducational Battery–Revised.* Allen, TX: Developmental Learning Materials Teaching Resources.

World Health Organization. (1978). *A growth chart for international use in maternal and child care: Guidelines for primary health care personnel.* Geneva: Author.

World Health Organization. (1980). *International Classification of Impairments, Disabilities and Handicaps (ICIDH).* Geneva: Author.

World Health Organization. (2001). *International Classification of Function, Disability, and Health (ICF).* Geneva: Author.

Wunsch, M.J., Conlon, C.J., & Scheidt, P.C. (2002). Substance abuse: A preventable threat to development. In M.L. Batshaw (Ed.), *Children with disabilities* (5th ed., pp. 107–122). Baltimore: Paul H. Brookes Publishing Co.

Ylippo, A. (1919). Das Wachstum der Fruhgeborenen von der Geburt bis zum Schulalter. *Z Kinderheilkd, 24.*

Zahr, L.K., & Balian, S. (1995). Responses of premature infants to routine nursing interventions and noise in the NICU. *Nursing Research, 44,* 179–185.

Zeskind, P.S., Marshall, T.R., & Goff, D.M. (1996). Cry threshold predicts regulatory disorder in newborn infants. *Journal of Pediatric Psychology, 21,* 803–819.

Zimmerman, I.L., Steiner, V.G., & Pond, R.E. (1991). *Preschool Language Scale–3 (PLS-3): Examiner's manual.* San Antonio, TX: The Psychological Corporation.

Zimmerman, I.L., Steiner, V.G., & Pond, R.E. (2002). *Preschool Language Scale, Fourth Edition (PLS-4).* San Antonio, TX: The Psychological Corporation.

Glossary of Abbreviations

A	apnea
Ab	abortions (includes spontaneous)
ABG	arterial blood gas
AFDC	Aid to Families with Dependent Children
AGA	appropriate for gestational age
ANS	autonomic nervous system
APIB	Assessment of Preterm Infant Behavior
AROM	assisted rupture of membranes
A's & B's	apnea and bradycardia
ASD	atrial septal defect
B	bilateral *or* bradycardia
BAER	brainstem auditory evoked responses
BPD	bronchopulmonary dysplasia
BPM	beats per minute (heart rate)
BW	birth weight
CBC	complete blood count
CDH	congenitally dislocated hip
CHD	congenital heart disease
CHF	congestive heart failure
CLD	chronic lung disease
CMV	cytomegalovirus
CNS	central nervous system
CPAP	continuous positive airway pressure
CPS	child protective services

CPT	chest physical therapy
C/S	cesarean section
CSF	cerebral spinal fluid
CXR	chest X-ray
D_5W	5% glucose solution
$D_{10}W$	10% glucose solution
DIC	disseminated intravascular coagulation
DTGV	transposition of the great vessels
ECMO	extracorporeal membrane oxgenation
ELBW	extremely low birth weight (less than 1,000 grams [g])
EPSDT	early and periodic screening, diagnosis, and treatment
FEN	fluids, electrolytes, nutrition
FHR	fetal heart rate
FiO_2	fraction inspired oxygen (percentage of oxygen concentration)
FLC	functional lung capacity
FT	full term
FTT	failure to thrive
G	gravida
GA	gestational age
GBS	group B streptococcus
GER	gastroesophageal reflux
HAL	hyperalimentation
HC	head circumference
HFFI	high-frequency flow interruption
HFJV	high-frequency jet ventilation
HFOV	high-frequency oscillating ventilation
HFV	high-frequency ventilation
HIE	hypoxic-ischemic encephalopathy
HMD	hyaline membrane disease
HR	heart rate
HSV	herpes simplex virus
HTN	hypertension
ICH	intracranial hemorrhage

ICN	intensive care nursery
IDM	infant of diabetic mother
IDV	intermittent demand ventilation
IMV	intermittent mandatory ventilation
INF	intravenous nutritional feeding
INO	inhaled nitric oxide
I/O	intake/output
IPPB	intermittent positive pressure breathing
IRV	inspiratory reserve volume
IUFD	intrauterine fetal demise
IUGR	intrauterine growth restriction
IV	intravenous
IVDA	intravenous drug abuse
IVF	intravenous feeding *or* in vitro fertilization
IVH	intraventricular hemorrhage
kcal	kilocalories
L	living children
LA	left atrium
LBW	low birth weight (less than 2,500 g)
LGA	large for gestational age
LMP	last menstrual period
L/S ratio	lecithin/sphingomyelin ratio
LTGV	physiologically corrected transposition of vessels
LV	left ventricle
MAP	mean airway pressure
MAS	meconium aspiration syndrome
MCA	multiple congenital anomalies
MICU	maternal intensive care unit
MRSA	methicillin-resistant staphylococcccus aureus
NB	newborn
NBAS	Neonatal Behavioral Assessment Scale
NC	nasal cannula
ND	nasoduodenal

NEC	necrotizing enterocolitis
NG	nasogastric
NGT	nasogastric tube
NICU	neonatal intensive care unit
NIDCAP	Neonatal Individualized Developmental Care and Assessment Program
NJ	nasojejunal tube
NNNS	Neonatal Network Neurobehavioral Scale
NNS	nonnutritive sucking
NO	nitric oxide
NP	nasopharyngeal
NPCPAP	nasopharyngeal continuous positive airway pressure
NPO	nothing by mouth
NS	nutritive sucking
NTE	neutral thermal environment
O_2 sats	oxygen saturation
OD	oral duodenal *or* right eye
OG	orogastric
OGT	oral gastric tube
OS	left eye
P	para *or* pulse
P1	primipara (first birth)
$PaCO_2$	arterial partial pressure of carbon dioxide
PaO_2	arterial partial pressure of oxygen
PCA	postconceptional age
PDA	patent ductus arteriosus
PEEP	positive end expiratory pressure
PerQ	percutaneous catheter
PFC	persistent fetal circulation
PIE	pulmonary interstitial emphysema
PIP	pulmonary insufficiency of the preterm *or* peak inspiratory pressure
PKU	phenylketonuria
PPD	packs per day (cigarettes)
PPHN	persistent pulmonary hypertension of the newborn

PO	by mouth
PROM	premature rupture of membranes
PS	pulmonic stenosis
PT	preterm
PTL	preterm labor
PVL	periventricular leukomalacia
q	every
qh	every hour
qid	four times per day
RA	right atrium
RBC	red blood cell
RDS	respiratory distress syndrome
ROM	rupture of membranes
ROP	retinopathy of prematurity
RPR	rapid plasma reagent (test for syphillis)
RR	respiration rate
RRR	rate, rhythm, respiration
RSV	respiratory syncytial virus
RV	right ventricle
sats	oxygen saturation levels
SGA	small for gestational age
SIMV	synchronized intermittent mandatory ventilation
s/p	status post
SROM	spontaneous rupture of membranes
SVD	spontaneous vaginal delivery
TA	truncus arterious
TAPVR	total anomalous pulmonary venous return
TCM	transcutaneous monitor
$TcPCO_2$	transcutaneous carbon dioxide pressure
$TcPO_2$	transcutaneous oxygen pressure
TLC	total lung capacity
TOF	tetralogy of Fallot

TORCH	congential viral infections (toxoplasmosis, other infections, rubella, cytomegalovirus, herpes)
TPF	toxoplasmosis fetalis
TPN	total parenteral nutrition
TPR	temperature, pulse, respiration
TRDN	transient respiratory distress of the newborn
TTN	transient tachypnea of the newborn
UAC	umbilical artery catheter
UAL	umbilical artery line
URI	upper respiratory infection
US	ultrasound
USG	ultrasound
UTI	urinary tract infection
UVC	umbilical venous catheter
VEP	visual evoked potential
VLBW	very low birth weight (less than 1,500 g)
VSD	ventricular septal defect
WBC	white blood cells
WBD	weeks by dates
WBE	weeks by examination

Index

Page numbers followed by *f* indicate figures; numbers followed by *t* indicate tables.